1

Color Atlas of Pediatric Diseases

With Differential Diagnosis

Fourth Edition

Color Atlas of Pediatric Diseases

With Differential Diagnosis

Fourth Edition

Written by

Claus Simon
Children's Clinic of the University of Kiel
Kiel, Germany
and
Michael Jänner
Dermatology Clinic of the University of Hamburg
Hamburg, Germany

English Edition Edited by

Roger F. Soll, M.D.
Associate Professor of Pediatrics
University of Vermont College of Medicine
Burlington, VT

Translation by Olga Karkalas
Transcription by Karen Steinhaus

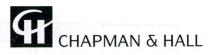 CHAPMAN & HALL

 International Thomson Publishing
Thomson Science
New York • Albany • Bonn • Boston • Cincinnati • Detroit • London • Madrid • Melbourne
Mexico City • Pacific Grove • Paris • San Francisco • Singapore • Tokyo • Toronto • Washington

Cover Design: Andrea Meyer, Emdash, Inc.

Copyright © 1998
Chapman & Hall

Printed in the United States of America

For more information, contact:

Chapman & Hall
115 Fifth Avenue
New York, NY 10003

Chapman & Hall
2-6 Boundary Row
London SE1 8HN
England

Thomas Nelson Australia
102 Dodds Street
South Melbourne, 3205
Victoria, Australia

Chapman & Hall GmbH
Postfach 100 263
D-69442 Weinheim
Germany

International Thomson Editores
Campos Eliseos 385, Piso 7
Col. Polanco
11560 Mexico D.F.
Mexico

International Thomson Publishing-Japan
Hirakawacho-cho Kyowa Building, 3F
1-2-1 Hirakawacho-cho
Chiyoda-ku, 102 Tokyo
Japan

International Thomson Publishing Asia
221 Henderson Road #05-10
Henderson Building
Singapore 0315

1 2 3 4 5 6 7 8 9 10 XXX 01 00 99 98

Library of Congress Cataloging-in-Publication Data

Simon, Claus.
    [Farbatlas der Pädiatrie. English]
    Color atlas of pediatric diseases with differential diagnosis / by Claus Simon and Michael Jänner. —
4th ed., rev. and expanded.
        p. cm.
    Includes index.
    ISBN 0-412-08131-8 (alk. paper)
    1. Children—Diseases—Diagnosis—Atlases.   2. Diagnosis, Differential—Atlases.
    3. Pediatrics—Atlases.   I. Jänner, Michael.   II. Title.
    [DNLM: 1. Pediatrics—atlases.   2. Diagnosis, Differential—atlases.   WS 17 S594f 1997a]
    RJ50.S57613   1997
    618.92′0075—dc21
    DNLM/DLC   97-3047
    for Library of Congress   CIP

British Library Cataloguing in Publication Data available

To order this or any other Chapman & Hall book, please contact International Thomson Publishing, 7625
Empire Drive, Florence, KY 41042. Phone: (606) 525-6600 or 1-800-842-3636.
Fax: (606) 525-7778, e-mail: order@chaphall.com.

For a complete listing of Chapman & Hall's titles, send your requests to
Chapman & Hall, Dept. BC, 115 Fifth Avenue, New York, NY 10003.

Contents

Preface to the Fourth English Edition

It continues to be a pleasure to help edit the English Edition of the Color Atlas of Pediatric Diseases. The authors continue to update the book in ways which are relevant and make this a valuable resource in the diagnosis of pediatric diseases.

I would like to thank Lauren Enck for her assistance in organizing this Fourth English Edition. I would also like to thank my sons, Gregory and Benjamin, for reminding me daily how important it is that we cherish our children and maintain them in good health.

Burlington, September 1997   Roger F. Soll

Preface to the Fourth German Edition

In comparison with the third edition, we have expanded the illustrations with 93 figures. I would especially like to thank Mrs. Hanna Lüthje-Reimers (Photography Department of the Children's Clinic of the University of Kiel) for her valuable assistance and great personal dedication. I would also like to thank the Ophthalmology, Dermatology, Otolaryngology, and Orthopedics Clinic, Dental and Orofacial Clinic of the University of Kiel, the Municipal Children's Clinic in Kiel, the Children's Clinic of the University of Lübeck, the Ophthalmology Clinic of the University of Zurich (Klara Landau, M.D.), and Professor Andreas Rett, M.D., (Vienna) for graciously providing numerous photographs. The text was updated and expanded to include new information on the etiology and pathogenesis of various childhood diseases. Translations into English, Italian, Portuguese, and Indonesian have been published in the interim. We hope that the new edition of the Color Atlas will continue to be helpful in the diagnosis of rare diseases and to enable medical students to become familiar with the major clinical syndromes.

Sadly, my co-author, Professor Michael Jänner, M.D., who was very instrumental in the production of the Color Atlas, passed away in 1991. I deeply regret his death and will always remember him with heartfelt appreciation.

C. Simon

Foreword to the Second German Edition

The success of the First Edition and its English and Italian translations prompted us to prepare an up-to-date Second Edition. We have added 96 illustrations and revised the text to reflect current knowledge and research. Several illustrations were improved with better photographs. We hope that the Color Atlas will remain a reliable reference work in the diagnosis and differential diagnosis of pediatric diseases.

In preparing the Second Edition, we received considerable help from Ms. Hanna Lüthje-Reimers (Photography Department at the University of Kiel Children's Clinic). We would like to thank her and Dr. K. Heyne (Children's Clinic-University of Lübeck) for their assistance.

Kiel, September 1989   C. Simon and M. Jänner

Preface to the Second English Edition

It is a pleasure to help with the 2nd Edition of the Color Atlas of Pediatric Diseases. The addition of 96 new figures will help this book continue to be a valuable resource in the diagnosis of pediatric diseases.

I would again like to note the contribution of Jake Barickman in translating the German text, Dr. Alan Guttmacher for his assistance in tracking down the more obscure syndromes, Nancy Moreland for her preparation of the manuscript, and my family for their patience.

Burlington, October 1989   Roger F. Soll

Foreword to the First German Edition

The color figures of this atlas demonstrate symptoms of illnesses observed mostly in the medical treatment of children, as well as in other specialties of medicine. Therefore, the atlas will be of interest not only to pediatricians and general practitioners, but also to midwives, surgeons, and other specialists. Medical students can use the book as a supplement to a basic text, which will allow them to become familiar with diseases rarely dealt with in clinical instruction. The figures chosen for their rarity of symptoms seemed most valuable; other figures were chosen with certain instructional points in mind. A comprehensive discussion of every conceivable symptom was not our intent and would have made the atlas unnecessarily cumbersome and expensive. Rather, the accompanying text consists of short descriptions of each figure and offers possible differential diagnoses. Only those figures illustrating rare diseases receive a more detailed discussion along with important points for clinical diagnostic interpretation. The carefully compiled index facilitates the location of illustrated symptoms as well as diseases; this can be important with regard to differential diagnosis. For the most part, the figures originate from the Photography Department at the University of Kiel Children's Clinic, directed by Ms. Herta Dibbern, whom we thank in particular for her assistance. Other photographs were made available to us courtesy of the Dermatology Clinic at the University of Hamburg and other clinics and institutes of the University of Kiel (Orthopedics, Dermatology, Ophthalmology, Otolaryngology, Craniofacial Clinic, as well as the Institute for Human Genetics and the Pathology Institute). We owe a debt of thanks to the doctors there as well as to many colleagues at other institutions who have loaned us photographs, especially Dr. O. Braun (City Children's Clinic of Pforzheim) and Professor V. von Loewenich (University Children's Clinic in Frankfurt/Main). Finally, we thank our publisher, F. K. Schattauer, and in particular Professor P. Matis, for their openness to our objectives and for their active support.

Kiel, September 1981

C. Simon
M. Jänner

Preface to the First English Edition

Much has been said about the relative worth of pictures over words. Perhaps nowhere is this cliché more true than in the practice of medicine where the recognition of the disease process is essential to diagnosis and treatment. It was, therefore, a pleasure to help with the English edition of Drs. Simon and Jänner's *Color Atlas of Pediatric Diseases*. The excellent photographs and accompanying text should aid in the recognition of a broad range of pediatric problems.

In preparing the English edition, I would like to thank Jake Barickman for the translation of the German text, Brian Decker for his advice, Nancy Moreland for her expert preparation of the manuscript, and both Nancy and my wife Roberta for their patience.

Roger F. Soll, M.D.

Living with an illness is a task that many people, including children, must face. The value judgments of the healthy must not apply to the ill. Illness is a part of human existence and, even when prolonged, should not be perceived as a defect. On the contrary, an illness can raise a person's esteem when one rises above suffering and shapes one's life according to one's own standards.

Kiel, September 1981

C. Simon
M. Jänner

1.1 Erythroblastosis Fetalis

Hydrops fetalis (generalized edema and ascites) without jaundice in a 2-hour-old newborn. The 35-year old Rh-negative mother had already given birth to two children with symptoms of Rh-incompatibility. Erythroblastosis fetalis can occur through transplacental passage of anti-D antibody in sensitized mothers. The infant was profoundly anemic at birth. Peripheral blood smear showed an increase in nucleated red blood cells (erythroblastosis) and reticulocytosis. Cord bilirubin was 3.7 mg/dl, and the result of the direct Coombs test was strongly "positive" for antibodies. The infant was treated with exchange transfusion.

Differential Diagnosis—Previously, erythroblastosis fetalis was the most common cause of hydrops fetalis. With the widespread use of Rhogam, fewer cases of hydrops fetalis secondary to isoimmunization are seen, and nonimmune causes are increasing in frequency. Hydrops fetalis can occur in conditions where there is increased intravascular hydrostatic pressure, either from primary myocardial failure (cardiac malformation or cardiac arrhythmia), high output failure (anemia or arteriovenous malformation), or obstruction of venous return (neoplasm). Decreased plasma oncotic pressure seen in liver failure or congenital nephrosis can present as hydrops. Increased capillary permeability (seen with anoxia or congenital infection) and obstruction of lymph flow (seen in Turner syndrome) may also cause hydrops fetalis.

1.2 Kernicterus

Erythroblastosis fetalis led to kernicterus in this 6-day-old newborn. The infant's peak bilirubin level was 36 mg/dl. The early signs of lethargy and loss of Moro reflex were followed by rigidity and opisthotonos. Death occurred on the eighth day due to respiratory complications.

Differential Diagnosis—Opisthotonos may also occur in association with intracranial (infratentorial) bleeding and bacterial meningitis. Neck stiffness and opisthotonos have also been observed in association with retropharyngeal abscess due to severe pain.

1.3 Bronze Baby Syndrome

Bronze baby syndrome noted in a 10-day-old premature infant with hyperbilirubinemia. Gray-brown discoloration of the skin is a side effect of phototherapy administered to infants with elevated direct-reacting bilirubin. The natural skin color returned after 4 months. Other side effects of phototherapy include loose stools, skin rash, hyperthermia, and dehydration.

1.1

1.2

1.3

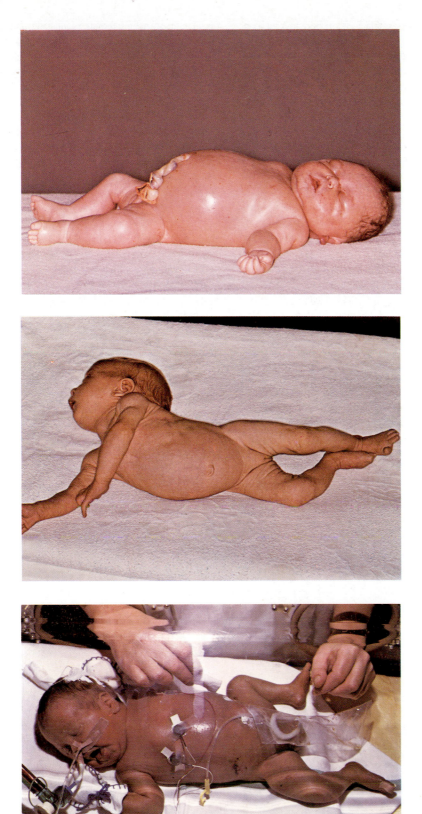

1.4 Infant of Diabetic Mother

Macrosomic infant (birthweight 5,200 g) born to a diabetic mother whose blood glucose was poorly controlled during pregnancy. Polyhydramnios is frequently seen in pregnancies complicated by diabetes. The infant is remarkably puffy and plethoric. Polycythemia was noted (hematocrit: 75%). Dextrose infusions given immediately after birth and early enteral feedings successfully prevented hypoglycemia.

Diagnosis—Macrosomic infants are prone to hypoglycemia due to the effects of maternal diabetes. Intrauterine growth retardation is possible in cases where there is uteroplacental insufficiency due to long-standing diabetes with vascular involvement. Infants of diabetic mothers have a higher incidence of birth asphyxia, birth injury, metabolic imbalance, respiratory distress, and congenital anomalies.

Differential Diagnosis—Macrosomia may be seen in Beckwith-Wiedemann syndrome (macrosomia with macroglossia), celebral gigantism (Soto syndrome), or as a variant of normal. Hypoglycemia (blood glucose < 30 mg/dl) may be seen in infants with intrauterine growth retardation, erythroblastosis fetalis, galactosemia, leucine sensitivity, and glycogen storage disease. Resistant hypoglycemia may be caused by nesidioblastosis or islet cell adenoma.

1.5 Congenital Nephrotic Syndrome (Infantile Microcystic Disease)

A 2-week-old boy with generalized edema that steadily increased after birth. Laboratory investigations revealed proteinuria and hypoproteinemia as well as low serum complement levels. Renal biopsy demonstrated cystic dilatation of the proximal tubules. Since congenital nephrosis is always resistant to steroids, therapy was limited to restriction of sodium intake and provision of adequate nutrition. The child died 6 months later with severe pneumonia.

Differential Diagnosis—For the differential diagnosis of edema in the newborn, see Figure 1.1.

1.6 Turner Syndrome

A 2-day-old infant (birthweight 2,600 g) with extensive edema of the dorsum of the foot, loose skin (cutis laxa), low posterior hairline, widely spaced nipples, and deeply set hypoplastic finger- and toenails; karyotype: 45,XO. The swelling of the soft tissue in the dorsum of the foot and hand is lymphedema, which occurs in approximately 40% of cases. Turner syndrome is associated with short stature, cardiac abnormalities (coarctation of the aorta), cubitus valgus, renal abnormalities, and ovarian dysgenesis.

Differential Diagnosis—Noonan syndrome may share many of the features of Turner syndrome; however, individuals with Noonan syndrome have a normal karyotype and may be of the male sex. Cardiac abnormalities (pulmonary stenosis) are more common in Noonan syndrome. Congenital hereditary lymphedema (Milroy's disease), is usually restricted to the lower extremity and may be progressive.

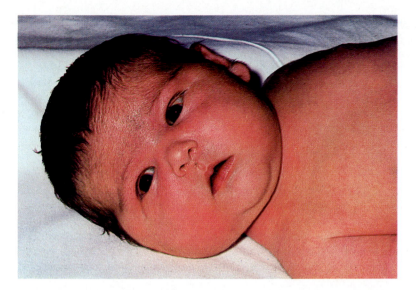

1.4

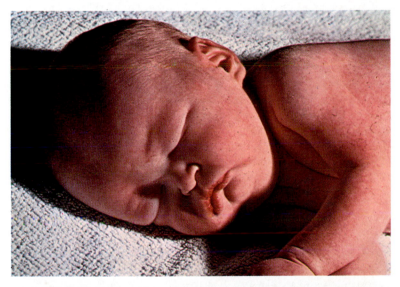

1.5

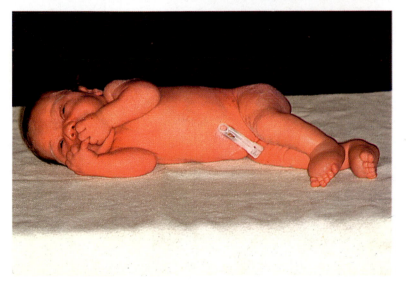

1.6

1.7

**Intrahepatic
Bile Duct
Hypoplasia**

Conjugated hyperbilirubinemia in a 2-month-old boy. Findings included jaundice due to an elevated direct-reacting bilirubin (4 mg/dl), acholic stools, hepatomegaly, and failure to thrive. The child became increasingly jaundiced after birth (maximum serum bilirubin: 17 mg/dl). Laboratory studies revealed elevated total and direct bilirubin as well as an elevated transaminase and γ-glutamyl transferase. The diagnosis of intrahepatic biliary hypoplasia was confirmed by liver biopsy. Histologic examination revealed an inflammatory process involving the intralobular bile ducts. The outcome of these children is variable; the disease may slowly progress toward biliary cirrhosis or may stabilize without obvious progression. Conjugated hyperbilirubinemia may also occur in extrahepatic biliary atresia, choledochal cyst, neonatal hepatitis, congenital infections, and metabolic disorders, including galactassemia and α-antitrypsin deficiency.

1.8

Physiologic Jaundice

Mild jaundice in a 3-day-old baby girl. Jaundice was first noticed on the second day of life and was resolved by the sixth day of life. Indirect bilirubin reached a peak level of 6.8 mg/dl. Mild elevation of indirect bilirubin is common in the newborn because of the immaturity of hepatic enzymes and increased intrahepatic circulation. Pathologic conditions causing hyperbilirubinemia in the newborn can be differentiated from physiologic jaundice by their early onset (before 24 hours of age), persistence beyond 1 week of age, and greater elevation of either total or direct bilirubin.

Differential Diagnosis—Differential diagnosis includes fetomaternal blood group incompatibility (isoimmunization), closed space hemorrhage, impaired hepatic uptake (Gilbert syndrome), or impaired conjugation (Crigler-Najjar syndrome).

1.9

**Extrahepatic
Biliary Atresia**

Cirrhosis of the liver, ascites (due to portal hypertension), and hepatosplenomegaly in an 8-month-old boy. The diagnosis of extrahepatic biliary atresia was confirmed by documenting interrupted bile flow and performing a liver biopsy to rule out an intrahepatic process. The child underwent a hepatic portoenterostomy (Kasai procedure) at 4 months of age. The operation was unsuccessful, and severe conjugated hyperbilirubinemia and cirrhosis of the liver developed. Despite supportive care, the child died at 1 year of age.

Differential Diagnosis—See text accompanying Figure 1.7 for causes of conjugated hyperbilirubinemia. Severe abdominal distension may be seen in ileus, intraabdominal tumors, hemoperitoneum, or fecal impaction. Ascites may be seen in congestive heart failure, malnutrition, malignancy, nephrotic syndrome, pancreatitis, and urinary obstruction.

1.10

**Alpha-1-Antitrypsin
Deficiency**

A 5-month-old boy with abdominal distention, hepatomegaly, ascites, and cirrhosis. Serum measurements of α-1-antitrypsin levels were low. Typical PAS-positive granules were detected in the cytoplasm of hepatocytes on liver biopsy. Liver disease in children who are homozygous for this disorder (pi-type ZZ), may develop but the majority present with pulmonary complications.

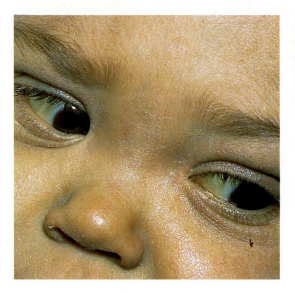

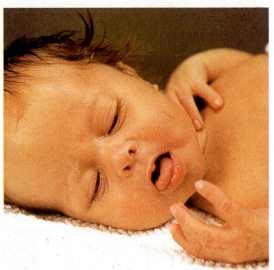

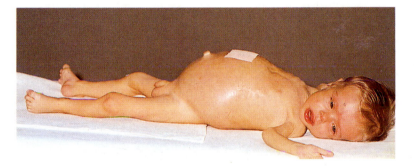

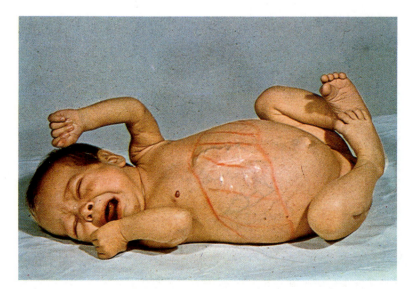

1.11–1.13
Prematurity

Figures 1.11 and 1.12 show a 2-day-old, 900-g, premature infant born at 28 weeks gestation. Physical findings include thin, red skin with little subcutaneous fat, abundant lanugo, large head relative to body size, and soft pinna due to the lack of cartilage. Figure 1.13 shows the same infant at 97 days of age, weighing 3,000 g; no striking neurologic sequelae were noted at this time. The child was discharged from the hospital and sent home.

Differential Diagnosis—All low-birthweight infants are not premature. Dysmature infants reach a birthweight lower than that expected for the corresponding gestational age, and may have dry, peeling skin, little subcutaneous fat, and meconium staining. Although their birthweight is low, head growth in these infants may be normal, and they do not usually show signs of immature organ development.

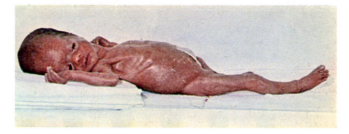

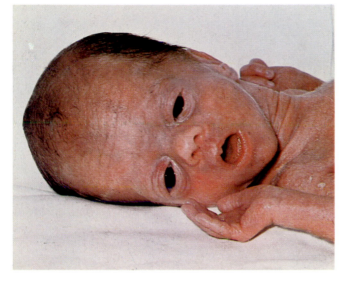

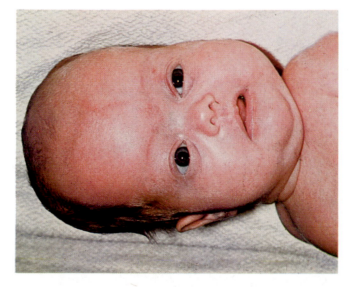

1.14
Feto-fetal Transfusion Syndrome

Feto-fetal transfusion syndrome seen in prematurely born identical twins. The syndrome is due to vascular anastomosis in the monochorionic placenta. Of greatest pathologic significance is the arteriovenous anastomosis (due to the pressure differential). Transfusion syndrome may complicate 15% of identical twin pregnancies. Discordance, defined as a 20% difference in birthweight, or a difference in hemoglobin of greater than 5 mg/dl may result between the twins.

These twins were discordant. The pale donor twin had a hematocrit of 36%, as well as hypovolemia, respiratory distress, and anemia, which required blood transfusions. The recipient twin had hyperbilirubinemia and required phototherapy. Polycythemia may also be seen in uteroplacental insufficiency, delayed cord clamping, and materno-fetal transfusion.

1.15
Dysmaturity

A disproportionately low weight (2,800 g) relative to length (48 cm) in a 2-day-old neonate. The findings included decreased subcutaneous fat, dry desquamating skin with poor turgor, and meconium-stained skin and nails. Numerous

causes can be considered, including placental insufficiency, fetal alcohol syndrome, intrauterine infection, and chromosomal abnormalities.

1.16
Postmaturity

Postmature 1-day-old neonate born 2 weeks after expected date of confinement. The infant's birthweight was 3,300 g, and his length was 58 cm. Findings included dry, desquamating skin, decreased subcutaneous fat, "washerwoman's

hands," long nails, and yellow discoloration of both the nails and the skin due to meconium staining. Additional signs included the absence of lanugo and vernix caseosa.

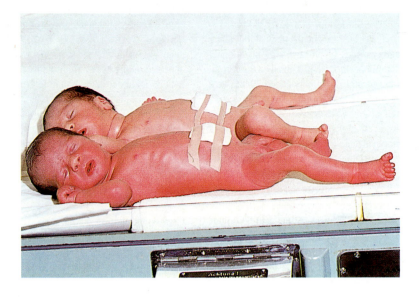

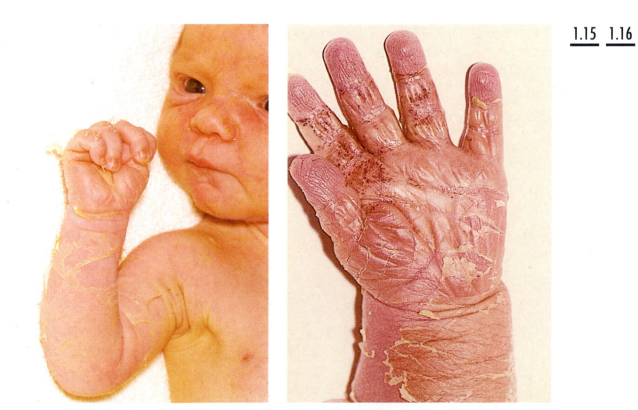

1.17

Isoimmune Thrombocytopenia

Petechial and purpuric skin lesions in a 1-day-old girl. Lesions were observed over the face and the body of the infant. There were no clinical signs of prenatal viral infection or bacterial sepsis. Thrombocytopenia was noted on the peripheral blood smear, but no other laboratory abnormalities were seen. The thrombocytopenia was caused by the transplacental passage of maternal isoantibodies directed against the child's platelets. The most common platelet antigen involved in isoimmune thrombocytopenia is the Pl^{A1} antigen present in 98% of the general population. There were no signs of intra-cranial hemorrhage, a major risk of thrombocytopenia in the newborn. Over the first month of life, the infant's platelet count gradually returned to normal, and no more skin lesions appeared. Other causes of thrombocytopenia in the newborn include maternal autoimmune thrombocytopenia, inherited disorders of platelet production (thrombocytopenia with absent radius, Wiskott-Aldrich syndrome), prenatal or postnatal infection, maternal medications, and platelet consumption in a cavernous hemangioma (Kasabach-Merritt syndrome).

1.18

Birth Trauma

Severe birth trauma seen in a 6-day-old newborn. Findings included superficial skin hemorrhages over the extremities and torso. The infant experienced severe fetal distress in utero (demonstrated by a slow, irregular fetal heart rate) and postpartum asphyxia (cyanosis, bradycardia, respiratory distress, and cardiogenic shock shortly after birth). The infant died from complications of birth trauma on the ninth day. Autopsy revealed an infratentorial hemorrhage as well as pulmonary hemorrhage with edema and atelectasis of both lungs.

1.19

Neonatal Sepsis

Sepsis due to *Escherichia coli* in a 2-day-old boy born after prolonged rupture of membranes. Petechial skin lesions were the first sign of sepsis in this infant. Other clinical signs of sepsis include poor feeding, lethargy, hypothermia, respiratory distress, and apnea. Bacteria were isolated from both the blood and cerebrospinal fluid. Although thrombocyto-penia was noted, the typical findings of disseminated intra-vascular coagulation were not seen. The infection apparently began in utero due to maternal chorioamnionitis. Coagulation problems in the newborn can also be caused by vitamin K deficiency, hepatic dysfunction, or hereditary coagulation disorders.

1.20

Birth Trauma

Ecchymotic skin lesions in a 1-day-old premature infant born after face presentation. Note the deep blue discoloration and swelling of the face.

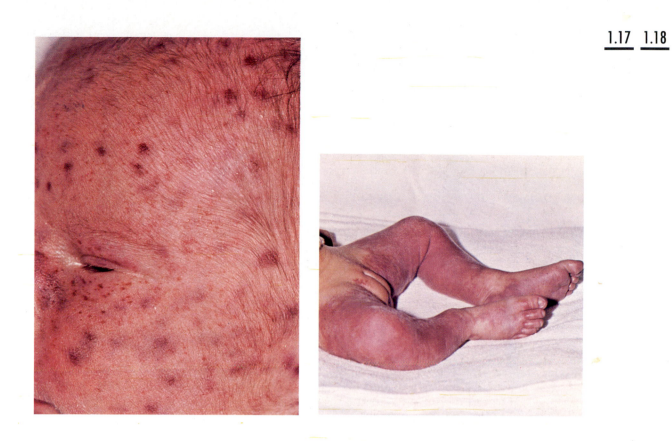

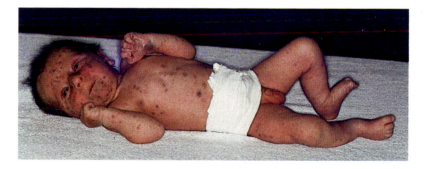

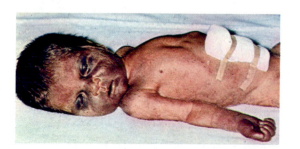

1.21
Birth Trauma

Pseudoparalysis of the legs due to traumatic epiphyseal fracture after a difficult delivery. Radiographic studies demonstrate a lateral shift of both femoral epiphyses. Patellar and Achilles tendon reflexes were absent. The infant died on the sixth day of life due to a large subdural hematoma. The epiphyseal fracture of the femur with extensive subperiosteal hematomas was confirmed on autopsy.

Differential Diagnosis—Traumatic proximal epiphyseal fracture must be distinguished from traumatic or congenital hip joint subluxation. In epiphyseal fracture, the radiographic studies reveal typical callus formation after 1 week; callus formation is not seen in subluxation. Fracture of the shaft of the femur can be easily ruled out. Genuine paralysis is possible due to traumatic vertebral fracture and damage to the spinal cord. Pseudoparalysis of Parrot is seen with congenital syphilis and can present with similar symptoms. Other conditions that may appear as reduced spontaneous movement include muscular hypotonia caused by Werdnig-Hoffmann disease and the temporary hypotonia caused by intracranial hemorrhage.

1.22
Umbilical Cord Furrows

Umbilical cord furrows with skin ulcerations in the flank of a prematurely born twin. The skin lesions were caused by the binding of the hip of one twin with the umbilical cord of the other twin who had died in utero. Because of uterine myomatosis, the delivery was done by cesarean section. The skin lesion gradually healed after antibiotic treatment.

Differential Diagnosis—Similar skin lesions may be seen with amniotic bands. Intrauterine rupture of the amnion may cause entrapment in fibrous bands, leading to skin lesions or, in severe cases, amputation of the extremity (Figures 2.96 and 2.106).

1.23
Hematoma of the Umbilical Cord

Large hematoma of the umbilical cord resulting from the rupture of the umbilical vein. The hematoma was present at birth and was surgically removed on the second day of life.

Differential Diagnosis—The differential diagnosis of a large umbilical mass include congenital omphalocele, umbilical cord tumors such as angioma, enteroteratoma, dermoid cysts, myosarcoma, and persistence of the omphalomesenteric duct or urachus.

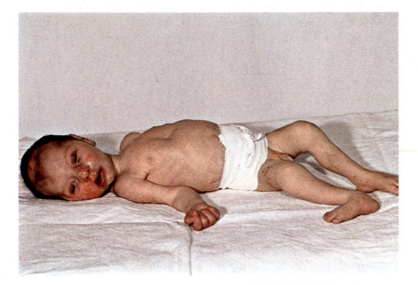

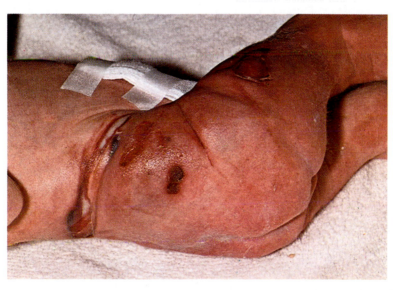

1.22

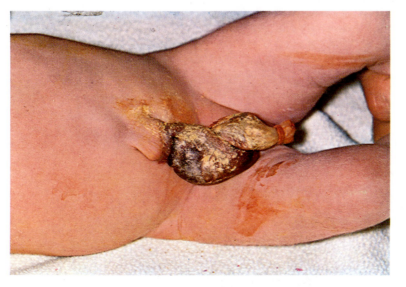

1.23

1.24
Congenital Facial Paresis

Facial paresis in a 1-day-old newborn with multiple deformities (dysplastic pinna and tympanic canal, bilateral radial aplasia, and congenital heart disease). When the infant cried, only the nonparalyzed side of the face would move. On the affected side, the forehead was smooth, the eye could not be closed, the nasolabial fold was absent, and the mouth drooped. The other cranial nerves were intact. Meningitis and encephalitis were ruled out. The facial paresis was probably attributable to traumatic damage to the peripheral portion of the facial nerve at birth. Eventually, complete recovery from the paresis was achieved. No single syndrome that encompassed the other deformities was identified.

In cases of traumatic facial paresis, usually only the peripheral portion of the facial nerve is affected. In central facial paralysis, the two lower branches are affected, allowing for movement of the forehead. With central lesions, there are usually other signs of brain damage (e.g., simultaneous abducens paralysis). In Mobius syndrome (malformation of the cranial nerve nuclei) facial paralysis starts at birth, but is usually bilateral and incomplete. Abducens paralysis of one or both sides is always present. Children affected with Mobius syndrome have a noticeably expressionless face and a constant flow of saliva. Other deformities are present, including micrognathia, talipes equinovarus, and Poland's sequence (absence of pectoralis muscle). Older children can have facial paralysis due to tumors of the brainstem, basilar skull fracture, acute or chronic otitis media, or Bell's palsy. Facial paresis is seen in Melkersson syndrome associated with edema of the eyelids.

1.25
Congenital Facial Paresis

Congenital facial paresis in a 3-day-old boy. The right corner of the mouth was turned down and the nasolabial fold was flattened. The temporofacial branch was intact because the right eye could be closed and the forehead could move symmetrically. In this case, only the fibers supplying the cervicofacial branch were damaged due to traumatic forceps delivery.

Similar facial appearance occurs in asymmetric crying facies caused by unilateral absence or hypoplasia of the angular depressor muscles. In this syndrome, the nasolabial fold is normal, and the affected side will not move when the infant cries. The syndrome may be associated with cardiovascular abnormalities.

1.26
Subgaleal Hemorrhage

Subgaleal hemorrhage in a 1-day-old infant born with the aid of vacuum extraction. Edematous swelling, subcutaneous hematoma, and skin abrasion were noted over the scalp. There was no evidence of skull fracture or intracranial bleeding. Subgaleal hematoma occurs between the periosteum and the epicranial aponeurosis. The hematoma often goes beyond the cranial suture line and may spread over the entire scalp. Significant blood loss may occur.

Differential Diagnosis—A cephalhematoma lies below the periosteum, and is confined by the cranial sutures. Caput succedaneum refers to edematous or ecchymotic swelling of the scalp and may cross over suture lines.

1.27
Cephalhematoma

Cephalhematoma in a 9-day-old infant. A spherical fluctuant mass, which did not cross the suture line, was noted over the right parietal bone. No other scalp defect was noted. There was no radiographic evidence of a parietal skull fracture. Calcification of the lesion occurred, giving the lesion an "eggshell" feel.

Differential Diagnosis—Other extracranial hematomas, including caput succedaneum and subgaleal hemorrhage, must be excluded. An encephalocele can be differentiated by pulsation during crying and by radiographic studies demonstrating a skull defect.

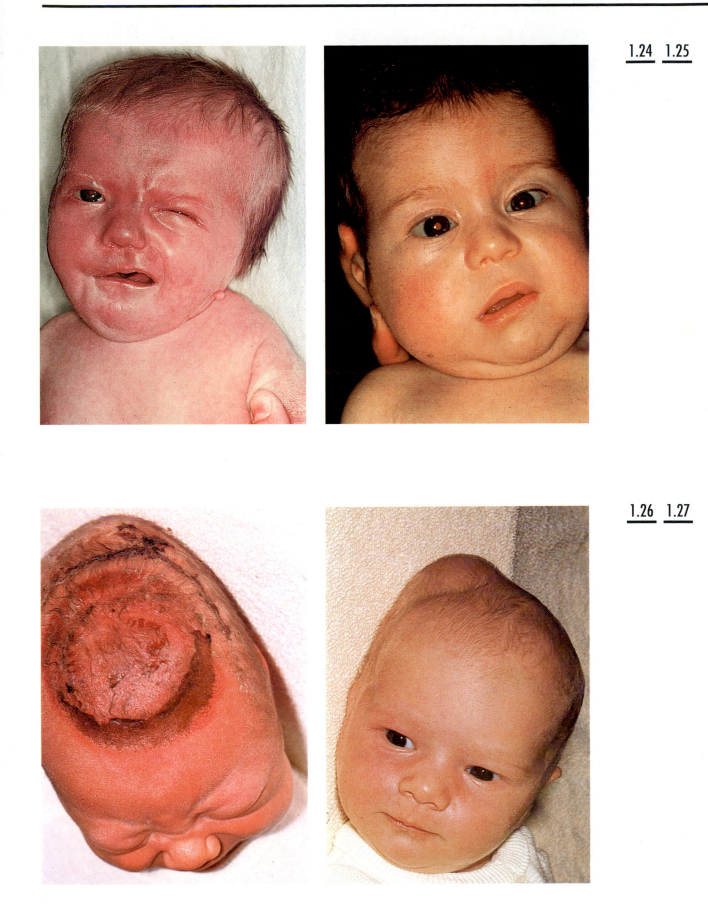

1.28

Omphalocele

A walnut sized omphalocele in a 6-week-old boy. An omphalocele occurs when there is herniation of abdominal contents through a defect in the base of the umbilical cord. The defect is covered only by peritoneum without overlying skin. Intestinal contents were noted in the hernial sac. The child was treated conservatively with frequent brushing of the hernial sac with a 2% Merthiolate solution, leading to epithelialization and shrinking of the hernial sac, retraction of the bowel contents, and closure of the hernial opening. Malrotation was diagnosed by barium enema but was not associated with any clinical manifestations. Conservative therapy is successful in only some of the cases of omphalocele; others require surgical correction.

1.29   1.30

Omphalocele

A 1-day-old infant with omphalocele. The omphalocele lay at the base of the umbilical cord, covered by peritoneum fused with amniotic membrane. Liver, spleen, and bowel could be seen through the thin membranous covering. Malrotation, a finding frequently associated with omphalocele, was recognized after appropriate radiographic studies. Due to the size of the omphalocele, immediate operative repair was not undertaken. With conservative treatment (brushing the surface of the omphalocele with a 2% Mercurochrome solution), the hernial sac gradually decreased in size, and the everted viscera returned to the abdomen. Within 4 weeks, the hernial sac had shrunk to half the original size and was fully epithelialized (Figure 1.30). Treatment with organic mercurial antiseptic is controversial, as infants may develop potentially toxic levels of mercury. In general, early operative repair is desirable if it is required.

Differential Diagnosis—Omphalocele must be distinguished from umbilical hernia. Umbilical hernia occurs with incomplete closure or weakness of the umbilical ring and is often associated with diastasis recti. An umbilical hernia is covered with skin, protrudes when the child cries, and can be easily reduced.

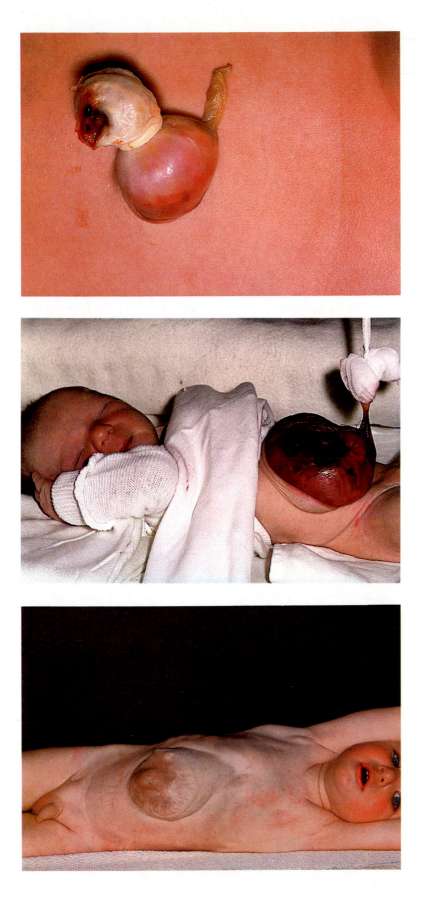

1.31

Harlequin Skin Changes

A 5-day-old newborn with harlequin skin changes (due to vasomotor instability). The child is pictured lying on one side. The left lateral aspect of the child is pale; the right side is deep red. The color change lasted only a few minutes and disappeared when the child's position was changed. Sometimes, the skin changes were noted only on the torso or face. Movement of the infant would occasionally cause a generalized temporary redness.

1.32

Cutis Marmorata

Cutis marmorata with harlequin skin changes in a 2-week-old newborn. The lightly reticulated skin became pale on the right side when the infant lay on the left side; the left side became livid and red. The opposite changes were noted when the infant lay on the right side. The infant was referred to the clinic because of unilateral "cyanosis." When the child was picked up, the color change disappeared. Congenital heart disease was ruled out. By the time the child was 4 weeks old, this phenomenon could no longer be observed.

1.33

Cutis Marmorata

Cutis marmorata in a 4-month-old child. A fine reticulated network of superficial vessels could easily be appreciated due to the paucity of subcutaneous fat. The relatively frequent finding of cutis marmorata may later become idiopathic livedo reticularis (gray-blue skin discoloration with characteristic reticulated pattern). Livedo reticularis may first present with exposure to the cold, but later may become a more persistent finding. Frequently, it begins on the arms and legs, but it can also spread to the torso. Livedo reticularis may occur secondary to vascular disease such as periarteritis nodosa or systemic lupus erythematosus.

1.34

Cutis Marmorata Telangiectasia Congenita

Congenital cutis marmorata telangiectasia (congenital livedo reticularis) in a 6-week-old girl. Dilated superficial capillaries and veins were noted from birth. The skin appeared as a fine reticulated network with white insulae. The light red markings of the skin increased in response to crying or cooling. The affected skin seemed thinner than normal due to a deficiency in subcutaneous fat. These skin changes were found predominantly on the legs, face, and back.

Congenital livedo reticularis usually persists throughout life, but may improve with increasing age. Small areas of superficial ulceration may develop in some patients. Nevi araneous (p. 162) and angiokeratomas can also be present.

1.31

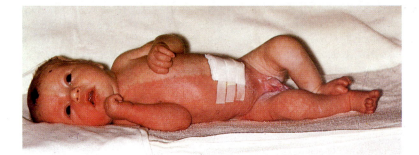

1.32

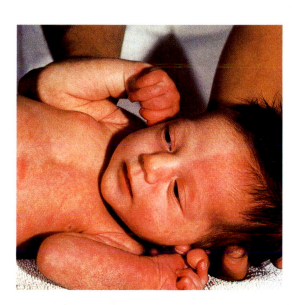

1.33 1.34

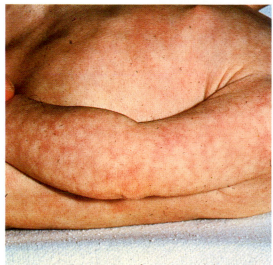 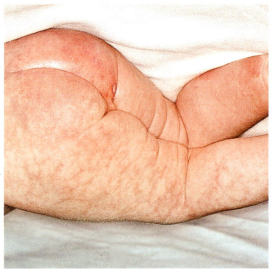

1.35

Cavernous Hemangioma

Cavernous hemangioma (strawberry nevus) in a 5-month-old girl. The soft, spherical, compressible growth was noted over the right parietal bone, measuring 3 × 4 cm. The mass was red-blue and not painful. Radiographic studies demonstrated normal cranial bones underneath the lesion. By age 4 years, the hemangioma had spontaneously disappeared.

Most (90%) cavernous hemangiomas are noted within the first month of life; the remainder develop within the first 9 months. They may go through a growth phase in the first 6 to 9 months, but will then begin a period of involution at 1 to 2 years of age. After 5 years, 50% have involuted. After 7 years, 70% disappear. During the growth phase, complications may occur if the hemangioma impinges upon vital structures. Larger hemangiomas can cause thrombocytopenia and hemorrhage (Kasabach-Merritt syndrome). Steroids may be used to induce involution.

1.36

Congenital Dermoid Cyst

A 2-day-old newborn with a cystic growth in the midline of the scalp over the parietal bone. The lesion was erythematous with a central tuft of hair. The mass grew slowly over a 2-week period and required surgical removal. Histologic examination revealed a cyst comprised of an outer surface of squamous epithelium and containing hair, fatty material, and keratin. Dermoid cysts usually develop from sequestered cells in embryonic rests and are most common in the area of the eyes, nose, mouth, or neck.

Differential Diagnosis—Meningoencephaloceles are associated with an underlying bony defect and, in general, are pulsatile.

1.37

Cutis Aplasia

Congenital cutis aplasia in an 8-month-old boy. At birth, the child had a sharply delineated solitary skin defect. The lesion crusted and healed within a few weeks leaving an oval, hairless, atrophic gray scar (1 × 2 cm) located on the head, slightly displaced from the midline. No other malformations were noted. Trisomy 13 (Patau syndrome, p. 74) was ruled out.

Differential Diagnosis—Birth trauma (forceps marks), nevus sebaceous (p. 168, 264), and certain forms of alopecia, including oculomandibulofacial syndrome (abnormal cranium, microphthalmia, cataracts, micrognathia), must be ruled out.

1.38

Scalp Abscess

Scalp abscess in an 8-day-old prematurely born infant. The infant was delivered by cesarean section after prolonged rupture of membranes and maternal amnionitis. The abscess was successfully treated by surgical incision and drainage followed by antibiotic therapy. Skin abrasions caused by forceps or scalp electrodes for fetal monitoring may often be the site of similar lesions. The parietal area is a frequent site for scalp abscesses, and often these lesions are bilateral. The infection is usually caused by *Staphylococcus*.

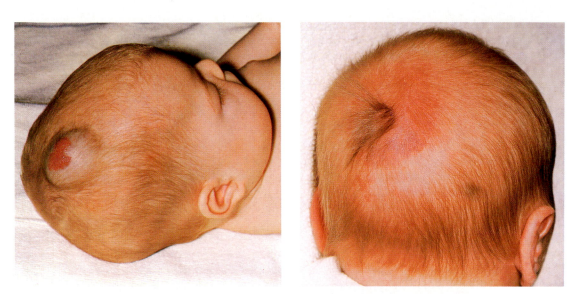

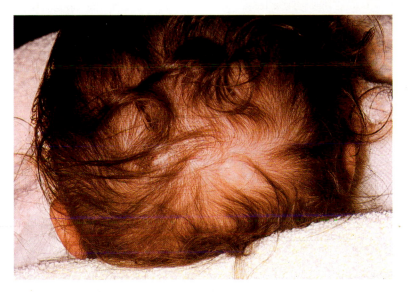

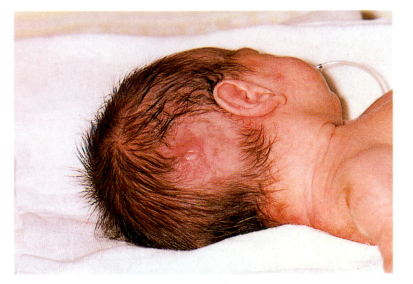

1.39

Milia

Numerous tiny, yellow papules on both sides of the cheeks, as well as the nose, upper lip, and chin of a 7-day-old boy. Milia are small superficial inclusion cysts containing keratin, occurring in 40% of all newborns. In addition to the face, milia may be found over the upper body and limbs, but seldom on the genitals. They disappear by the third or fourth week of life. Persistent and numerous milia may be seen in orofacial-digital syndrome type I (cleft palate, flat mid-face, brachydactyly).

1.40

Mongolian Spot

Mongolian spots in a 6-month-old Korean girl. Several oval, poorly defined, gray-blue pigmented spots of varying size were noted in the lumbosacral area. Mongolian spots frequently occur in Oriental and African infants (80%), while the frequency in the European Caucasian population is only 1% to 5%. They are usually located on the flanks and shoulders and fade during childhood. They seldom persist into adulthood. Unlike mongolian spots, the blue nevus (p. 168) is slightly raised, is located on the arms, legs, or face, and lasts throughout life.

1.41

Erythema Toxicum

Erythema toxicum in a 1-day-old girl. Numerous, irregularly defined erythematous areas (0.3 to 3.0 cm in diameter) were noted over the torso as well as the arms and legs. In response to pressure, the erythema faded, and the underlying skin appeared slightly thickened. After a few hours, the rash could no longer be detected.

The cause of erythema toxicum is unknown; its occurrence is relatively frequent in full-term infants, but is seldom seen in premature infants. The rash may present at birth, but usually begins on the first or second day of life and is rarely seen after the 14th day of life. In more severe cases, the erythema evolves into a papular, vesicular exanthem. The rash will usually disappear within 2 to 4 days.

1.42

Erythema Toxicum

Erythema toxicum in a 2-day-old full-term girl. Small vesicles and pustules on an erythematous base were noted over the trunk and the extremities, but spared the palms of the hands and the soles of the feet. Wright stain of the contents of the vesicles demonstrated eosinophils and no bacteria.

Differential Diagnosis—Staphylococcal skin infection can be ruled out. In staphylococcal infections, neutrophils and bacteria may be demonstrated in the pustule. Miliaria crystallina (caused by superficial blockage of the secretory ducts of sweat glands) can be confused with erythema toxicum. Miliaria crystallina can be recognized by characteristic tiny diaphanous retention "cysts," which can easily be wiped away. Miliaria rubra (caused by deeper blockage of the sweat gland ducts) is associated with red "pinhead" papules over the trunk, which are pruritic and somewhat painful. Candidal skin infections may be acquired congenitally from ascending maternal colonization or infection. In generalized cutaneous candidiasis, a scaly erythematous rash as well as small pustules are noted on an erythematous base. The palms and soles are also affected. *Candida albicans* is detected microscopically or through culture. Systemic disease is rare, but, if present, is frequently fatal.

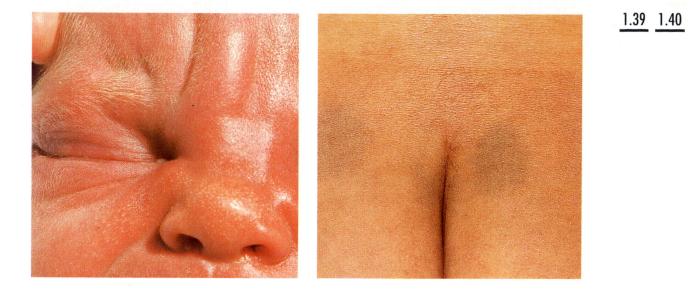

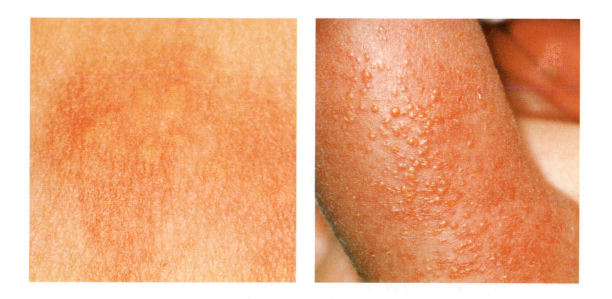

1.43
Congenital Syphilis

A 3-week-old girl with diffuse erythematous maculopapular rash over the soles of her feet and legs due to congenital syphilis. The rash was also noted on the torso, arms, and palms of the hands. Areas of the rash were consistent with a bullous eruption. Hepatosplenomegaly was noted. Serologic testing was positive for syphilis in both mother and child. The infant was treated with penicillin G for 2 weeks.

Differential Diagnosis—Since the appearance of a rash in congenital syphilis can be extremely variable, many different skin diseases must be ruled out, including bullous impetigo, pemphigoid, exfoliative dermatitis, dermatitis herpetiformis, epidermolysis bullosa, intercontinentia pigmenti syndrome, urticaria pigmentosa, acrodermatitis enteropathica, and congenital bullous ichthyosiform erythroderma.

1.44
Congenital Syphilis

A 6-week-old child with an erythematous rash and vesicles and bullae on the toes and the soles of the feet. The infant also had serous coryza (snuffles). The mother was not tested for syphilis during her pregnancy, but subsequent serologic testing was positive for syphilis in both mother and child. The child was successfully treated with penicillin G.

Differential Diagnosis—Syphilitic dactylitis (osteochondritis of the hand) must be differentiated from tuberculous dactylitis, dactylitis associated with sickle cell anemia or coccidioidomycosis, and distal dactylitis with blister formation due to streptococcal infection.

1.45
Congenital Syphilis

Although asymptomatic at birth, this 4-week-old girl slowly acquired heepatomegaly and direct hyperbilirubinemia. Radiographic studies demonstrated the typical bony changes (an area of periosteal calcification at the tibial diaphysis and a radiolucent band below the metaphyseal plate).

Differential Diagnosis—Hepatomegaly and direct hyperbilirubinemia occur in biliary atresia, choledochal cysts, other prenatal or postnatal infections, galactosemia, and α-1-antitrypsin deficiency.

1.46
Congenital syphilis

Abnormal dentition in a 15-year-old girl. The teeth have the typical changes associated with congenital syphilis (Hutchinson's teeth, barrel-shaped upper incisors with half-moon-shaped indentations due to a defect in the enamel). The girl also had hearing loss and chorioretinitis. The diagnosis of congenital syphilis was not recognized until the girl was 13 years old. After serologic confirmation, she was treated with penicillin G for 15 days.

Differential Diagnosis—Tooth anomalies are present in ectodermal dysplasia, intercontinentia pigmenti, and cleidocranial dysplasia (Scheuthauer-Marie-Sainton syndrome).

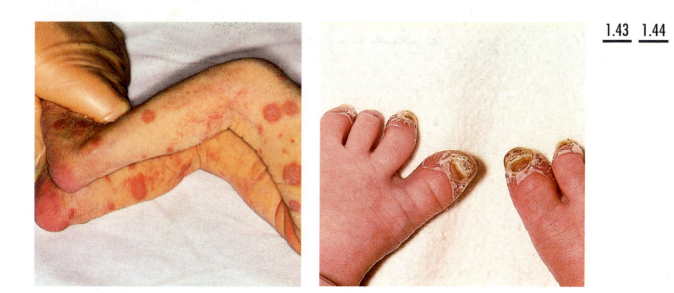

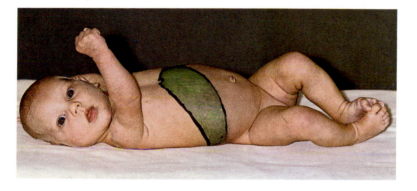

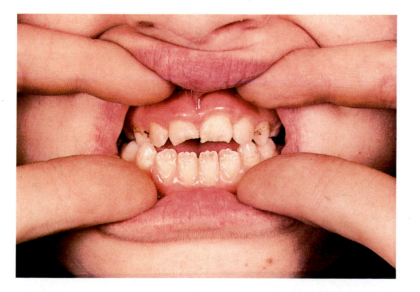

1.47

Congenital Rubella Syndrome

Congenital rubella syndrome in a 1-day-old term newborn. The infant had thrombocytopenic purpura and bilateral lens opacification (cataracts). A patent ductus arteriosus was noted shortly after birth. Rubella virus was cultured from the infant's throat. IgM antibody specific for rubella was detected in the serum. Bilateral hearing loss was diagnosed in the second year of life. The child's unvaccinated mother had contact with a child with German measles (rubella) in the third month of pregnancy.

1.48

Scrotal Hematoma

Scrotal hematoma in a 1-day-old newborn who was born by breech delivery. The dark blue discoloration of the enlarged scrotum was caused by birth trauma. There were no other hematomas noted. Testicular torsion (usually unilateral and very painful) was ruled out by Doppler ultrasound imaging.

1.49

Neonatal Sepsis

Neonatal sepsis in a 2-day-old term newborn with ecchymosis and petechiae over the entire body. These skin lesions were noted in association with fever, hypotension, and poor perfusion. The infant was born to an afebrile mother who had prolonged rupture of membranes (5 days before delivery). Thrombocytopenia (platelet count: 3,000/µl), neutropenia, and a predominance of bands was noted. *Escherichia coli* was cultured from the blood. The infant was successfully treated with early institution of antibiotic therapy because of suspected maternal chorioamnionitis.

1.50

Waterhouse-Friderichsen Syndrome

Patchy purpuric lesions were evident on the face and over the rest of the child's body. This child had a fulminant course of meningococcemia with widespread purpura and shock associated with adrenal hemorrhage (Waterhouse-Friderichsen syndrome).

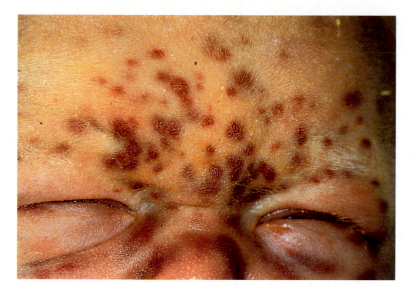

1.47

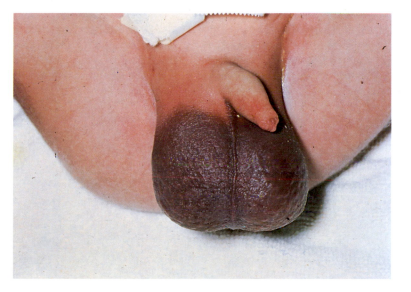

1.48

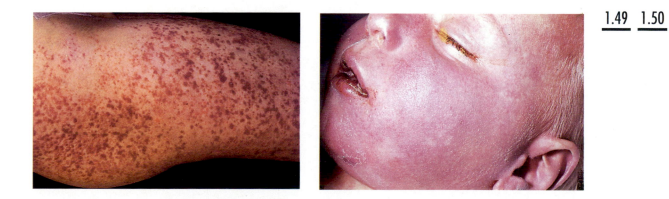

1.49   1.50

2.1

Brachycephaly

Flattening of the occiput (brachycephaly) in a 3-week-old boy with Down syndrome. Brachycephaly also occurs in Brachmann-de Lange syndrome, hypochondroplasia, cleido- cranial dysplasia, Apert syndrome, Carpenter syndrome, and other clinical conditions where there is premature closure of the coronal suture.

2.2

Craniofacial Dysostosis

Craniofacial dysostosis (Crouzon's disease) in a 6-year-old girl. Findings included deformed skull (acrocephaly), short- ened occiput, exophthalmos, external strabismus, hypoplastic maxilla, short upper lip, and protruding lower lip. Radio- graphic studies of the skull demonstrated premature synosto- sis with shortening of the base of the skull and narrow optic foramina. Due to signs of early optic atrophy, cranial surgery, including decompression and maxillary advancement, was undertaken.

2.3

Microcephaly

Microcephaly in a 6-month-old boy. The cranium was small (OFC 39 cm), the fontanel closed, and the ears low-set. The child had convergent strabismus and severe developmental delay. The underlying cause of the microcephaly was unclear. Congenital microcephaly occurs with intrauterine infections (rubella, toxoplasmosis, cytomegalovirus), with chromo- somal abnormalities (cri du chat syndrome, Wolf-Hirschhorn syndrome, trisomy 13), with toxic drug effects (fetal alcohol syndrome, fetal aminopterin syndrome), and with Fanconi Syndrome.   P KU

2.4

Anencephaly

A 6-day-old newborn with anencephaly (just before death). The infant had a major congenital skull and central nervous system defect, including the absence of the skull bones, cranial vault, and incomplete development of the brain. Fa- cial features included protruding eyes and prominent nose. Malformation of other organs may occur in association with anencephaly, including adrenal hypoplasia and genitourinary abnormalities. Children with anencephaly are frequently stillborn or die within a few days after birth.

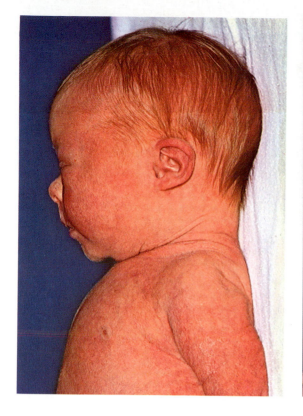 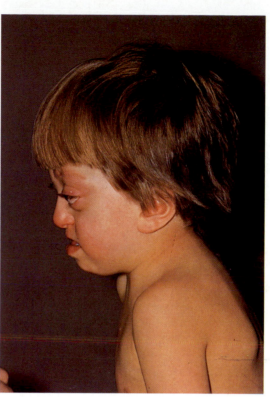

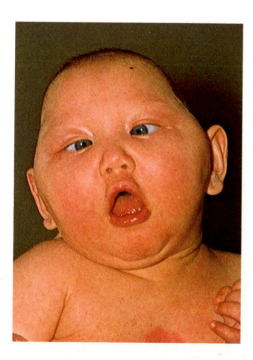 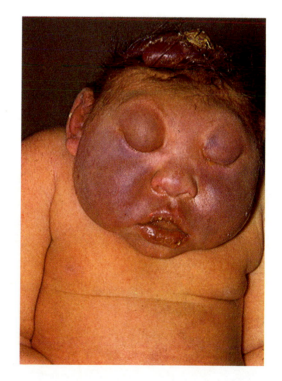

2.5–2.7

Apert Syndrome

Apert syndrome (acrocephalosyndactyly) in a 5-day-old newborn. Findings included acrocephaly (due to bilateral congenital coronal craniosynostosis) and facial dysmorphism (protruding forehead, small nose, maxillary hypoplasia, high arched palate). Soft tissue syndactyly of both hands and feet was noted. Osseous syndactyly of the third and fourth phalanges was demonstrated radiographically. No other abnormalities were noted. The child underwent early surgical treatment even though there were no symptoms of increased intracranial pressure. Although mental retardation is frequent in Apert syndrome, mental development was normal in this case. Surgical correction of the syndactyly began at 6 months of age. Apert syndrome follows an autosomal dominant pattern of inheritance. Since both parents of this child are unaffected, this case was thought to be due to a new mutation.

Acrocephaly (turribrachycephaly) occurs in:

1. Other acrocephalosyndactylic syndromes, such as Saethre-Chotzen syndrome, Mohr syndrome (oro-facio-digital syndrome type II), and Pfeiffer syndrome
2. Acrocephalopolysyndactylic syndromes, such as Carpenter syndrome and Noack syndrome
3. Crouzon's disease (craniofacial dsyostosis), associated with craniosynostosis, midface hypoplasia, and exophthalmos.

2.8   2.9

Apert Syndrome

Apert syndrome (acrocephalosyndactyly) in a 6-year-old girl. Physical findings included acrocephaly, maxillary hypoplasia, exophthalmos (more prominent on the right than on the left), hypertelorism, and external strabismus. Radiographs of the skull taken before surgery demonstrated closed coronal sutures, pronounced shortening of the front of the skull, and enlargement of the orbits. Computed tomography of the skull demonstrated findings consistent with increased intracranial pressure. Surgical intervention included repair of a cleft palate, surgical correction of syndactyly, surgery for cranial synostosis, and maxillary advancement (at age 5). After cranial surgery, intracranial pressure returned to normal, and vision improved.

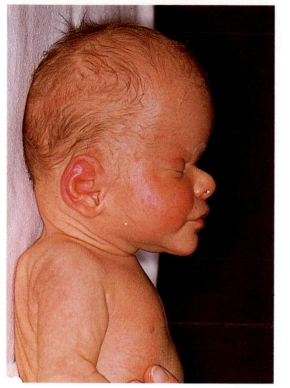

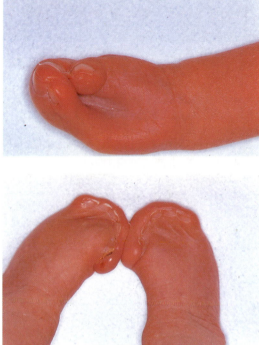

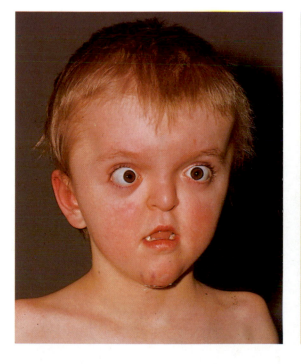

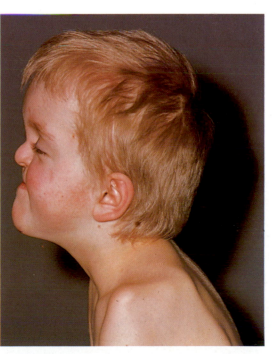

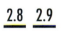

2.10 2.11

C Syndrome

C syndrome (Opitz (trigonocephaly) syndrome) in a 3-month-old boy. Physical findings included abnormal skull shape (skull tapering to a point at the forehead), protruding glabella, hypertelorism, and upward-slanting palpebral fissures. The right hand had postaxial syndactyly with cutaneous synostosis and clinodactyly of the fifth finger. Radiographic studies of the hand demonstrated brachymesophalangia. Physical findings also included a patent ductus arteriosus. The child's physical and mental development was severely retarded.

2.12 2.13

Cloverleaf Skull Syndrome

Cloverleaf skull syndrome (Kleeblattshädel) in a 6-day-old boy. Findings included the cloverleaflike skull deformity (with indentations in the center and in the temporal regions), low-set ears, depressed nasal bridge, and pronounced shortening of all extremities (micromelia). The cranial abnormalities are due to premature cranial synostosis. Cloverleaf skull syndrome is often associated with skeletal dysplasia. The infant's length was 47 cm. Cranial ultrasound imaging demonstrated significant hydrocephalus and absence of the corpus callosum. The child died on the sixth day of life.

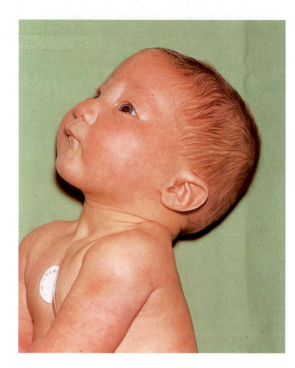

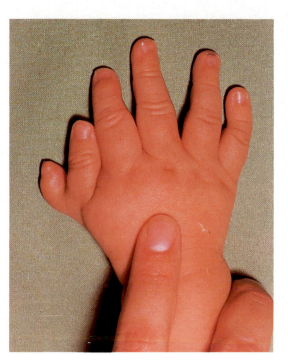

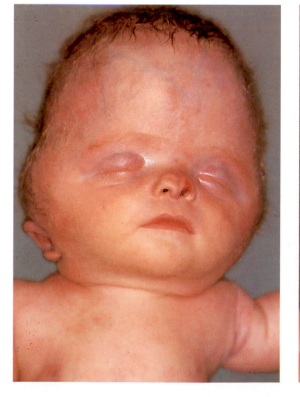

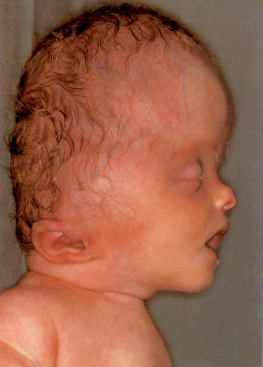

2.14
Cleft Lip and Palate

Complete unilateral cleft lip, alveolar process, and palate in a 1-week-old newborn. The nose was flattened and the right nostril shifted laterally. Cleft palate occurs when the lateral palatine process fails to fuse with either the median palatine process, the nasal septum, or the primary palate. Because of difficulties with feeding, gavage feedings were initially used.

After the infant was 7 weeks old, bottle feeding was possible. In the second week of life, the infant developed acute otitis media, a frequent complication of cleft lip and palate. Other complications include failure to thrive, pneumonia due to milk aspiration, recurrent otitis media, abnormal dentition requiring orthodontic procedures, and speech disorders.

2.15
Cleft Lip

Incomplete unilateral cleft lip in a 4-week-old boy. The upper lip was indented to the left of the philtrum, but the defect did not extend into the alveolar process or palate. Defects are described as "complete" if the cleft reaches the nostril on the affected side. Unilateral cleft lip occurs when the maxillary process on the affected side fails to merge with the medial nasal elevations. Cleft lip may occur in conjunction with clefts of the alveolar process or palate. Isolated cleft palate (either the soft palate, the hard palate, or both) occurs more frequently in females and is frequently associated with other abnormalities. Isolated cleft palate is a frequent finding in the Robin sequence.

2.16   2.17
Cleft Lip, Alveolar Process, and Palate:

Child with complete unilateral cleft lip, alveolar process, and palate seen before (Figure 2.16, age 4 months) and after (Figure 2.17, age 8 months) corrective surgery. Cleft lip and alveolar process with or without cleft palate occurs in approximately 1:1,000 births and is more frequent in males. Cleft lip and palate occur in conjunction with many syndromes including trisomy 13 (Patau syndrome), trisomy 18 (Edwards syndrome), Wolf-Hirschhorn syndrome (partial deletion of the short arm of chromosome 4), cri du chat syndrome (partial deletion of the short arm of chromosome 5), and certain of the ectodermal dysplasia syndromes, including ectrodactyly-ectodermal dysplasia-clefting syndrome (EEC syndrome).

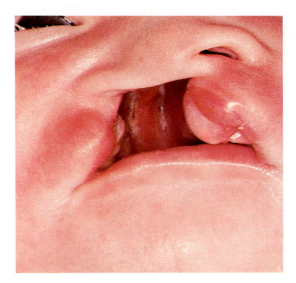
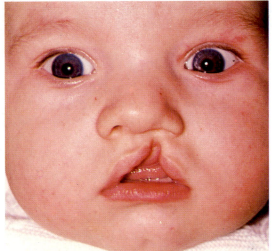

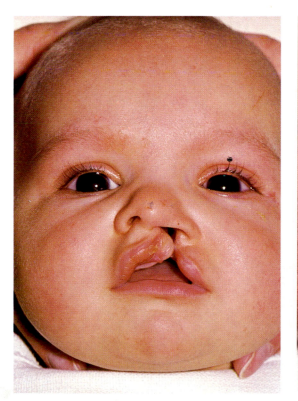
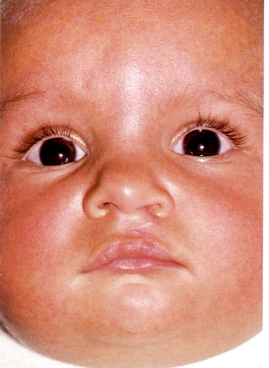

2.18

Bifid Uvula

Bifid uvula in a 5-year-old girl. Bifid uvula represents the most minimal expression of a cleft palate. A bifid uvula can be seen in association with a submucous cleft palate, which at times may be overlooked on initial physical examination.

2.19

Incomplete Cleft Palate

Cleft of the soft palate and the posterior third of the hard palate in a 7-month-old girl. This finding was not associated with other malformations (e.g., Robin sequence, fetal alcohol syndrome).

2.20

Complete Cleft Palate

Complete cleft palate in a 6-year-old boy. A wide cleft of the soft and hard palates was noted as a result of failure of the palatal shelves to fuse. The cleft extended into the nasal cavity. The child experienced frequent tonsillitis, middle ear infections, and speech disorders. Initial treatment generally includes placement of a plastic obturator to separate the oral and nasal cavities; surgical correction is usually attempted within the first year of life.

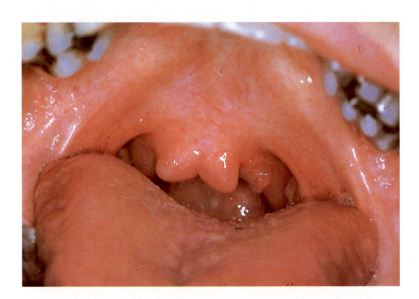

2.18

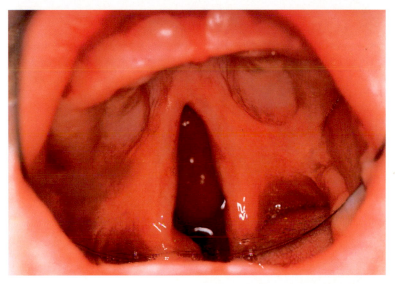

2.19

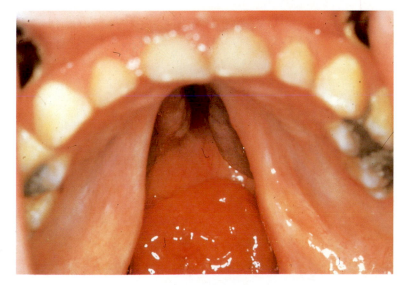

2.20

2.21

Lateral Cleft

Congenital lateral or transverse facial cleft of the mouth in a 2-week-old boy. The asymmetrical mouth with the right lateral cleft is due to malformation of the mandibular arch (failure of the lateral maxillary and mandibular processes to merge). The defect may be unilateral or bilateral and is associated with deformities of the outer ear, hypoplasia of the mandible or maxilla, and median cleft palate.

2.22

Oblique Facial Cleft

A 4-week-old boy with a unilateral oblique facial cleft or orbital facial fissure extending from the left upper lip to the medial aspect of the orbit. Oblique facial clefts are often bilateral and may involve the orbit, leading to colobomas or microphthalmos. The deformity may involve the nose, the tear ducts, the ears, or the central nervous system. Surgical correction may involve several stages.

2.23

Ankyloglossia

A 4-week-old boy with ankyloglossia (tongue-tie). The lingual frenulum is shortened and lies close to the tip of the tongue. Movement of the tongue may be limited. Generally, this anomaly is of no pathologic importance. Surgery, if necessary, should not be performed before the child is 8 months old.

2.24

Microstomy

A 2-week-old girl with microstomy (small mouth). Congenital microstomy is due to excessive merging of the maxillary and mandibular processes of the mandibular arch. In this case, microstomy was an isolated finding. Congenital microstomy is seen in Ruvalcaba syndrome, Hallermann-Streiff syndrome, and craniocarpotarsal dysplasia. Acquired microstomy may occur in older children with progressive scleroderma (as a result of hardening and shrinking of the skin around the mouth).

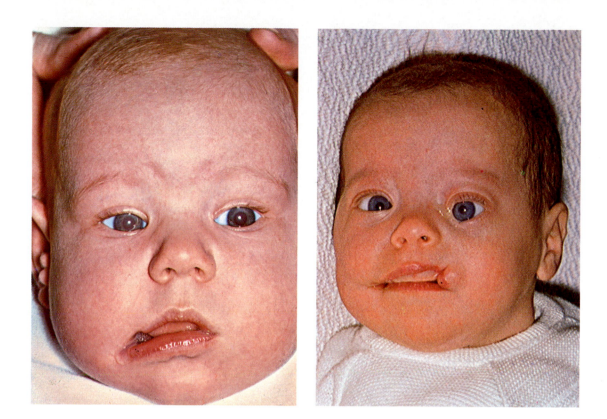

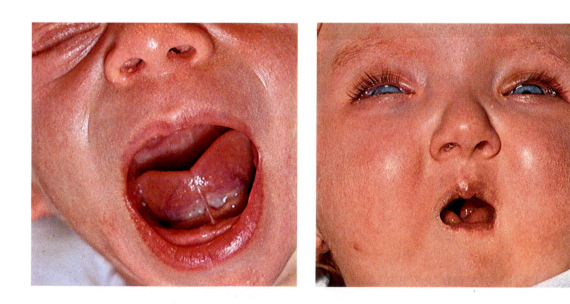

2.25

Ankyloglossia

Ankyloglossia (tongue-tie) in a 6-year-old boy. The shortened lingual frenulum lies close to the tip of the tongue limiting movement. This is a congenital developmental defect of the tongue, in contrast to the acquired form, which is caused by scarring and adhesions of the tongue to the floor of the mouth.

2.26

Frenulum of the Lip

Frenulum of the lip between the two permanent maxillary central incisors in a 5-year-old girl, associated with medial diastema (space between the maxillary central incisors). Initially, no treatment was needed. Removal of the low-set frenulum occurred only after eruption and stabilization of the permanent incisors enabled orthodontic closure.

2.27

True Medial Diastema

True medial diastema (space between the maxillary central incisors not caused by tooth loss) in the permanent dentition of a 16-year-old girl. Similar medial diastema can occur in agenesis of the lateral incisors, nasopalatine cyst, or mesiodens. False medial diastema in the primary dentition can occur if the lateral incisors and canines close the space after eruption of divergent central incisors. This frequent event allows for space to be reserved in the primary dentition for the broader permanent incisors.

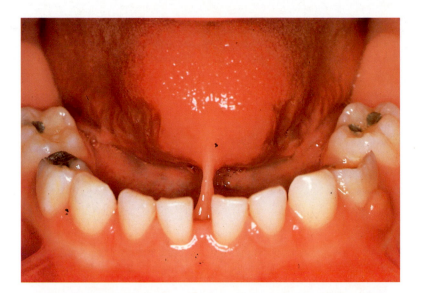

2.25

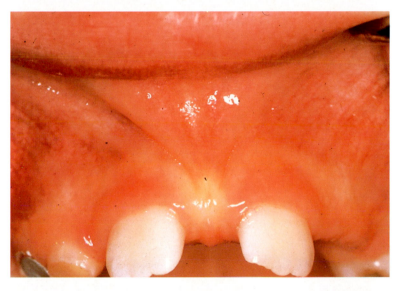

2.26

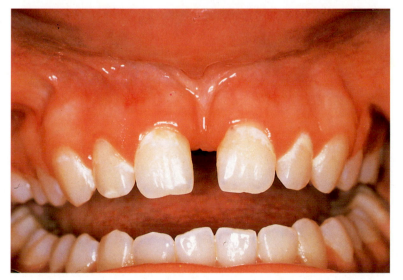

2.27

2.28

Congenital Hypodontia

Congenital hypodontia (oligodontia) in the primary dentition of a 3-year-old boy with anhidrotic ectodermal dysplasia (X-linked recessive form). The maxillary central incisors are conical and all mandibular teeth are missing. Radiographs demonstrate the absence of a primordium for the corresponding permanent teeth as well.

2.29

Hyperdontia

Supernumerary teeth (hyperdontia) in the permanent dentition of a 10-year-old boy. Supernumerary teeth are not uncommon, occurring in approximately 3% of the normal population. Supernumerary teeth occur more frequently in the region of the anterior palate. Supernumerary teeth may undergo a variety of problems, including impaction, crowding of normal dentition, and cystic change.

2.30

Mesiodens

Mesiodens in a 7-year-old boy. Supernumerary, conical anterior teeth were noted in the midline. These supernumerary teeth could impede the eruption of the permanent maxillary central incisors. If delay in anterior tooth eruption occurs, radiographs are necessary to clarify whether or not mesiodens is the cause.

2.31

Open Frontal Bite

Open frontal bite (vertical nonocclusion of the anterior teeth) in a 12-year-old girl. During occlusion, the rows of teeth in the front are 7 mm apart. Open bite can have a variety of causes, including familial pattern, early rickets, finger sucking, macroglossia, and habits such as tongue pressing or biting of the cheeks.

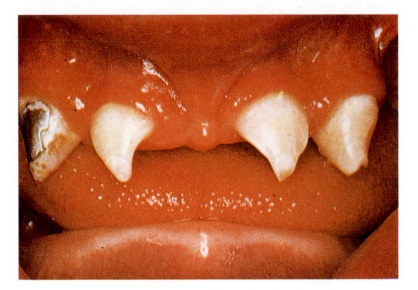

2.28

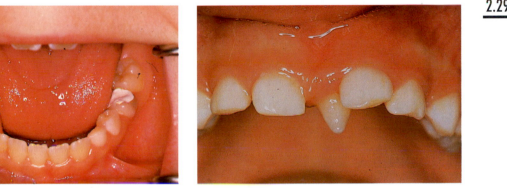

2.29   2.30

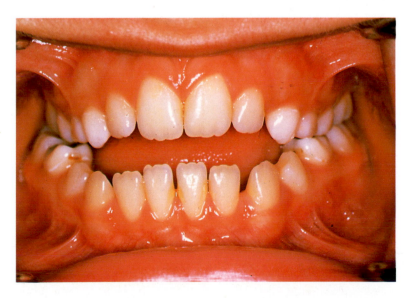

2.31

2.32

Dentinogenesis Imperfecta

Dentinogenesis imperfecta (hereditary dentin hypoplasia) in a 15-year-old boy. The "glass teeth" are blue in color and have an opalescent sheen. The primary teeth are more affected than the permanent dentition. Radiographic studies demonstrate that the roots are shortened and the pulp cavity is calcified.

2.33

Enamel Dysplasia

Enamel dysplasia in a 7-year-old boy with yellow-brown discoloration of the tooth enamel.

2.34

Ameliogenesis Imperfecta

Ameliogenesis imperfecta in a 10-year-old girl with yellow-brown discoloration of all teeth, including primary and permanent dentition. Ameliogenesis imperfecta involves the enamel of the primary and the permanent teeth without affecting dentin, pulp, or cementum. Ameliogenesis imperfecta is an inherited disorder of mineralization. The remnants of the surface of the permanent teeth are evident: The teeth were highly sensitive due to the loss of enamel caused by abrasion and erosion. Radiographic studies were unable to differentiate enamel from dentin due to the decreased density of the enamel.

2.32

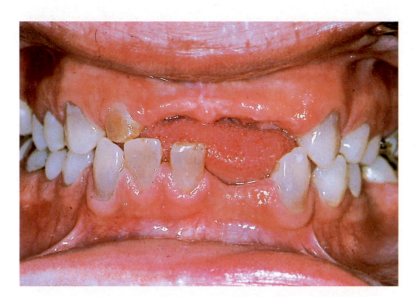

2.33

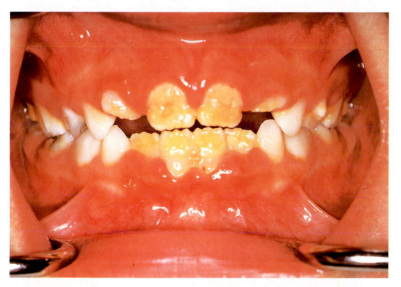

2.34

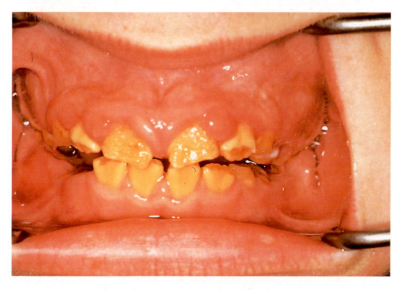

2.35 Exophthalmos

Unilateral exophthalmos due to a retrobulbar cavernous hemangioma in a 5-month-old girl. In the few weeks before presentation, the parents noted enlargement, prominence, and limited motion of the right eyeball. Sonography and computed tomography were used to locate the tumor. Because of imminent danger to the optic nerve, the retrobulbar hemangioma was removed surgically by using a transfrontal approach.

Differential Diagnosis—Exophthalmos includes:
1. Intraorbital tumors, such as rhabdomyosarcoma, metastatic neuroblastoma, dermoid cyst, teratoma, glioma of the optic chiasm, intraorbital glioma, orbital cyst, and leukemia
2. Inflammatory processes, such as orbital cellulitis and thrombophlebitis
3. Malformations, such as anterior meningiocele or encephalocele and vascular anomalies
4. Trauma leading to basilar skull fracture, fracture of the orbital wall, and retroorbital hemorrhage
5. Orbital pseudotumor (unilateral chronic inflammatory process amenable to steroid therapy)

2.36 Torticollis

Congenital muscular torticollis in a 10-year-old girl. Shortening of the right sternocleidomastoid muscle caused the head to tilt toward the affected side and turn toward the opposite side. A ropelike hardening of the sternocleidomastoid muscle was noted. Over time, the face became increasingly asymmetric. The cause of torticollis, which had persisted since 1 year of age, was unknown. Unlike torticollis secondary to strabismus (ocular torticollis), correction by means of active or passive physical therapy was not possible; surgical treatment was required.

Differential Diagnosis—Torticollis persisting from birth may be due to malformation of the cervical vertebrae (seen in Klippel-Feil syndrome). Acquired torticollis may occur after fracture or dislocation of the cervical vertebrae, or in association with pharyngitis, cervical lymphadenitis, intraspinal tumors, and juvenile rheumatoid arthritis.

2.37 Facial Hemiatrophy

A 5-year-old boy with atrophy of the right side of the face (absent subcutaneous tissue, musculature, and bone). Atrophy developed gradually over the course of a year. Facial asymmetry was clearly evident when the boy opened his mouth. There was no sign of hyper- or hypopigmentation of the skin on the affected side of the face (Russell-Silver syndrome) or alopecia (Hallermann-Streiff syndrome). The cause in this case was unknown.

Differential Diagnosis—Facial hemiatrophy occurs in conjunction with scleroderma (frontoparietal involvement "en coup de sabre") and inflammation or traumatic injury to the mandible.

2.38 Hemihypertrophy

Left-sided hemihypertrophy in an 8-year-old girl. As an infant, she was incorrectly diagnosed as having congenital hip dislocation. From birth onward, enlargement of the entire left side of the body occurred; at the age of 8, the left leg was 4 cm longer than the right leg, the left arm was 2 cm longer than the right arm, the mass of the left side of the body was obviously greater, and a right convex scoliosis of the spine was noted. Hemihypertrophy may be associated with aniridia, neoplasms, genitourinary abnormalities, hemangiomas, and nevi. In this girl, a cavernous hemangioma of the right upper lip, and a small capillary hemangioma above the sacrum were noted; otherwise, no anomalies were detected.

Differential Diagnosis—In Klippel-Trenaunay-Weber syndrome there is usually no true hemihypertrophy but localized hypertrophy of a limb. Angiography (to detect vascular anomalies that occur in Klippel-Trenaunay-Weber syndrome) was not performed in this case. Hemihypertrophy is found in Beckwith-Wiedemann syndrome (in 15% of cases) and in Russell-Silver syndrome (skeletal asymmetry with prenatal growth disturbance and abnormal sexual development).

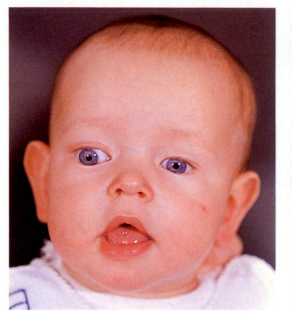

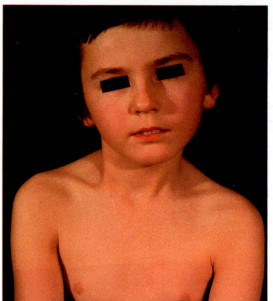

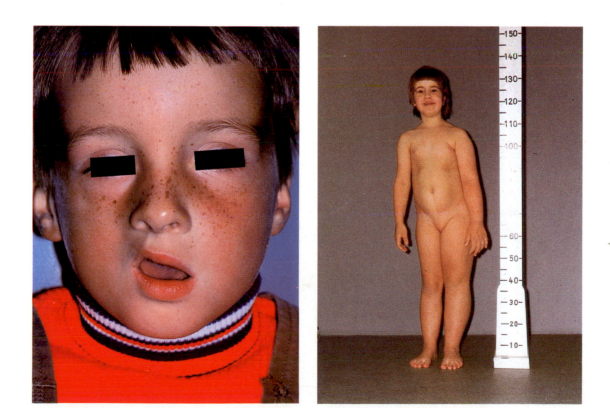

2.39   2.40

Robin Anomaly (Pierre Robin Syndrome)

A 2-month-old boy with micrognathia (Figure 2.39, hypoplasia of the mandible) and glossoptosis (Figure 2.40, retraction of the tongue, which may lead to stridor and upper airway obstruction). No cleft palate was noted. The child had a variety of problems including upper airway obstruction, poor nutritional intake, frequent vomiting, and growth failure. Due to respiratory difficulty, the child had to lie prone and be fed by a gavage tube. These problems improved after the first few months of life due to growth of the mandible. In certain circumstances, the tongue tip may be sutured forward or a tracheostomy may be required.

Differential Diagnosis—Micrognathia and glossoptosis may be part of Smith-Theiler-Schachenmann syndrome (along with hypoplasia of tracheal cartilage) as well as hypoglossia-hypodactylia syndrome (in combination with limb anomalies). Micrognathia also occurs in conjunction with mandibulofacial dysostosis, certain deletion syndromes (including cri du chat syndrome, Wolf Hirschhorn syndrome, antimongolism 21q-), trisomy 18, Bloom syndrome, and Brachmann-de Lange syndrome.

2.41

Mandibulofacial Dysostosis

A 6-month-old child with mandibulofacial dysostosis (Treacher Collins or Franceschetti-Klein syndrome). Findings include downward-slanting palpebral fissures, coloboma of the lower eyelid, hypoplastic malar bones, hypoplasia of the mandible, deformities of the auditory canal as well as conductive hearing loss. Other cases may include malformation of the outer and middle ear, large beak-like nose, micrognathia, and deformities of the eye. Intelligence is usually normal. Plastic and orthodontic surgery may improve appearance.

Differential Diagnosis—Downward-slanting palpebral fissures ("antimongolism") may be seen with partial deletion of the long arm of chromosome 21, with G-monosomy, and with other syndromes including Coffin-Lowry syndrome, Sotos syndrome, and Apert syndrome.

2.42

Potter Syndrome

Bilateral renal agenesis in a 2-day-old male infant. Birthweight was 2,100 g. Of note was the typical Potter facies: wrinkled facies (with a prominent skin fold extending from the inner corner of the eye laterally to the cheek), wide-set eyes, beaklike nose, and low set dysplastic ears. Oligohydramnios (decreased amniotic fluid) was noted at birth, and the infant was anuric until he expired on the second day of life. The autopsy demonstrated bilateral renal agenesis with agenesis of the ureters, a rudimentary bladder, and bilateral pulmonary hypoplasia, confirming the diagnosis of Potter syndrome. No anomalies of the spine or lower extremities were noted.

Differential Diagnosis—Physical findings virtually identical to those seen in bilateral renal agenesis may occur in any situation where amniotic fluid is severely decreased (oligohydramnios sequence).

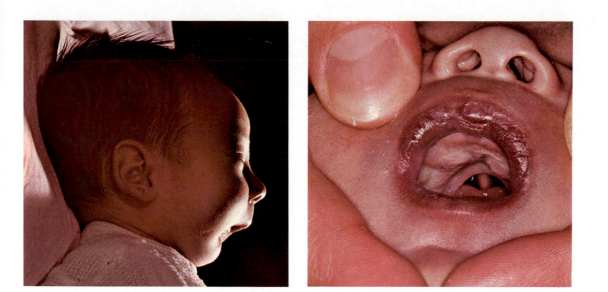

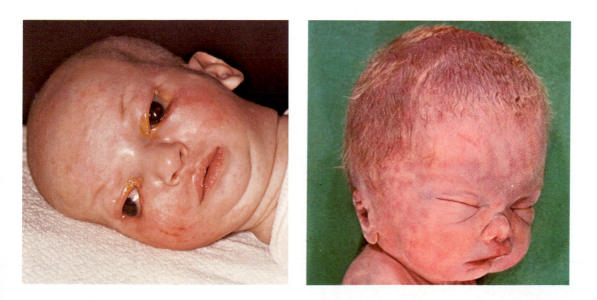

2.43

Williams Syndrome

Williams syndrome (idiopathic hypercalcemia syndrome) in a 10-month-old mentally retarded child. Findings included "elfin facies" (full cheeks, slightly upturned nose, depressed nasal bridge, long philtrum, prominent lips) and growth deficiency. Postnatal growth was poor due to anorexia and obstipation. Microcephaly (OFC 29 cm) and muscular hypotonia were noted. Metabolic abnormalities included hypercalcemia, decreased serum alkaline phosphatase, and decreased renal function (elevated BUN, decreased creatinine clearance). Cardiac catheterization demonstrated supravalvular aortic stenosis. Clinical and laboratory improvement was noted after 1 year on a low calcium diet.

2.44

Brachmann-de Lange Syndrome

Brachmann-de Lange syndrome in a 15-year-old girl. Mental retardation was noted since early childhood and epilepsy was diagnosed at the age of five. The child had the typical facies seen in Brachmann-de Lange syndrome: synophrys, downward-slanting palpebral fissures, low hairline, long eyelashes, long philtrum, and downturned corners of the mouth. Other findings include microcephaly, mental retardation, and limb abnormalities (small hands and feet, short digits, single flexion creases, and limb reduction).

2.45

Sturge-Weber Syndrome

Sturge-Weber syndrome (encephalotrigeminal angiomatosis) in a 4-month-old boy. Of note was a nevus flammeus (port-wine nevus) on the left side of the face in the distribution of the trigeminal nerve (ophthalmic distribution).

At 6 months of age, right-sided spastic hemiplegia was noted (contralateral to the hemangioma). Radiographs of the skull revealed unilateral, curvilinear double-contoured lines of calcification in the cerebral cortex. These radiographic findings are pathognomonic of Sturge-Weber syndrome.

2.46

Bloom Syndrome

Bloom syndrome in a 7-year-old girl. Findings include telangiectatic erythematous lesions in a butterfly distribution over the face (noted since 1 year of age). Lesions were also noted on the volar surface of the arm. The rash was photosensitive (sunlight intensified the erythema, causing blister formation particularly on the eyelids or mouth). Short stature and microcephaly were present; intelligence was normal. This syndrome is an autosomal recessive trait causing defective chromosomal repair (increased exchange in homologous chromatids). Children affected with Bloom syndrome have an increased tendency toward malignancy (including leukemia and lymphomas).

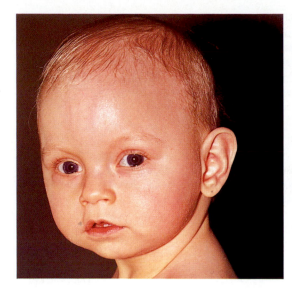
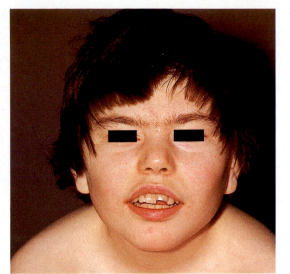

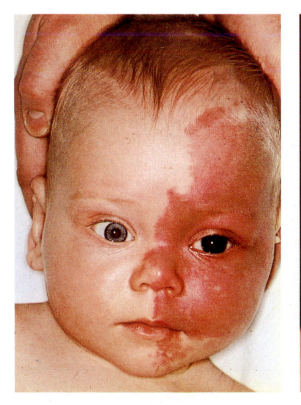
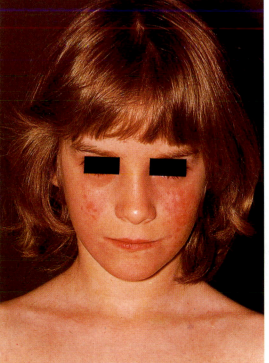

2.47   2.48

Rubinstein-Taybi Syndrome

Rubinstein-Taybi syndrome in a 2-month-old boy. The infant's birthweight was 1,200 g. The infant had a characteristic face with beaked nose, long nasal septum, broad nasal bridge, hypertelorism, slanted palpebral fissures, external strabismus and low set ears (Figure 2.47). Broad thumbs with radial angulation were noted (Figure 2.48). Mental retardation and failure to thrive associated with retarded bone age are characteristic of this syndrome. Rubinstein-Taybi syndrome can be differentiated from other syndromes by the peculiar appearance of the nose as well as the broadening and shortening of the thumbs and large toes. Affected children will have mental retardation and failure to thrive.

2.49   2.50

Blepharophimosis

Blepharophimosis in a 6-year-old boy. Physical findings include short, narrow palpebral fissures and low-set ears (Figure 2.49) as well as clinodactyly (inward curving of the fifth finger), flexion contraction of the middle fingers (camptodactyly) (Figure 2.50) and contraction of the toes. The child was of normal intelligence.

Blepharophimosis is described in many syndromes (in association with ptosis, deafness, failure to thrive, and mental retardation). However, no specific diagnosis was made in this child's case.

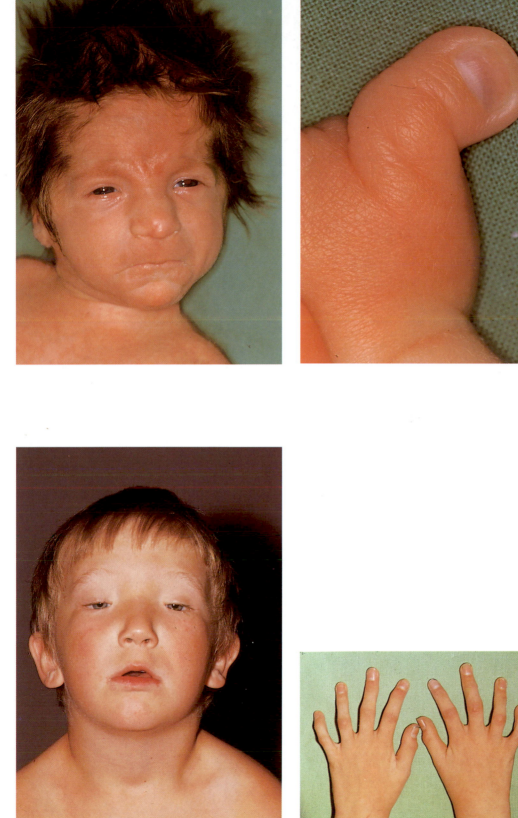

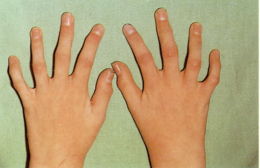

2.51

Miescher Syndrome

Miescher syndrome in a 13-year-old boy. The physical findings included benign acanthosis nigricans as well as type I diabetes mellitus. The figure demonstrates the brown, symmetric skin changes that give the skin a velvety appearance. These changes are caused by papillomatosis and hyperkeratosis. Skin changes were noted in the area of the neck and axilla. Similar changes were found in the groin area, on the inside of the upper thigh, and on the palms of the hands and soles of the feet. The child was diagnosed with diabetes mellitus and treated with subcutaneous insulin. Other physical findings included dental deformities, fissured tongue, and low-set ears.

Acanthosis nigricans appears in other syndromes, including Seip-Lawrence syndrome (generalized lipodystrophy with increased growth and diabetes mellitus).

2.52

Cherubism

Cherubism in a 4-year old boy. Physical findings included swelling of the upper and lower jaw, malalignment of the teeth, and upturning of the eyes. Both the mother and the sister were similar in appearance. The cause was fibrous dysplasia of the upper and lower jaw with upward displacement of the zygomatic arches. These changes were radiographically apparent.

2.53

Facial Hemiatrophy

Facial hemiatrophy in an 8-year-old boy. Hypoplasia of the soft tissues and bones of the left side of the face were noted. There were no other associated anomalies.

2.54

Van der Woude Syndrome

Van der Woude syndrome (Demarquay-Richet syndrome) in a 14-year-old girl. Physical findings included paramedian fistula of the lower lip and cleft soft palate. Two incisors of the upper jaw were absent. The lower lip fistula had small accessory salivary glands that secreted a watery mucoid substance. The glands were surgically removed, and the cleft of the soft palate was repaired.

Van der Woude syndrome, an autosomal dominant disorder, is associated with lip fistula, cleft palate, cleft lip, defective dentition, and skeletal abnormalities. The range of symptoms in affected individuals can vary considerably.

2.55

Goldenhar Syndrome

Goldenhar syndrome in an 8-month-old boy. Physical findings included a diagonal crease in the right cheek and facial asymmetry (hypoplastic right mandible and narrowing of the right palpebral fissure) associated with bilateral preauricular appendages and lipodermoid of the right eye. Characteristic of Goldenhar syndrome is the combination of unilateral facial hypoplasia, epibulbar dermoid, ocular abnormalities, preauricular appendages, and unilateral dysplasia of the auricle.

2.51

2.52

2.53

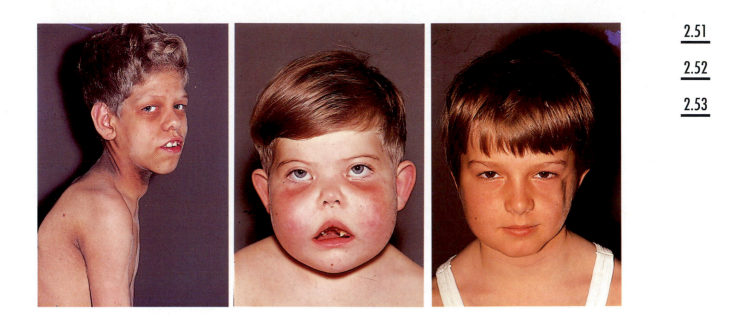

2.54

2.55

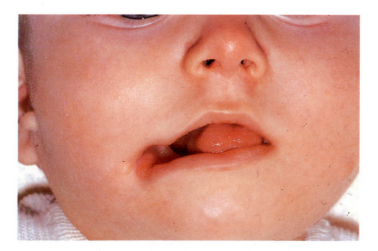

2.56
Hypochondroplasia

Hypochondroplasia in a 4-year-old boy. Short-limbed short stature was noted in this child. His length was 93 cm. Growth was asymmetric with a relatively large head and short arms and legs. The hands and feet were shortened and widened. The length at birth was 50 cm (25th percentile), but at 6 months of age was noted to be in the 3rd percentile. His bone age was commensurate with chronologic age. Radiographs of the long bones were typical of hypochondroplasia. Mental development was normal for age.

The physical findings of achondroplasia are noted at birth. These findings may include a small torso, large head, and shortening of the limbs. The radiographic findings are more pronounced than those of hypochondroplasia. Disproportionate growth occurs in other hereditary osteochondrodysplasias, such as lethal dwarfism, chondroplasia punctata (rhizomelic type), and diastrophic dysplasia.

2.57
Robinow Mesomelic Dysplasia

Robinow mesomelic dysplasia in a 15-year-old boy. Disproportionate growth was noted in this child; length was 126 cm (30 cm under the 3rd percentile) and shortening of the lower arms and thighs (mesomelic shortening) was noted. Bone age was delayed 2 years. Other findings included microphallus and hypertelorism. Radiographs revealed a short ulna and radius and brachymesophalangia. Typical facial dysmorphism was not present. The typical facies in Robinow syndrome include a flat facial profile, hypoplastic mandible, prominent forehead, and hypertelorism.

Aarskog syndrome presents with similar facial dysmorphism, failure to thrive, and shortening and widening of the hands and feet.

2.58
Russell-Silver Syndrome

Russell-Silver syndrome in a 3-year-old boy. Physical findings included disproportionate dwarfism (noted since birth) with relatively short proximal extremities and long distal extremities. The child's length was 77 cm (11 cm under the 3rd percentile). The head was disproportionately large relative to the length of the body. Also noted were genital hypoplasia, hypospadias, and cryptorchidism. No specific endocrine abnormalities were noted. The child's intelligence was normal for his age.

2.59
Russell-Silver Syndrome

Russell-Silver syndrome in a 7-year-old boy. Disproportionate dwarfism was noted since birth with typical facial features (triangular face, hypertelorism, hypognathia). Also noted was a high-pitched squeaky voice.

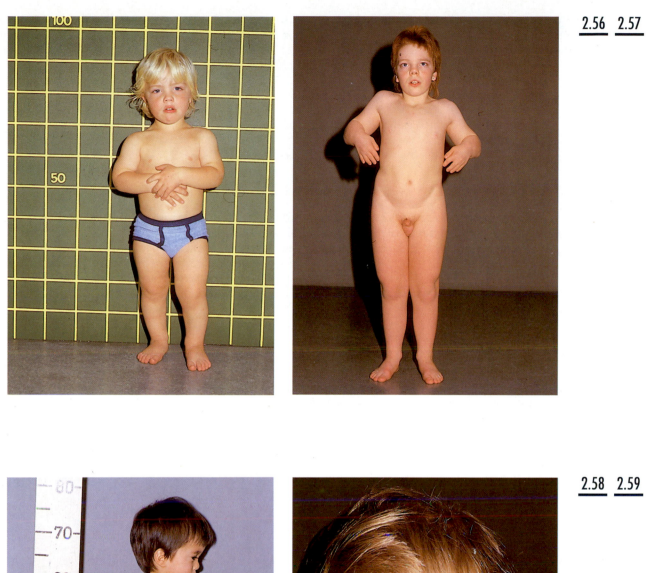

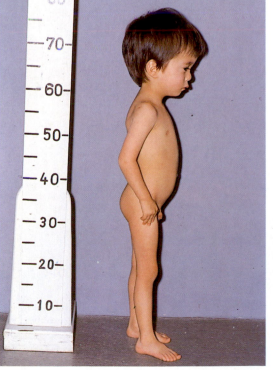

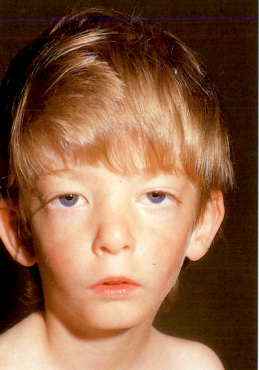

2.60

Talipes Equinovarus

Bilateral congenital clubfoot (talipes equinovarus) in a 3-month-old boy. Findings included inversion and adduction of the forefoot, inversion of the heel, and plantar flexion of the foot. The foot could not be dorsiflexed to the neutral position, and the heel was fixed in the varus deformity. Congenital clubfoot is a structural deformity that has a familiar predisposition and occurs more often in male children. The skeletal changes observed radiographically occur because of medical and plantar deviation of the anterior talus. Clubfoot is associated with congenital hip dysplasia, spina bifida, and other neuromuscular conditions. Early treatment is warranted in cases of talipes equinovarus. Conservative management consists of manipulation and casting; if not successful, surgical treatment is necessary.

Differential Diagnosis—Talipes equinovarus must be differentiated from talipes calcaneovalgus and metatarsus varus (or metatarsus adductus). In the two latter conditions the foot can be dorsiflexed and the heel is in valgus (when observed from behind). Both are considered positional defects.

2.61

Talipes Equinovarus

Talipes equinovarus (clubfoot) in a 2-day-old newborn with an open thoracolumbar meningomyelocele. The infant was paralyzed from the level of T8 downward and had progressive hydrocephalus as well as other malformations. No operative repair was performed. The child died at 2 months of age due to increased intracranial pressure. In spina bifida apperta (with meningomyelocele), neurologic defect may lead to paralysis of the lower limbs, dislocated hips, and talipes equinovarus. Without treatment, increasing deformity may occur. Specific therapy for clubfoot may be conservative (braces or support devices) or operative (tendon release or transfer, arthrodesis, or osteotomy).

2.62

Pes Cavus

High arched foot (pes cavus) and clawlike big toe in an 8-year-old girl with progressive neuromuscular atrophy associated with Charcot-Marie-Tooth disease. This motor neuropathy was first suspected when the child walked with an abnormal gait.

Differential Diagnosis—The development of pes cavus can be seen in other neurologic disorders, including Friedreich's ataxia.

2.60

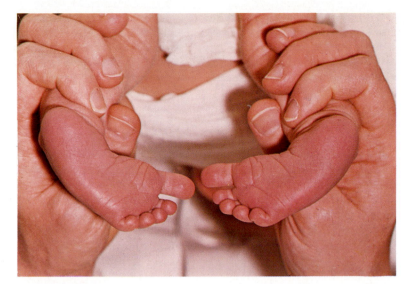

2.61

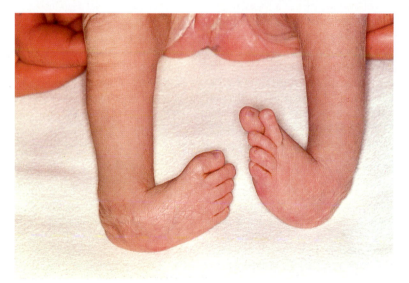

2.62

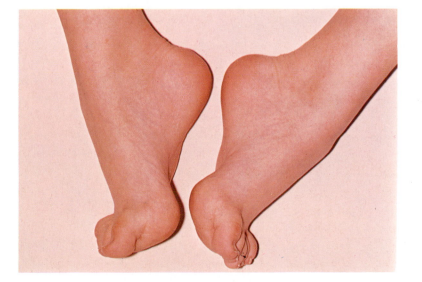

2.63
Amniotic Band Disruption Complex

Autoamputation and furrows of the fingers in a 1-day-old newborn. These findings probably originated during fetal development due to amniotic bands. Cutaneous syndactyly developed between the second and third finger. The infant died at 2 days of age due to other severe malformations.

Amniotic bands may cause major disruptions in the newborn that lead to defects in the extremities (constriction or amputation) or to craniofacial disruption. Disruption from amniotic bands may be differentiated from genetic causes of craniofacial or limb anomalies by the lack of symmetry of these lesions.

2.64
Osteogenesis Imperfecta

Osteogenesis imperfecta in a 2-month-old boy. Physical findings included shortening and deformity of the legs, which had been noted since birth. These findings were due to multiple fractures of the upper and lower femur. The radius and ulna were also broken in several places. The cranial bones were soft and impressionable. The sclerae were blue. Radio-graphs of the skeleton revealed multiple deformities and fractures, a thin cortex, minimal skull ossification, and generalized osteoporosis. Osteogenesis imperfecta is caused by a disturbance in collagen synthesis, leading to imperfect formation and calcification of bone.

2.65
Crescent Foot

Unilateral crescent foot (pes adductus) in a 1-year-old boy. The left foot was in the adduction position so that the anterior portion of the foot was medially displaced relative to the vertical axis of the leg. Radiographs demonstrate an arch-shaped angulation of the forefoot axis and bony deformities. Because of the danger of contracture in advancing forefoot adduction, appropriate therapy was initiated. The foot was cast in the correct position and frequent cast changes were made over several months. Therapy later included braces and special shoe inserts.

Crescent foot (pes adductus) must be distinguished from the harmless, congenital pes supinatus (climber's foot) in which the whole foot is suppinated at the ankle joint. This loose dislocation can be easily corrected with lateral pressure against the back of the foot. Heel and forefoot deviation are usually not present. The radiograph is normal. Because of the rapid, spontaneous correction of pes supinatus, further treatment is not necessary.

2.66 2.67
Congenital Subluxation of the Hip

Unilateral congenital hip subluxation in a 3-year-old girl. Physical findings included distortion of the anal and vulvar openings, asymmetry of skin folds, and shortening of the right leg. Abduction of the right thigh was only possible to 45 degrees; on the left, abduction was possible to 90 degrees. In abduction, the empty acetabulum opposite the lesser trochanter could be felt. The diagnosis was confirmed by sonography and treatment was begun immediately.

Acetabular dysplasia is more frequent than hip subluxation. It can be either unilateral or bilateral and is usually detected on physical examination (limited hip abduction), but confirmed radiographically or sonographically. Therapy for acetabular dysplasia is accomplished with restraining trousers or bandages that hold the hip in adduction, usually for 3 to 6 months. When untreated, acetabular dysplasia may lead to hip subluxation.

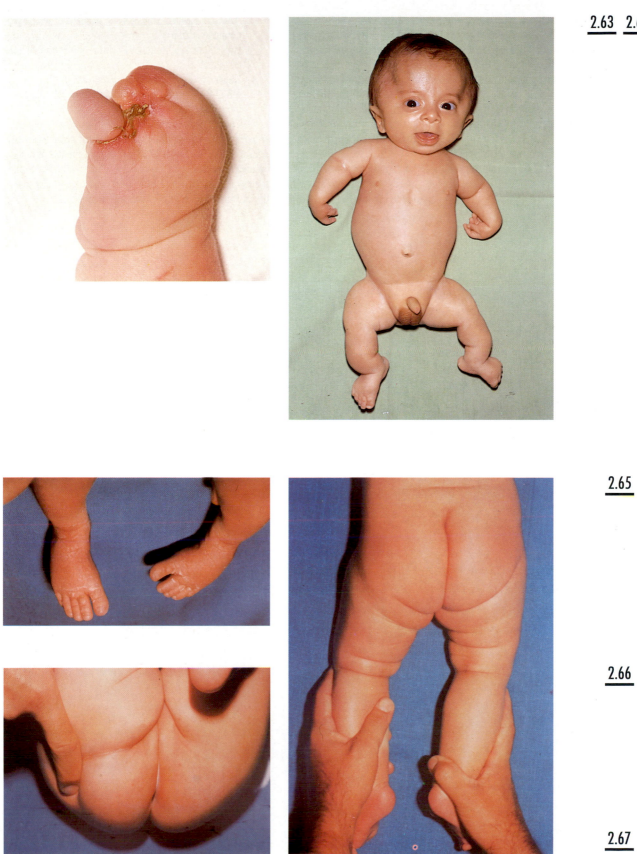

2.68—2.70
Fanconi Syndrome (Pancytopenia)

Fanconi syndrome (pancytopenia) in a 3-year-old boy. The boy had multiple congenital anomalies, including hypoplastic thumbs, hypoplastic radius, hypogenitalism, microsomia, microcephaly, and abnormally dark skin pigmentation. Laboratory investigations revealed pancytopenia (anemia, neutropenia, and thrombocytopenia), evidence of chromosome breaks, and elevated fetal hemoglobin. Radiographic examinations demonstrated bilateral radial hypoplasia with absence of the first metacarpal. Bone marrow failure leading to pancytopenia typically appears after 7 years of age.

Differential Diagnosis—Hypoplasia or aplasia of the radius or thumb also occurs in conjunction with the following:
1. Thrombocytopenia absent radius syndrome
2. Aase syndrome (hypoplastic anemia-triphalangeal thumb syndrome)
3. Holt-Oram syndrome (with atrial or ventricular septal defect)
4. Nager syndrome (acrofacial dysostosis)
5. VATER association (associated with vetebral, gastrointestinal or renal anomalies)
6. Thalidomide embryopathy

Hypogenitalism (hypoplasia of the external genitalia) is also seen in Laurence-Moon-Biedl syndrome, Prader-Willi syndrome, Froehlich syndrome, Klinefelter syndrome, Smith-Lemli-Opitz syndrome, LEOPARD syndrome (multiple lentinges syndrome), and hypophyseal dwarfism.

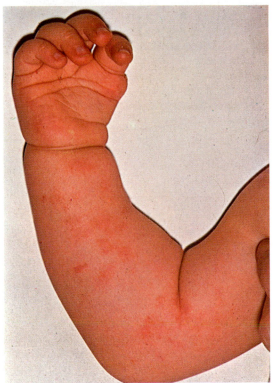
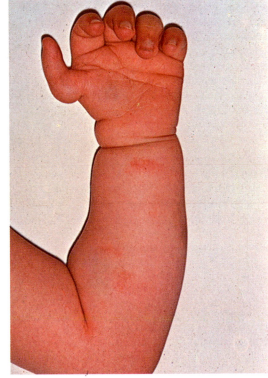

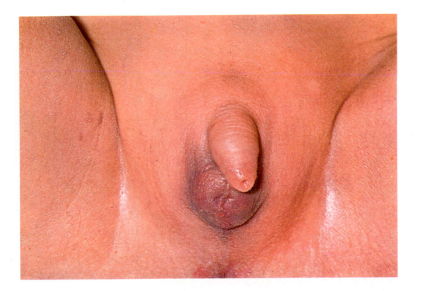

2.71

Smith-Lemli-Opitz Syndrome

Smith-Lemli-Opitz syndrome in a 1-year-old boy. The findings included osseous and cutaneous syndactyly of the third and fourth fingers of the left hand. Other features typical of this syndrome include microcephaly, facial dysmorphism (ptosis, broad upturned nose, and low-set ears), hypogenitalism (hypospadias, cryptorchidism), and severe mental retardation. Other malformations of the hand may include single palmar crease, brachydactyly, clinodactyly, and polydactyly (particularly ulnar hexadactyly). Syndactyly occurs frequently in conjunction with other syndromes including:

1. Apert syndrome (acrocephalosyndactyly)
2. Carpenter syndrome (acrocephalopolysyndactyly)
3. Poland's anomaly (with ipsilateral aplasia of the pectoralis muscle)
4. Oculodentoosseous dysplasia (with microphthalmia, abnormal tooth enamel)
5. Cryptophthalmos syndrome

2.72

Clubhand

Clubhand in a 3-year-old child. Of note was the absence of the radius and thumb of the right forearm and hand. The left forearm was also shortened due to an ulnar defect, and movement at the elbow joint was restricted.

Clubhand may be a unilateral or bilateral defect, and may be seen as an isolated finding or in association with other anomalies (cleft lip and palate, costal or vertebral defects) or syndromes. A variety of conservative and operative procedures have been developed, which must be carried out in a timely fashion if function is to be preserved.

2.73

Amniotic Band Disruption Complex

Bilateral amputation of the distal fingers and toes in a 12-day-old child. Of note were partial ring-shaped indentations and cutaneous syndactyly. These findings suggest that amniotic bands caused intrauterine amputation of the distal fingers and toes. The child had no other deformities and had normal mental development. Surgical treatment to correct the syndactyly was needed in order to improve function of the hands.

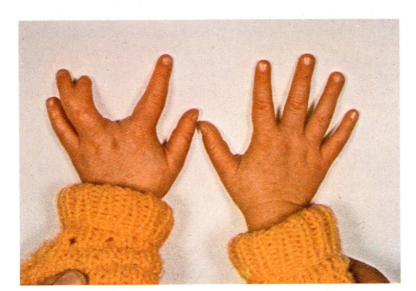

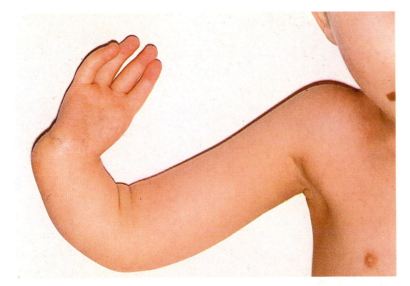

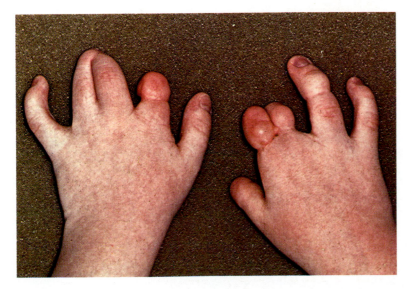

2.74

Phocomelia

Complete phocomelia in a 2-week-old newborn. The infant had a severe limb defect in which both arms were absent bilaterally (the hands emerged directly from the torso). Malformation of both hands was also noted (three phalangeal bones and three metacarpal bones only). The remainder of the skeletal examination was normal, and no further anomalies were noted. The cause of the deformities in this case was unknown. Phocomelia is a limb reduction defect in which there is concurrent lack of the humerus, radius, and ulna in the upper extremity, or absence of the femur, tibia, and fibula in the lower extremity. Sophisticated prosthetic devices are required if these children are to have a functional life. Phocomelia is seen in conjunction with thalidomide embryopathy.

2.75

Partial Hemimelia (Peromelia)

Partial hemimelia (congenital shortening of the limbs resembling amputation) in a 1-day-old newborn. The forearms and hands as well as the feet are absent bilaterally. Sophisticated prosthetic devices are required.

2.76

Amelia

Amelia (absence of the entire limb structure) in a 2-week-old newborn. The upper extremities were completely absent and both femurs were hypoplastic. The cause in this case is unknown. Extensive training to improve the grasping function of the foot as well as an arm-hand prosthesis was required.

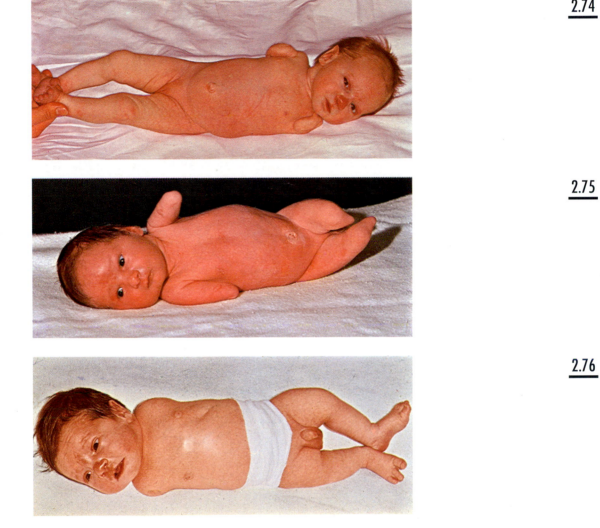

2.74

2.75

2.76

2.77

Cutaneous Syndactyly

Partial unilateral cutaneous syndactyly of the fourth and fifth fingers of the left hand in a 2-month-old girl. This was the sole deformity in this case and surgical correction was accomplished at 1 year of age.

In the event of osseous syndactyly, earlier operative repair would be advisable because persistence of the bony deformity can lead to secondary changes of the joints. Syndactyly is the most frequent form of hand deformity. It is often bilateral and may be associated with polydactyly, brachydactyly, ring-shaped indentations, or congenital finger amputations. Syndactyly of the index and middle finger is more frequent than syndactyly of the fourth and fifth fingers. Severe syndactyly (total fusion) is seen in Apert syndrome. Syndactyly also occurs with other syndromes including Poland's anomaly (unilateral syndactyly and ipsilateral absence of the pectoralis major muscle).

2.78

Clubhand

Bilateral clubhand in a 6-month-old boy. The findings included radial deviation of the hand, shortening of the forearm, and hypoplasia of the thumb. Radiographs demonstrated partial absence of the radius. No other anomalies were noted. Initially, the hands and lower arms were placed in a brace. After the child's first year of life, surgical correction took place. Clubhand can be either unilateral or bilateral and is caused by a complete or partial absence of the radius. Other bone or muscular anomalies are associated. Clubhand may be associated with cleft lip and palate, vertebral or costal anomalies, urogenital deformities, Franceschetti-Klein syndrome, Fanconi syndrome (pancytopenia), and thrombocytopenia (TAR syndrome).

2.79

Polydactyly

Polydactyly (in this case hexadactyly) in a 6-year-old girl. Findings included a hypoplastic sixth digit on the ulnar side of the left hand with partial syndactyly. The rudimentary finger was removed surgically. In polydactyly, the additional digit may consist solely of soft tissue, may contain bone, or may be complete (including a metacarpal bone). The extra digit is usually found on either the radial or ulnar side of the hand. Double thumb or triple phalangeal thumb may be seen. Polydactyly occurs with certain syndromes, including Ellis-van Creveld syndrome, Bardet-Beidl syndrome, Carpenter syndrome, and trisomy 13 or 18.

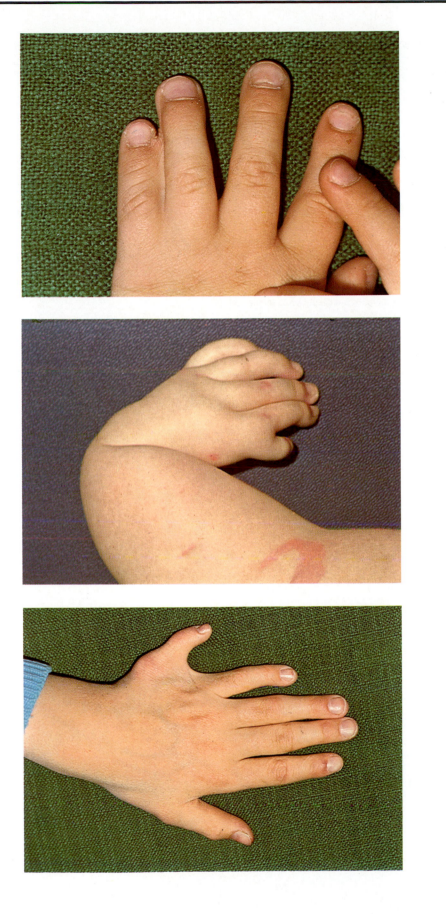

2.77

2.78

2.79

2.80

Cleft Hand

Cleft hand in a 6-month-old girl. Physical findings included absence of the third finger of the right hand. Gripping function of the hand was normal.

2.81

Duplication of the Thumb

Duplication of the thumb (preaxial hexadactyly) in a 3-year-old girl. Physical findings included additional bony structures of the first finger of the right hand, which was joined to the larger normal thumb. The extra digit was removed surgically. No other anomalies were noted. No other family members were similarly affected.

2.82

Freeman-Sheldon Syndrome

Freeman-Sheldon syndrome (whistling face syndrome) in a 7-month-old boy. Physical findings included bilateral ulnar deviation of the third, fourth, and fifth fingers, and low-set thumbs. Other findings included a small puckered mouth and congenital clubbed feet. The contractures of the fingers were noted from birth and improved through physical therapy. The child's intelligence was normal.

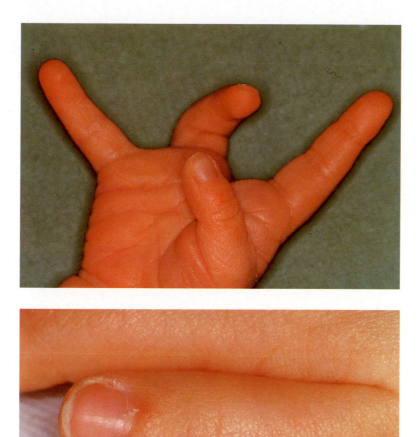

2.80

2.81

2.82

2.83
Cleidocranial Dysostosis

Cleidocranial dysostosis in a 7-year-old girl. Findings included hanging, narrow shoulders, narrow pectus, and abnormal shoulder movement due to the bilateral absence of the clavicles. The cranium was notable for frontal bossing and a large open fontanel. Skull radiographs demonstrated widening of the cranial sutures. In addition, the child had delayed ossification of the pubic bone. The hands had short distal phalanges and a long second metacarpal bone. Except for a minor gait problem, the child had no other problems.

2.84
Pectus Excavatum

Pectus excavatum in a 3-year-old boy. The lower third of the sternum was abnormally depressed. There was no obstruction to breathing. Operative correction of pectus excavatum is controversial and should be undertaken only if lung function is restricted. Pectus excavatum may occur in conjunction with Marfan syndrome, homocystinuria, and Coffin-Lowry syndrome.

2.85
Joint Contractures

Bilateral flexion contracture of the knee and hip with compensatory lordosis of the lumbar spine in a 5-year-old boy. These findings have been noted since the age of 1 year. The contractures are a result of cerebral palsy, specifically spastic diplegia. Other causes, such as neuromuscular disease or skeletal dysplasia, were ruled out.

Contractures in children with cerebral palsy are due to the predominantly flexed posture assumed by these children. Treatment involves extensive physical therapy with stretching exercises and operative correction if necessary.

2.86
Congenital Hip Subluxation

Bilateral congenital hip subluxation in a 9-year-old boy. The child walked with a waddling gait and was noted to have severe lordosis of the lumbar spine. Unfortunately, subluxation of the hip was identified late in this case. Therapy should be instituted as soon as possible. Therapy may consist of either conservative measures (casting) or operative measures to correct the subluxation and osseous malformation.

2.87
Hemihypertrophy

Hemihypertrophy (partial gigantism) of the left leg of a 9-year-old girl. The girl was treated for a seizure disorder and mental retardation (due to encephalopathy). On physical examination the left leg was 2 cm longer, the pelvic stance was slanted, and scoliosis of the lumbar spine was noted. There were no nevi or other vascular abnormalities. Fundoscopic examination of the eye was normal. No Wilms tumor could be detected. The discrepancy in leg length was treated with appropriate orthopedic shoes.

Differential Diagnosis—Partial gigantism may have the following causes:

1. Congenital malformations such as congenital hip subluxation and other skeletal diseases
2. Specific syndromes such as Klippel-Trenaunay-Weber syndrome or Beckwith-Wiedemann syndrome
3. Infection (such as osteomyelitis)
4. Arthritic processes (juvenile rheumatoid arthritis)
5. Trauma (fracture or damage to the epiphyseal plate)
6. Neuromuscular conditions (cerebral palsy or poliomyelitis)
7. Tumors (neurofibromatosis, Wilms tumor)
8. Avascular necrosis of the femoral head.

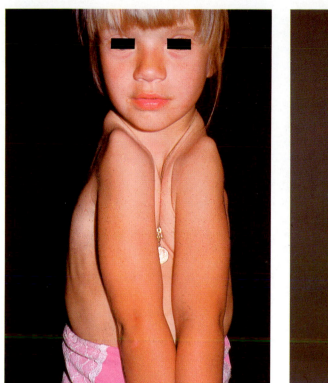
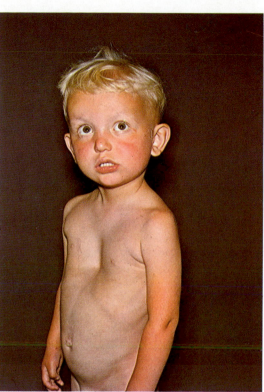

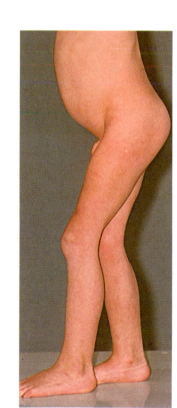
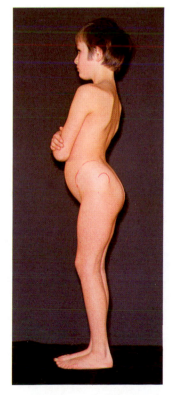
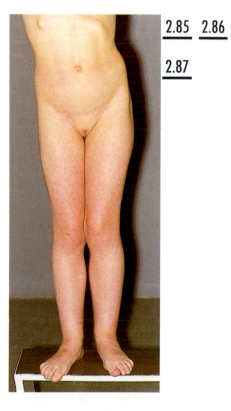

2.88

Sprengel Deformity

Sprengel deformity in a 6-year-old girl. Congenital elevation of the left shoulder blade was noted. Abduction of the left arm was only minimally affected. Radiographs demonstrated hemivertebrae in the upper thoracic and lower cervical spine as well as rib synostoses on the affected side.

2.89

Asphyxiating Thoracic Dystrophy

Asphyxiating thoracic dystrophy (Jeune syndrone) in a 15-month-old boy. Physical findings included an abnormally long and narrow thorax with limited chest wall movement. Shortening of the arms and legs was noted as well as the inability to extend the forearm at the elbow joint. The child required tracheostomy and continuous positive airway pressure due to pulmonary hypoplasia. Radiographs demonstrated shortening of the ribs, horizontal placement of the ribs, irregular costochondral junctions, and pelvic dysplasia. A rudimentary sixth finger was surgically removed. Abdominal ultrasound demonstrated renal enlargement; renal function was noted to be normal. The child's intelligence was normal.

Other short rib-polydactyly syndromes include
1. Majewsky syndrome (with cardiovascular defects and cleft lip or palate)
2. Saldino-Noonan syndrome (with severe bony changes)
3. Ellis-van Creveld syndrome (chondroectodermal dysplasia with congenital heart disease and ectodermal dysplasia)

2.90

Conjoined Twins

Conjoined twins (Siamese twins) before surgical separation on the first day of life. This ischiopagus pair was joined at the pelvis; both twins had male genitals located on the posterior aspect of the body. Two anal openings, which led into a common rectum, were noted. At 8 months, surgical separation was performed at the Children's Surgery Clinic at the University of Munich. The shared colon was divided between the twins. In addition, a colostomy was performed. Since the ureter of each twin emptied into the opposite twin's bladder, the ureters were separated and reattached appropriately. The postoperative period was without complication. Paralysis of the sciatic nerve was noted as a result of the operation.

2.91 2.92

Conjoined Twins

Conjoined twins (Siamese twins) after surgical separation at 15 months. Both twins had adequate bowel and bladder function. Leg movement was virtually normal in both children. They could sit without support and stand and run with support.

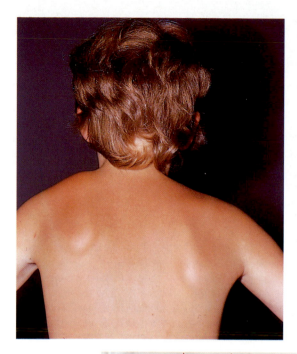

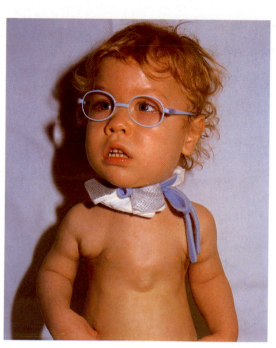

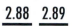

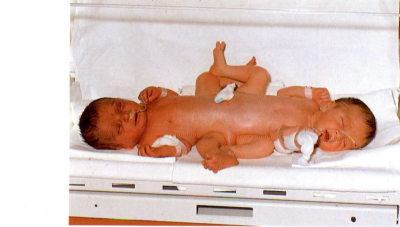

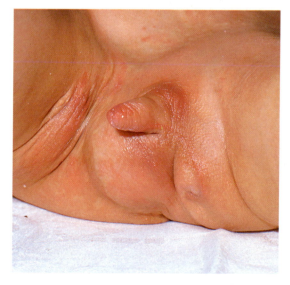

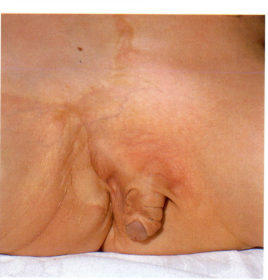

2.93

Lumbar Hernia

Hernia in the upper lumbar region in a 1-month-old girl. The physical findings included a cherry-sized white protrusion on the left upper lumbar region. The mass appeared to enlarge when the child cried. The hernia was easily reducible. When the hernia sac was surgically removed, it was noted to be filled with adipose tissue. The hernia apparently developed through a congenital defect in the trigonum lumbocostale.

Hernias may also exist in the lower lumbar area (caused by a defect in Petit's triangle). The hernial sac can hold retroperitoneal fat, ascending colon, descending colon, or kidney.

2.94

Teratoma

Benign teratoma in a 6-day-old boy. On physical examination, a tangerine-sized, coarse, nodular tumor was noted in the anterior aspect of the neck. The mass could be easily moved. The tumor was surgically removed without difficulty. Histologic examination demonstrated a differentiated teratoma consisting of various tissue components. No other therapy for this tumor was necessary.

2.95

Gastroschisis

Gastroschisis in a newborn before surgical repair. A large abdominal wall defect (10 cm in length) was noted, through which edematous small and large intestine protruded. No covering sac was noted, and the umbilical cord was normally inserted. A fibrinous material was found between the prolapsed intestines, which were dark red. Peristaltic activity of the bowel was not detected, and the mesentery was edematous and thickened. Neither intestinal atresia nor stenosis was present, although both may be seen with gastroschisis.

Immediately after birth, the abdomen and prolapsed intestines were wrapped in sterile gauze in order to prevent any ongoing damage or infection. The bowel was decompressed by means of a nasogastric tube. A staged reduction of the herniated viscera was accomplished by means of a silo constructed of mesh reinforced Silastic. Postoperative complication, which may include adhesions, ileus, malrotation, or volvulus, were not seen in this case. The child was initially given total parenteral nutrition, but by 2 weeks of age was feeding normally.

2.96

Ectopia Cordis

Ectopia cordis in a 2-week-old boy. Physical findings included a defect of the sternum and abdominal wall with protrusion of the heart and liver through the defect. The hernial sac consisted of fetal amniotic membrane. The child died at the end of the first month of life due to congestive heart failure secondary to congenital heart disease.

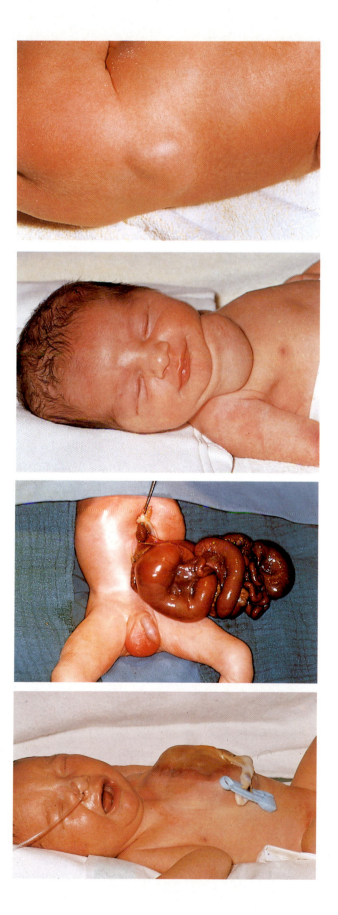

2.97

Fetal Alcohol Syndrome

Fetal alcohol syndrome in a 2-month-old girl. Intrauterine growth retardation (birthweight: 1,200 g) was noted. Physical findings included microcephaly and dysmorphic facial features. The face was remarkable for short palpebral fissures, hypoplasia of the midface, hypoplastic philtrum, and thin vermilion border of the upper lip. The prenatal history was remarkable for considerable alcohol abuse by the mother during pregnancy. The hospital course was unremarkable. Many of these children may have serious developmental delays, behavioral disorders, and continued failure to thrive.

2.98

Fetal Hydantoin Syndrome

Fetal hydantoin syndrome in a 13-year-old girl whose mother had taken anticonvulsants regularly during pregnancy. Physical findings included craniofacial abnormalities (microcephaly, low broad nasal bridge, short upturned nose, and hypertelorism), nail and digital hypoplasia, and failure to thrive. Mental retardation is also a part of fetal hydantoin syndrome. In this case, the girl had a seizure disorder requiring anticonvulsant therapy.

2.99 2.100

Coumarin Embryopathy

Coumarin embryopathy in a 6-year-old girl. Physical findings included a broad flat face and nasal hypoplasia, with a characteristic deep groove between the alae nasi and nasal tip. The mother, who was unaware of being pregnant, had been given a coumarin derivative during the first trimester of pregnancy. In addition to the dysmorphic facial features, the infant had pronounced chondrodysplasia punctata with stippling of the epiphyses. These findings were evident on radiographs, especially along the vertebral column, pelvis, and tarsal bones.

Coumarin embryopathy is phenotypically similar to hereditary chondrodysplasia punctata. Coumarin embryopathy leads to intrauterine growth retardation and nasal hypoplasia. It can occur in the sixth to ninth week of pregnancy, after the intake of a coumarin derivative. Coumarin embryopathy must be distinguished from different hereditary forms of chondrodysplasia punctata (Conradi-Huenermann form, autosomal recessive rhizomelic form, and an X-linked inherited form).

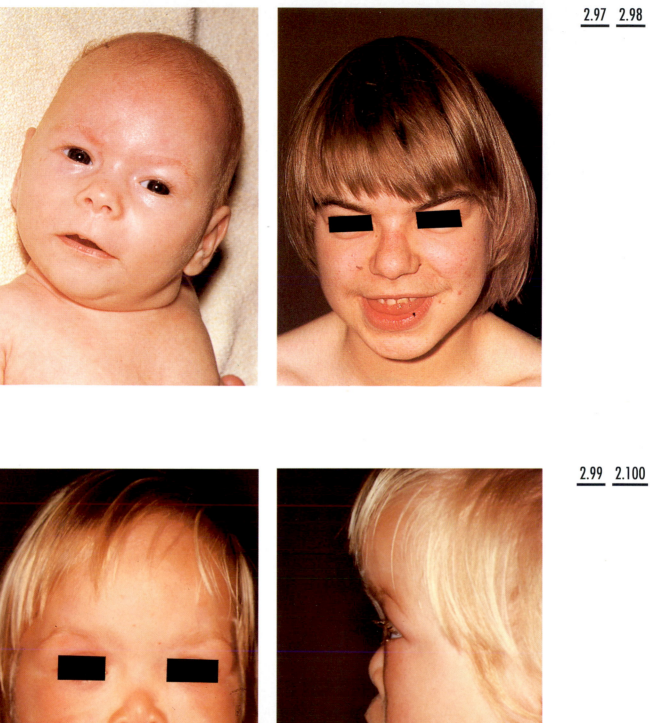

2.101

Down Syndrome

Down syndrome (trisomy 21) in a 4-year-old boy. Findings included a broad, flat face with small orbits and downward-slanting palpebral fissures. The ears were small and low set. The tongue protruded forward, and the mouth was held open.

Congenital heart disease, including ventricular septal defect with severe pulmonary hypertension, was diagnosed on cardiac catheterization.

2.102

Congenital Hypothyroidism

Congenital hypothyroidism in an 11-month-old girl. Of note was myxedema of the face, swollen lips, macroglossia, and an abnormally broad nose. The condition was noted due to developmental delay and abnormally quiet behavior. Laboratory examination revealed a low thyroxine level (T_4) and a high thyroid-stimulating hormone level (TSH).

Macroglossia is also seen in Down syndrome as well as Pompe's disease (type II glycogenosis) and Beckwith-Wiedemann syndrome.

2.103

Down Syndrome

Down syndrome in a 4-year-old boy. The posture is the so-called "jacknife" phenomenon (caused by muscular hypotonia, weak ligaments, and loose skin).

2.104

Down Syndrome

Down syndrome in a 1-year-old girl. The findings include a bilateral, transverse palmar crease (the so-called "simian crease"), brachydactyly, and clinodactyly.

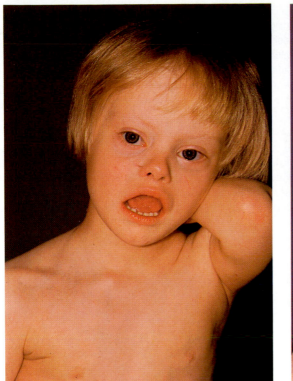
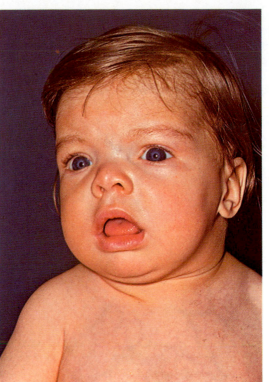

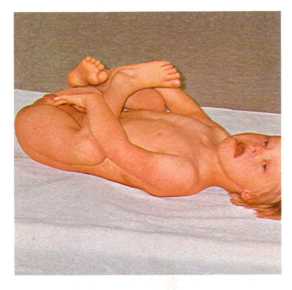
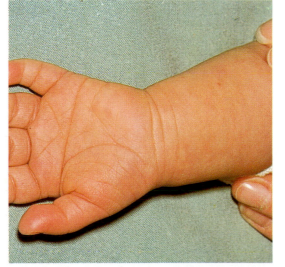

2.105   2.106

**Trisomy 13
(Patau Syndrome)**

Trisomy 13 in a 3-day-old boy, the ninth child of a 40-year-old mother. The child has characteristic craniofacial features of trisomy 13, including microcephaly, sloping forehead, microphthalmia, hypertelorism, and bilateral cleft lip and palate. Several ulcerlike scalp defects were found in the occipitoparietal area (cutis aplasia, Figure 2.106). In addition, the child had bilateral colobomas, numerous capillary hemangiomas, a transverse palmar crease, polydactyly, a large omphalocele, and congenital heart disease. The child's condition was incompatible with life and he died of bronchopneumonia on the ninth day. At autopsy, further findings included arhinencephaly, polycystic kidneys, and abdominal testes. Chromosome analysis confirmed the diagnosis of trisomy 13.

2.107   2.108

**Cri du Chat
Syndrome
(Deletion 5p-)**

Cri du chat syndrome. Findings included craniofacial dysmorphism with microcephaly, round face, dysplastic low-set ears, downward slanting palpebral fissures, hypertelorism, and micrognathia. During the first few months of life, the child had the characteristic high, shrill, catlike cry, which led to the presumptive diagnosis of cri du chat syndrome. Analysis of chromosomes revealed a partial deletion of the short arm of chromosome 5. Psychomotor development in this child was considerably delayed.

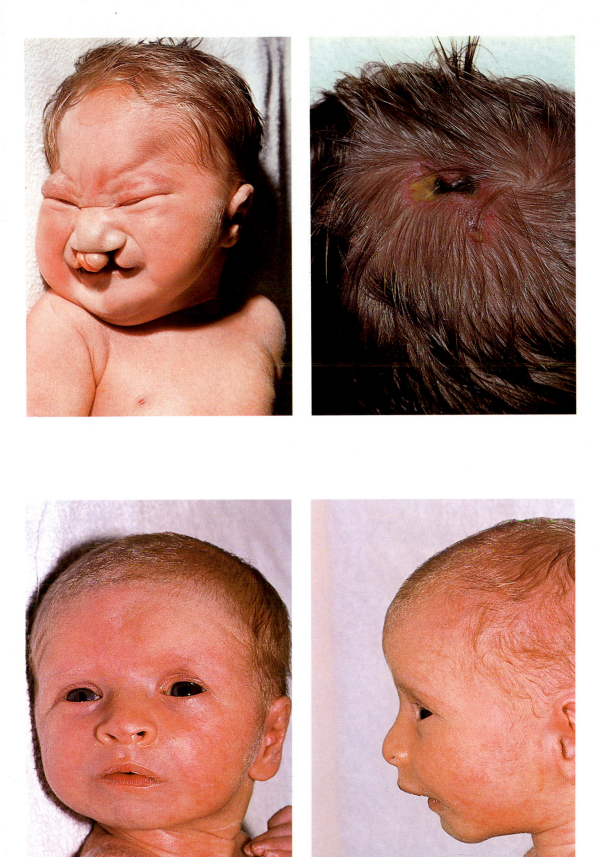

2.109
Polydactyly

Polydactyly (postaxial hexadactyly) in a 1-day-old girl. Physical findings included a rudimentary sixth finger on the right hand. The extra digit was attached to the hand by a narrow bridge of skin. The child also had a well-formed sixth toe on both feet. Similar findings were noted in the mother and the maternal grandfather. Complete duplication of the fifth finger or the fifth toe may follow an autosomal dominant pattern of inheritance with incomplete penetrance.

Postaxial hexadactyly is characterized by the duplication of a fifth finger or toe. The extra digits may be either membranous appendages or contain rudimentary bone. In preaxial hexadactyly, the thumb or big toe is duplicated. Hexadactyly can occur sporadically as an isolated anomaly or may be found in other family members. Hexadactyly occurs in several autosomal recessive hereditary syndromes, including Ellis-van Creveld syndrome (chondroectodermal dysplasia or short rib-polydactyly syndrome), Laurence-Moon-Biedl syndrome, and Patau syndrome (trisomy 13).

2.110
Trisomy 18

Trisomy 18 (Edwards syndrome) in a 1-month-old girl. Physical findings included a flexion deformity of the fingers (index and fifth fingers overlapping the third and fourth fingers, respectively). Short, dorsiflexed big toes were noted as well as congenital vertical talus (rocker-bottom feet).

2.111
Trisomy 18

Trisomy 18 (Edwards syndrome) in a 1-month-old girl. Physical findings include the typical facies with micrognathia, small mouth, narrow palpebral fissures, and low-set ears. The child was born to a 36-year-old mother and weighed 1,800 g at birth. The infant died at 1 month of age of cardiac failure due to underlying congenital cardiac malformation. Karyotype revealed trisomy 18.

2.112
Holt-Oram Syndrome (Cardiac Limb Syndrome)

Holt-Oram syndrome in a 2-month-old boy. The syndrome is characterized by absence or dysplasia of the thumb and radial abnormalities. Cardiac defects are associated with the syndrome. In this case, the left hand lacked both the radius and the thumb, and there was phocomelia on the right (three-finger rectomelia, a hand with three fingers directly connected to the shoulder). Atrial septal defect was detected on cardiac catheterization. The father had similar deformities of the extremities (bilateral aplasia of the thumb) and an atrial septal defect.

2.113
Triphalangeal Thumb

Triphalangeal thumb (five-fingered hand) in a 13-year-old girl. Physical findings included three phalanges comprising the thumb on the right hand, and a three-part contracted hypoplastic thumb on the left hand. Congenital hearing loss was also noted. No anemia or cardiac problems were seen.

Differential Diagnosis—Triphalangeal thumb (or hypoplasia or aplasia of the thumb) is seen in the autosomal recessive Fanconi syndrome (pancytopenia, hyperpigmentation of the skin, microcephaly, chromatid breaks, and increased risk of malignancy) or in the autosomal dominant Holt-Oram syndrome (with atrial or ventricular septal defect).

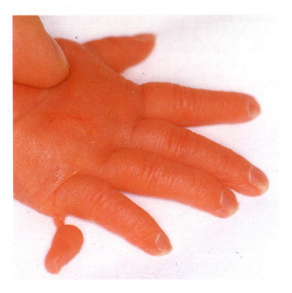

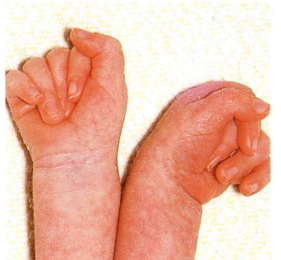

narrow palpebral fissure

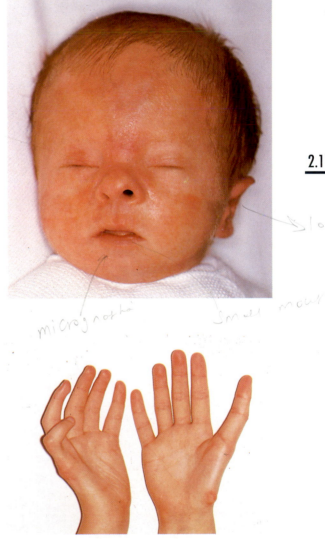

low set ears

micrognathia

small mouth

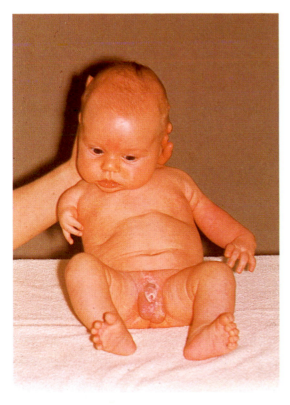

2.114 2.115

Turner Syndrome (XO Gonadal Dysgenesis)

Turner syndrome in a 15-year-old girl who had primary amenorrhea and lacked secondary sexual characteristics. On physical examination, a low hairline, redundant skin folds, webbing of the neck, and shieldlike chest with widely spaced nipples was noted. There was no breast development, and pubic hair was sparse. Analysis of chromosomes revealed X monosomy.

Differential Diagnosis—Noonan syndrome, in which there is short stature and Turner-like stigmata, must be ruled out. In Noonan syndrome, the karyotype is normal.

2.116

Turner Syndrome

Turner syndrome in a 12-year-old girl. This girl lacked breast development, had widely spaced nipples, and a shield-shaped thorax. Chromosome analysis revealed XO karyotype. Laparotomy demonstrated gonadal dysgenesis (streaks of connective tissue without follicles).

2.117

Noonan Syndrome

Noonan syndrome in a 10-year-old girl with normal karyotype. Findings included facial abnormalities (broad forehead, downward-slanting palpebral fissures, hypertelorism, micrognathia), shield-shaped thorax, widely spaced nipples, pigmented nevi on the lower abdomen, microsomia, skeletal abnormalities, and developmental delay. Noonan syndrome may be associated with cardiovascular abnormalities, including valvular pulmonic stenosis, patent ductus arteriosus, and aortic stenosis. Typical Turner syndrome (XO karyotype) was ruled out. However, the girl could be a mosaic for Turner syndrome, which can be detected from chromosome analysis and fibroblast culture.

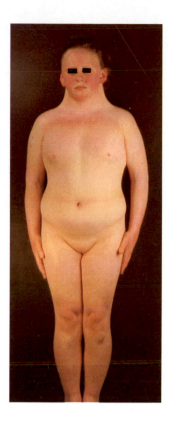

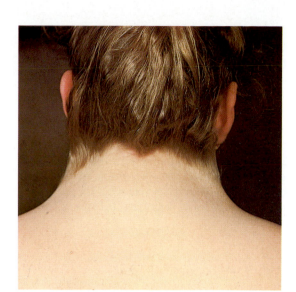

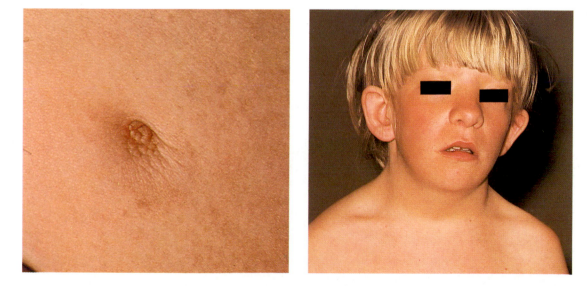

2.118

Klinefelter Syndrome

Klinefelter syndrome in a 14-year-old boy. Physical findings included tall stature (height 175 cm, greater than the 95th percentile), abnormally long legs, feminine distribution of pubic hair, absence of chest, axillary, or facial hair, and small penis and testes. The karyotype demonstrated 47XXY.

2.119

XYY Syndrome

XYY syndrome in an 18-year-old man. Physical findings included tall stature (209 cm). Sexual development was normal; no hypogenitalism or hypogonadism was noted. No other endocrine abnormalities were noted. The patient's intelligence was within the normal range. As a rule, tall stature is the only symptom of this chromosomal anomaly. Tall stature can have several causes, including familial gigantism, precocious puberty, preadolescent obesity, Klinefelter syndrome, Marfan syndrome, cerebral gigantism, and pituitary gigantism.

2.120

Fragile X Syndrome

Fragile X syndrome (Martin-Bell syndrome) in a 7-year-old boy. Physical findings included large protruding ears and prominent jaw. The child was mentally retarded (IQ: 50). Karyotype demonstrated a fragile site at the terminus of the long arm of the X chromosome (Xq 27 fra). The mother, sister, and maternal grandmother were carriers; the maternal uncle also had fragile X syndrome.

2.121

Mosaic Trisomy 8

Mosaic trisomy 8 in a 4-month old boy. Physical findings included deep flexion creases on the palms—a frequent finding in this syndrome that regresses with increasing age. In addition, the child also had deep plantar flexion creases and other findings typical for trisomy 8, including

1. Dysmorphic craniofacial features, including prominent forehead, short nose, broad nasal base, wide philtrum, thin upper lip, low-set ears, micrognathia, and cleft palate
2. Skeletal anomalies, including S-shaped clavicles, narrow pelvis, absent patella, and shortened metacarpals and metatarsals

At 10 months, the child's psychomotor development was noted to be delayed.

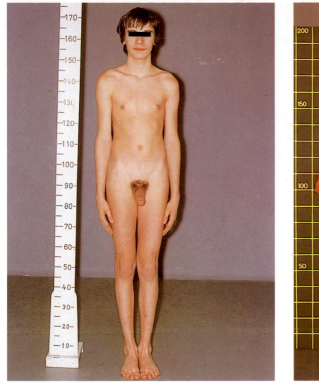
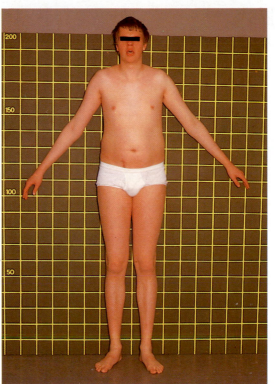

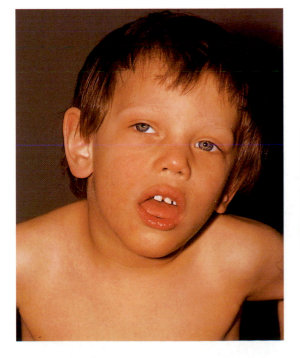
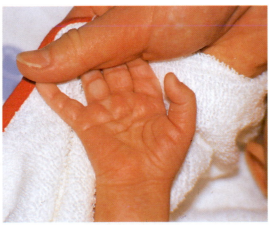

2.122   2.123

Pentasomy X

Pentasomy X (5X syndrome) in a 1½-year-old girl. Findings included slight mongoloid slant of the palpebral fissures and short neck (Figure 2.122). Growth retardation and psychomotor retardation were noted. A patent ductus arteriosus was surgically closed at the age of 5 months. Other anomalies included simian crease and clinodactyly (Figure 2.123). The external genitalia were normal for a female infant. Chromosome analysis revealed 5 X chromosomes.

2.124

Zellweger Syndrome

Zellweger syndrome (cerebrohepatorenal syndrome) in a 2-month-old boy. Findings included the characteristic face with the high prominent forehead, epicanthal folds, and hypoplasia of the supraorbital ridges and midface. The anterior and posterior fontanels were widely open. In addition, the child had severe generalized muscular hypotonia and marked hepatomegaly. Proteinuria and aminoaciduria with normal plasma amino acid levels indicated renal involvement. However, renal cysts were not detectable by ultrasonography. Radiographic examination of the knee demonstrated stippled calcifications in the patella (similar to chondrodysplasia punctata).

Electron microscopy of liver biopsy specimens revealed reduction in peroxisomes. Plasma levels of very long-chain fatty acids were elevated. The child, like his older brother, died at the beginning of the second year of life.

Zellweger syndrome is an inherited peroxisomal disease characterized by the reduction or absence of peroxisomes in the cells of all organs. Enzymes found in the peroxisomes are involved in the production and decomposition of hydrogen peroxide was well as lipid and amino acid metabolism. It is unclear how defects in peroxisome function lead to the widespread clinical manifestations.

2.125

Williams Syndrome

Williams syndrome in a 14-year-old boy. Findings included the typical facial features of the rounded face with a broad upper jaw, full prominent upper lip, and low-set ears. The boy also had cardiac findings of supravalvular aortic stenosis as well as growth and mental retardation.

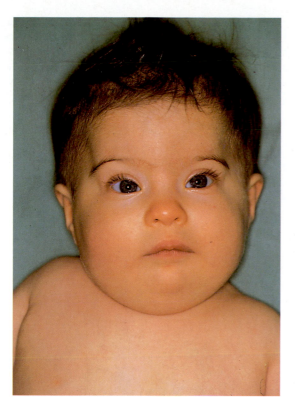
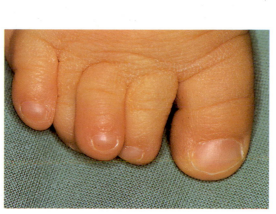

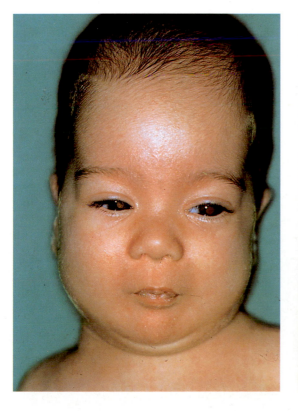
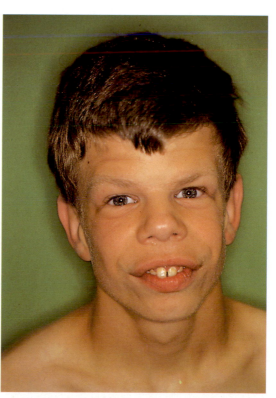

3.1 3.2

Tetralogy of Fallot

Tetralogy of Fallot in a 4-year-old boy. Physical findings included generalized cyanosis, dyspnea, clubbing of the fingers, and polycythemia. In order to relieve the symptoms, the child would assume the typical squatting position (Figure 3.2). The findings in tetralogy of Fallot include obstruction of right ventricular outflow, ventricular septal defect, dextroposition of the aorta, and right ventricular hypertrophy. Initially, the child underwent palliative surgical procedures (aortopulmonary anastomosis) with improvement of cyanosis and dyspnea. Surgical correction was completed at age 7 years.

Differential Diagnosis—Clubbing of the fingers occurs in cyanotic congenital heart disease as well as in chronic pulmonary disease (cystic fibrosis), congenital bronchiectasis, and thyroid disorders. In the hereditary form of club fingers, symptoms usually develop at puberty or later in life.

3.3

Tetralogy of Fallot

Protuberance of the sternum after operative repair of tetralogy of Fallot in a 4-year-old boy.

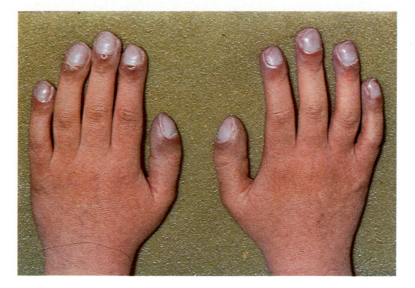

3.1

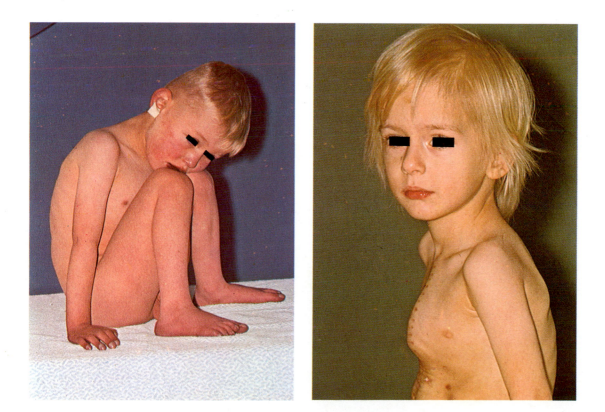

3.2 3.3

3.4
Transposition of the Great Vessels

Transposition of the great vessels in a 6-year-old girl. Physical findings included acrocyanosis, cyanosis of the lips, and clubbing of the fingers and toes. The child had mild dyspnea at rest and considerable dyspnea with exertion. The underlying cardiac lesion was identified by echocardiography and cardiac catheterization. In transposition of the great vessels, the aorta arises from the right ventricle, the pulmonary artery from the left ventricle, and the systemic veins drain into the right atrium.

3.5
Fetal Alcohol Syndrome

Fetal alcohol syndrome with congenital heart disease (ventricular septal defect and patent ductus arteriosus) in a 7-month-old child. The features of fetal alcohol syndrome included microcephaly, short palpebral fissures, hypoplastic midface, short nose, hypoplastic philtrum, thin vermilion border of the upper lip, micrognathia, and failure to thrive. Fetal alcohol syndrome may be associated with underlying congenital heart disease. The history of alcohol abuse during pregnancy was unclear, so other syndromes associated with congenital heart disease were evaluated. Because of a transverse palmar crease (simian crease) and mental retardation, a chromosome analysis was performed demonstrating a normal karyotype. Serologic examination ruled out intrauterine rubella infection.

3.6
Pericarditis

Constrictive pericarditis in a 12-year-old boy. Congestive heart failure led to protuberance of the abdomen due to ascites and hepatomegaly. Pericarditis may cause impairment of diastolic ventricular filling, and compromise cardiac contractility. The child was treated with thoracotomy and pericardiectomy with regression of symptoms afterward. The underlying cause of the pericarditis was unknown. Possible causes of pericarditis include tuberculous pericarditis, viral pericarditis, or pericarditis secondary to irradiation or trauma.

3.7
Marfan Syndrome

A 10-year-old girl with Marfan syndrome. The findings included tall stature (15 cm taller than average for age), long extremities, long fingers (arachnodactyly), hyperextensible joints, ectopia lentis, and flat feet. Marfan syndrome is associated with underlying cardiac defects including aortic and mitral insufficiency.

Differential Diagnosis—Classic homocystinuria (cystathionine synthetase deficiency) must be ruled out. In homocystinuria there may be tall stature, long extremities, arachnodactyly, and similar eye problems. Usually the homocystinine and methionine levels are elevated, and the cyanide nitroprusside test of the urine is positive. Other conditions, including congenital contractural arachnodactyly and Ehlers-Danlos syndrome, must be ruled out.

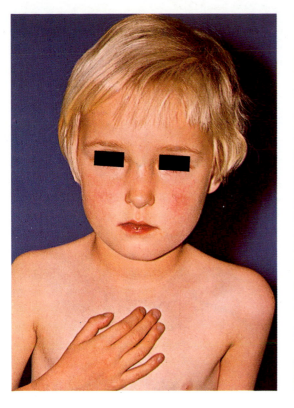
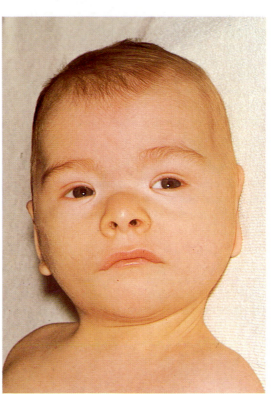

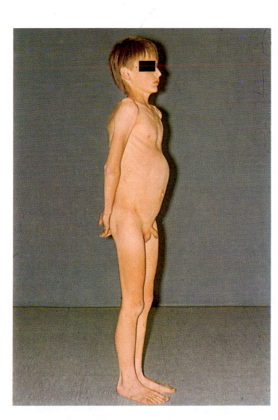
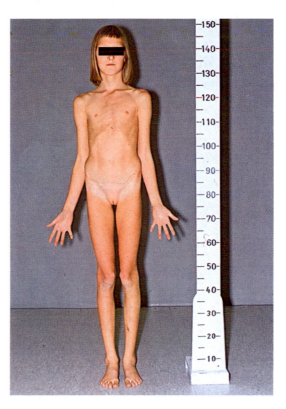

4.1

Endonasal Glioma

Endonasal glioma in a 2-week-old boy. The pea-sized, red, solid tumor was located in the left nasal cavity extending into the nasopharynx. At the time of surgical resection, it was noted to be fused with the nasal septum and lateral nasal wall. There was no recurrence. Histologically, the tumor was a benign nasal glioma (islands of glial tissue embedded in loose connective tissue).

Nasal gliomas are rare mesenchymal tumors that are usu-ally diagnosed soon after birth. The gliomas can be extranasal or intranasal; in 60% of the cases they are easily apparent, in 30% of the cases they are found endonasally and are frequently confused with polyps. Nasal gliomas can block nasal breathing.

Differential Diagnosis—Differential diagnosis of nasal gliomas include dermoids, hemangiomas, and menin-goencephaloceles.

4.2

Crooked Nose

Crooked nose in a 1-day-old boy. A crooked nose is usually due to decreased fetal movement and will resolve spontane-ously within a few days of birth. A crooked nose can also be caused by birth trauma due to dislocation of the nasal septum; these cases may be corrected with immediate man-ual realignment.

4.3

Malherbe's Calcifying Epithelioma

Malherbe's calcifying epithelioma in a 2-year-old boy with a solitary, bean-sized, hard tumor of the subcutaneous tissue at the right upper canthus. Histologic examination revealed calcified connective tissue with basophilic cells and "ghost cells."

4.4

Tonsillar Hyperplasia

Tonsillar hyperplasia in a 4-year-old girl. Both tonsils were greatly enlarged and touched in the midline ("kissing ton-sils"). The tonsils were not noted to have exudate or be erythematous. Adenoidal hypertrophy and a sterile tympanic effusion were also present.

Tonsillar hyperplasia, particularly when associated with generalized nasopharyngeal lymphoid hyperplasia (adenoi-dal hyperplasia) may cause difficulty in swallowing, respira-tory obstruction, and chronic otitis media due to blockage of the eustachian tubes.

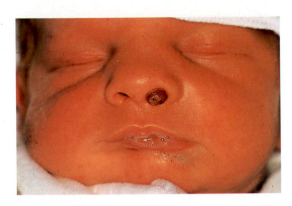

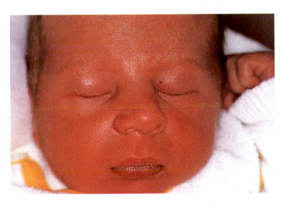

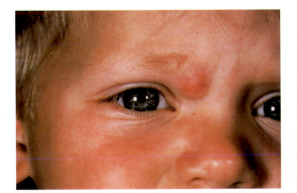

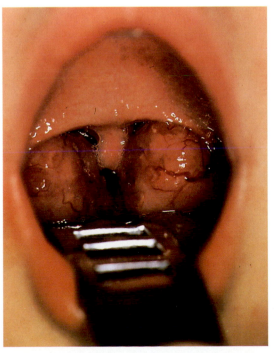

4.5

Acute Otitis Media

Acute otitis media in a 3-year-old boy. Otoscopic examination demonstrated a hyperemic, bulging tympanic membrane with poor mobility. Erythema and swelling were particularly notable in the region of the malleus (*arrow*). Children with acute otitis media may present with fever, generalized discomfort, and hearing loss.

4.6

Chronic Otitis Media

Chronic otitis media in a 16-year-old boy. Otoscopic examination revealed a retracted, sclerotic, tympanic membrane with perforation in the lower anterior and posterior portions of the tympanic membrane. Audiometry demonstrated normal bone conduction with conductive hearing loss (at about 30 db). After treatment for underlying infection, a tympanoplasty was performed. Normal hearing was restored.

4.7

Chronic Otitis Media

Chronic otitis media in a 10-year-old girl with cleft lip and palate. Tympanocentesis was performed and a tympanostomy tube was placed. The tympanostomy tube is visible in the figure. The attached wire allowed for easy removal of the tympanostomy tube. White sclerotic plaques are noted in the posterior region of the tympanic membrane. These represent calcium deposits in the tympanic membrane as a result of chronic recurrent infection. Myringotomy and the insertion of ventilation tubes allow for ventilation of the tympanic cavity. Ventilation tubes may prevent permanent structural damage to the middle ear. However, the efficacy of ventilation tubes in not well proven.

4.8

Mastoiditis

Mastoiditis in a 14-year-old girl. Physical findings included a cherry-sized, painful, erythematous swelling behind the left ear, which caused the pinna to protrude. Mastoiditis was the result of an acute bacterial otitis media 2 weeks earlier, which was not treated with systemic antibiotics. Antibiotics were initiated, and mastoidectomy was performed. Culture of the surgically drained fluid demonstrated pneumococcus.

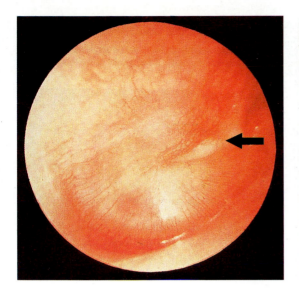

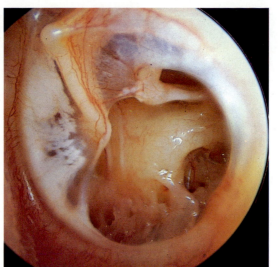

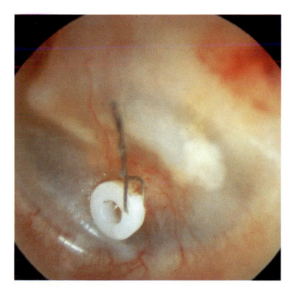

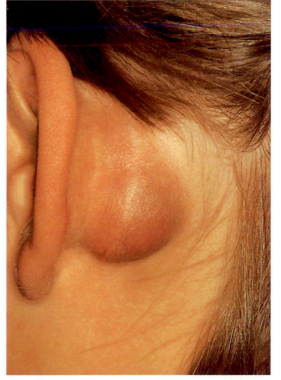

5.1

Florid Dental Caries

Florid dental caries in a 3-year-old boy who had frequently drunk sweetened tea from his bottle. Findings included partial destruction of the deciduous teeth and brown, bandlike defects on the labial surfaces of the maxillary incisors. "Baby bottle tooth decay" is an extensive form of tooth decay that occurs when infants are allowed to sleep with their bottle. This can be prevented with the appropriate parental counseling regarding nutrition and dental hygiene.

5.2

Dental Caries

Significant dental caries in a 4-year-old boy. All maxillary incisors, canines, and molars had extensive enamel defects with some pulp involvement. This may disrupt normal development of the successor permanent teeth.

5.3

Giant Cell Epulis

Benign giant cell epulis in a 17-year-old girl. The hemispherical red granulation tissue rested on the gingiva in the lower right incisor area; it had been present for several weeks and bled easily when touched. Excision and histologic examination demonstrated the diagnosis of giant cell epulis.

By contrast, epulis fibromatosa consists of mature connective tissue; it may be calcified and present as a pale, indurated gingival tumor at the gingival papillae that may recur after removal. Both giant cell epulis and epulis fibromatosa are inflammatory in origin.

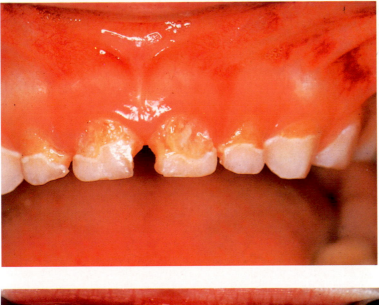

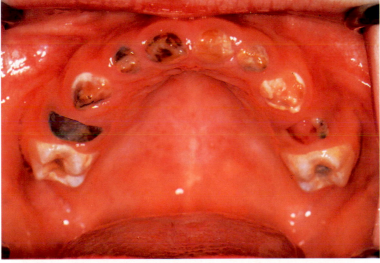

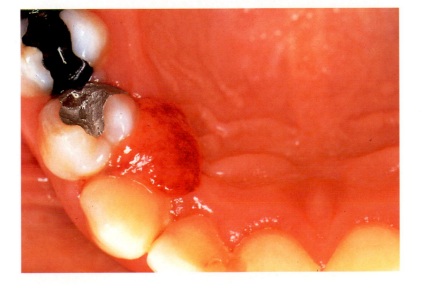

5.4

Benign Migratory Glossitis

Benign migratory glossitis (geographic tongue) in a 16-year-old girl. Findings included extensive, smooth, bright red areas of desquamation on the dorsum of the tongue (due to the absence of filiform papillae). These areas were surrounded by a yellow-gray margin. These lesions would heal spontaneously, only to be followed by the formation of similar lesions on other areas of the tongue. The etiology is unclear; however, benign migratory glossitis may be related to stress and allergies.

5.5

Dental Lamina Cysts

Dental lamina cysts in a 6-year-old boy. Findings included multiple pin-sized, white cysts on the upper alveolar ridge. These cysts contain remnants of the dental lamina epithelia. Dental lamina cysts require no treatment; they always regress spontaneously. Other causes of gingival cysts in the newborn include "Epstein pearls," keratin-filled cysts lined with stratified squamous epithelium occurring along the midpalatine raphe, and "Bohn nodules," small cystic lesions located along the mandibular and maxillary ridges containing remnants of mucous glands.

5.6

Herpetic Gingivostomatitis

Herpetic gingivostomatitis in a 10-year-old girl. Findings included multiple superficial vesicles surrounded by an erythematous halo on the mucosa of the lower lip. This was associated with gingival hyperemia and edema. These lesions were the result of a primary herpetic infection associated with systemic findings (fever). Other painful, ulcerated lesions were found on the buccal mucosa and on the tongue. Recurrent infection with herpex simplex virus is common. Thin-walled vesicles that rupture and become encrusted are commonly found with recurrent herpes simplex virus infection. Systemic symptoms are usually absent with recurrent infection.

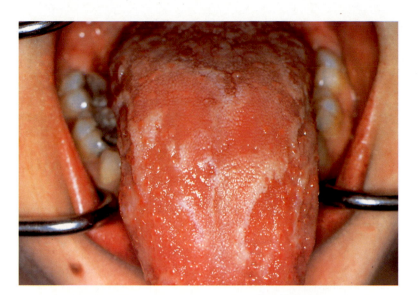

5.4

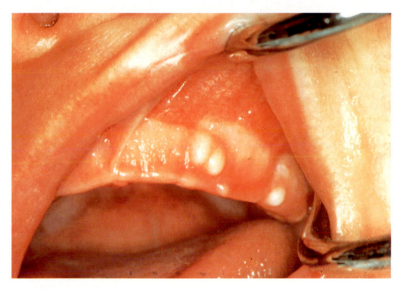

5.5

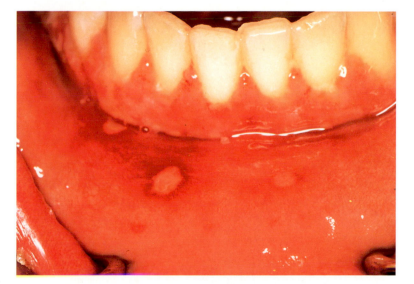

5.6

5.7
Acute Necrotizing Ulcerative Gingivitis

Acute necrotizing ulcerative gingivitis (Vincent's infection, trench mouth) in a 19-year-old man. Findings included red, painful ulcerations of the gingiva, which began in the interdental papillae. These areas of ulceration bled profusely at the slightest touch. Acute necrotizing ulcerative gingivitis is a fusospirochetal infection, which can be treated with improved oral hygiene and topical therapy. In severe cases, antimicrobial therapy is indicated. Acute necrotizing ulcerative gingivitis may occur in individuals who are immunocompromised or individuals who have very poor oral hygiene.

Differential Diagnosis—Acute necrotizing ulcerative gingivitis must be differentiated from simple gingivitis, which is a more superficial inflammation of the gingigiva and herpetic gingivostomatitis (caused by herpes simplex virus). In herpetic gingivostomatitis the vesicles may progress to small superficial ulcers. There is little tendency for these lesions to bleed.

5.8
Gingival Hyperplasia

Acquired gingival hyperplasia in a 16-year-old boy with chronic gingivitis secondary to gingival irritation and poor oral hygiene. Findings included extensive thickening and erythema of the gingiva, particularly in the maxillary area. Pseudopockets may form in the gingivae, which fill with plaque and result in secondary inflammation.

Differential Diagnosis—Extensive gingival hyperplasia may also occur with exposure to medication. Diphenylhydantoin and related compounds may lead to gingival hyperplasia with edema and erythema. A localized soft tissue tumor of the alveolar mucosa (epulis) may also occur.

5.9
Leukemic Gingival Infiltration

Leukemic gingival infiltration associated with gingivitis in a 19-year-old girl with acute myeloid leukemia. She presented with fever, lymphadenopathy, and swollen and erythematous gingiva, which bled easily. The diagnosis of acute myeloid leukemia was confirmed on bone marrow aspirate and complete blood count. The marked swelling, bleeding, and erythema of the gingiva resolved after 3 to 4 weeks of chemotherapy.

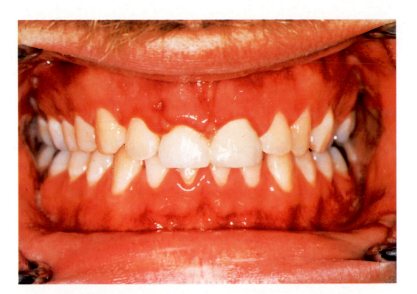

5.7

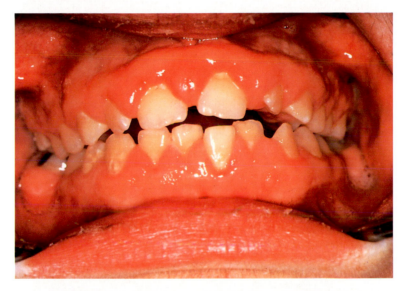

5.8

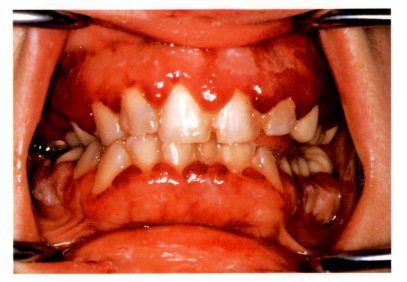

5.9

5.10 5.11
Imperforate Anus

Anal and rectal atresia with rectovaginal fistula in a 10-day-old girl. Stool was passed through the vagina. Radiologic examination indicated that this was a "high lesion" in which the rectum does not pass through the puborectalis muscle. Usually, there is an associated sacral malformation. In females, there is usually a rectovaginal fistula. The first step in an operative repair involves performing a colostomy and closing the rectovaginal fistula. At age 8 months, definitive repair was accomplished. Despite operative repair, this child remained incontinent.

5.12
Imperforate Anus

Anal and rectal atresia without fistula in a 3-day-old boy. No rectoperitoneal, rectovesicular, or rectourethral fistula could be detected. Radiographs taken with the infant held head down (Wangensteen-Rice technique) revealed the rectal fundus lying 3 cm from the perineal skin. Surgical repair was performed immediately due to symptoms of obstruction. In these "low" lesions, operative repair may be performed by using a perineal approach, with the fundus being pulled forward. Careful attention must be paid to avoid disrupting the anal sphincter. Postoperatively, dilatation must be performed in order to ensure patency.

5.13
Labial Adhesions

Labial adhesions in a 2-year-old girl. Physical findings included adhesions of both labia with a small ventrally placed opening through which urine could pass. The girl suffered from recurrent vulvitis. Appropriate hygiene and short-term application of estrogen cream resolved the adhesions. Complete closure resulting in urinary retention requires immediate separation of the labia.

5.14
Gluteal Abscess

Gluteal abscess (after incision and drainage) in a 4-month-old boy. The abscessed area was noted to be erythematous and swollen with purulent drainage. The child was afebrile. The abscess was treated with surgical incision and drainage and antimicrobial therapy.

5.15
Perianal Abscess

Perianal abscess in a 1-year-old boy. The figure demonstrates the completely healed perianal scar after spontaneous drainage. At the height of the illness, the child was febrile and experienced extreme pain when sitting or defecating. The underlying cause of the infection was anal fissures. Culture from the abscess revealed a mixed infection of aerobic and anaerobic bacteria (*Escherichia coli*, *Proteus*, and *Bacteroides fragilis*).

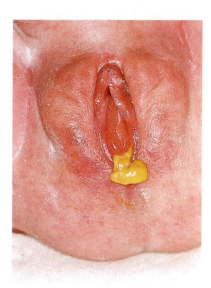
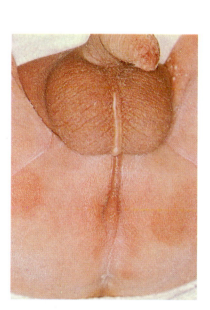

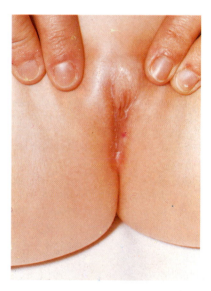

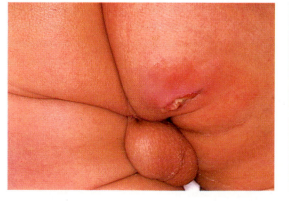
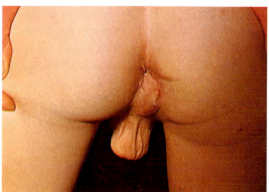
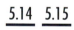

5.16
Cystic Fibrosis

Cystic fibrosis in a 1-year-old child with failure to thrive and a protuberant abdomen. Cystic fibrosis is caused by a dysfunction of exocrine glands. A wide spectrum of problems may occur including pancreatic insufficiency, nasal polyposis, pansinusitis, metabolic dysfunction, hepatic dysfunction, failure to thrive, and chronic lung disease. Growth failure is caused by malabsorption. Children have frequent, bulky, greasy stools and protuberant abdomens. The diagnosis can be made by pilocarpine iontophoresis (sweat test). This child was given pancreatic enzyme replacement, which led to a decrease in malabsorption and improved weight gain. However, chronic bronchitis and bronchopneumonia persisted.

Differential Diagnosis—The differential diagnosis of failure to thrive in the first year of life includes Schwachman-Diamond syndrome (congenital pancreatic insufficiency with neutropenia and bone abnormalities), celiac disease, protein-losing enteropathy, abetalipoproteinemia, cow's milk allergy, chronic intestinal infection (e.g., *Giardia lamblia*), and disaccharidase deficiency.

5.17
Celiac Disease

Celiac disease in a 21-month-old boy who had voluminous foul-smelling stools since the age of 3 months. Findings included sullen facial expression, protuberant abdomen, and malnutrition. The diagnosis of celiac disease was confirmed through a perioral suction biopsy of the small intestine. Histologically, the biopsy specimen demonstrated villous atrophy of the epithelium of the small intestine. When placed on a gluten-free diet, the steatorrhea ceased, and the child began to gain weight.

Other causes of malabsorption include chronic enteritis (especially in the developing world), short-gut syndrome, cow's milk protein intolerance, protein-losing enteropathy, abetalipoproteinemia, and intestinal infections such as giardiasis.

5.18
Cystic Fibrosis

Cystic fibrosis in a 10-year-old girl. Physical findings include an increase in the anteroposterior diameter of the chest ("barrel-shaped chest") and minimal chest wall movement. Chest radiographs demonstrated emphysematous changes. Severe dyspnea was noted after only minimal exertion. Other physical findings included clubbing of the fingers and nails, and failure to thrive. Chronic bronchitis, bronchiectasis, and frequent pneumonia were present from age 1 year onward. The condition worsened despite therapy.

Differential Diagnosis—The differential diagnosis of chronic bronchitis includes bronchial asthma, congenital bronchiectasis, lung anomalies, immotile cilia syndrome, primary or secondary immune deficiency, tuberculosis, and smoking.

5.19
Rectal Prolapse

Rectal prolapse in a 3½-year-old girl with cystic fibrosis. The rectal mucosa was prolapsed, inflamed, and swollen. Prolapse can usually be manually reduced and improves with pancreatic enzyme replacement therapy. Prolapse is due to increased intraabdominal pressure from pulmonary disease or malabsorption.

5.20
Cystic Fibrosis

Cystic fibrosis in a 10-month-old boy with cirrhosis of the liver. Findings included a protuberant abdomen (due to ascites) and dilatation of superficial veins. The child had biliary cirrhosis with secondary portal hypertension and esophageal varices. He presented with hematemesis, which was treated with vasopressin (Pitressin) and a Sengstaken-Blakemore tube. The child died 3 months later due to hepatic failure.

Multilobular biliary cirrhosis of the liver occurs in approximately 20% of individuals with cystic fibrosis and frequently leads to portal hypertension, esophageal varices, and hypersplenism.

The cirrhotic changes are most frequently localized leaving large parts of the liver parenchyma unaffected. Jaundice is usually absent and liver function may be minimally affected.

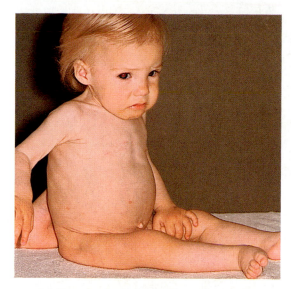

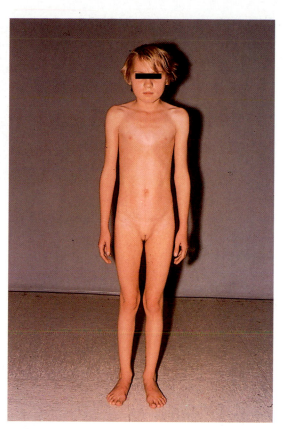

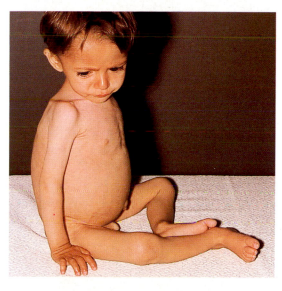

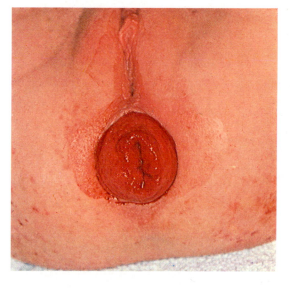

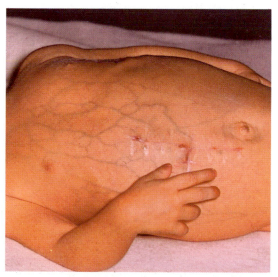

5.21

Hypertrophic Pyloric Stenosis

Hypertrophic pyloric stenosis in a 2-month-old boy. At 4 weeks of age the infant presented with nonbilious projectile vomiting after meals. Peristaltic waves proceeding from the left to the right were noted in the abdomen. The diagnosis was confirmed by sonography and subsequent surgery.

5.22

Perianal Lesion

Perianal lesion in a 9-year-old boy with Crohn's disease. A lentil bean-sized skin lesion was noted at the erythematous and swollen anus. Perianal disease is commonly seen with Crohn's disease (including tags, fistula, and abscess).

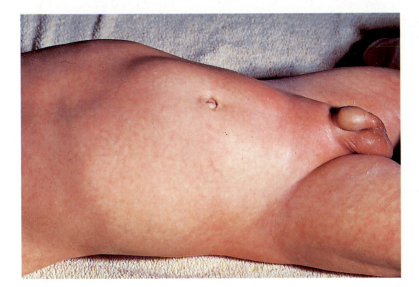

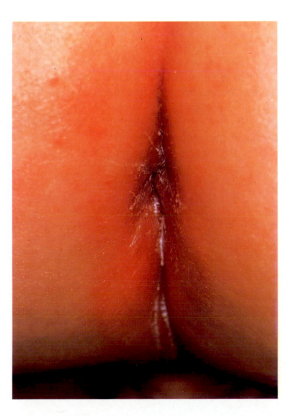

6.1

Hydrocele

Hydrocele in a 4-year-old boy. The left scrotum was enlarged due to a fluid collection in the tunica vaginalis. The hydrocele varied in size depending upon the posture of the boy.

A hydrocele can be differentiated from an indirect inguinal hernia by palpation and transillumination. Hydroceles may occur in combination with indirect inguinal hernia. Small hydroceles may resolve spontaneously in the first year of life. Larger hydroceles often persist and may require surgical treatment. In older children, torsion of the testes and testicular tumors must be ruled out.

6.2

Phimosis

Phimosis (narrowing of the opening of the foreskin preventing retraction) in a 3-year-old boy. The child complained of pain on urination and had a thin stream of urine. During urination the foreskin would inflate like a balloon. The disorder was corrected through circumcision.

Physiologic adhesions of the foreskin to the glans (without restriction of urinary flow) in small children requires no treatment. The adhesions normally resolve during the first 2 years of life, at which time the foreskin can be slightly retracted. Vigorous attempts to retract the foreskin can lead to acquired phimosis because of trauma and scarring. Paraphimosis occurs in children with mild phimosis when the foreskin in forcibly retracted over the glans penis. The retracted, edematous foreskin can strangle the glans and cause gangrene. Phimosis may also be caused by lichen sclerosus et atrophicus.

6.3

Gartner Duct Cyst

Gartner duct cyst in a 3-month-old girl. This saccular protrusion into the vestibule of the vagina was caused by a Gartner duct (mesonephric) cyst of the vaginal wall. A Gartner duct cyst must be differentiated from a müllerian (paramesonephric) duct cyst. Müllerian duct cysts may at first be asymptomatic, but at the time of menarche may fill with menstrual blood and become painful.

6.4

Retention Cysts

Retention cyst of the urethra in a 2-day-old newborn. A cyst was noted at the external opening of the penis, which hindered urinary flow. The cyst regressed during the first few days of life and no treatment was necessary. There were no other associated anomalies.

6.5

Balanitis

Balanitis (inflammation of the glans and foreskin) in a 4-month-old boy. Findings included diffuse erythema and swelling of the foreskin and glans with foul-smelling, cheesy secretion (which cultured positive for *Candida albicans*). A persistent diaper dermatitis was also noted.

Candidal balanitis occurs frequently in diabetics as well as in normal adults who have had sexual intercourse with an infected partner. In the circumcised child with candidal balanitis, the glans may be inflamed, and satellite lesions may be seen. Therapy involves local hygiene and topical treatment with antifungal agent (nystatin or miconazol).

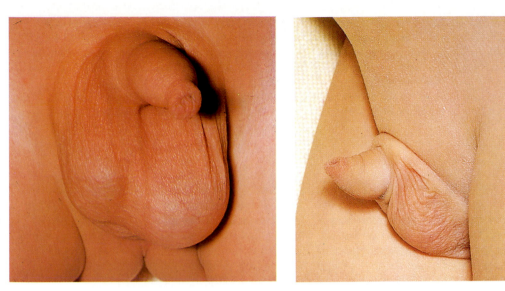

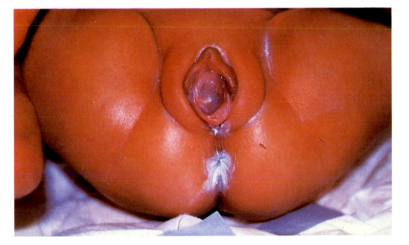

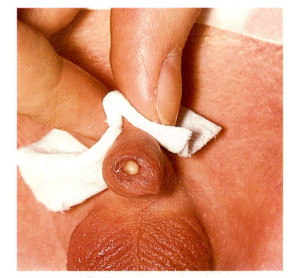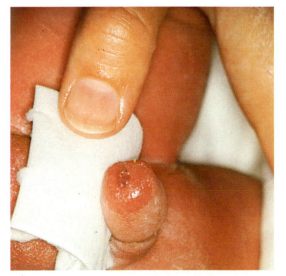

6.6

Lichen Sclerosus et Atrophicus Vulvae

Lichen sclerosus et atrophicus vulvae in a 7-year-old girl. Findings included a white discoloration and hardening of the vulval skin with early signs of atrophy of the external genitalia. Itching and burning were also noted. The condition improved with local application of corticosteroid cream.

The prognosis of lichen sclerosus in children is usually more hopeful than it is for adult patients. Girls have itching in 50% of the cases, and a vaginal discharge in 20%. In women, the skin around the anus is often involved. Lichen sclerosus can lead to considerable labial shrinkage and narrowing of the introitus. Adults may have extragenital lesions as well.

Differential Diagnosis—Morphea (page 166) and primary vulval atrophy (seen almost exclusively in adult patients).

6.7

Lichen Sclerosus et Atrophicus Penis

Lichen sclerosus et atrophicus penis in a 6-year-old boy. The foreskin could not be retracted over the glans (phimosis) and was noted to have a white discoloration with thickening of the tissue. Symptoms had been present for a year. Histologic examination of the tissue taken at the time of circumcision revealed a superficial hyperkeratosis in the atrophic epidermis with subepidermal sclerotic changes and lymphocytic infiltrate. With the exception of a brief application of corticosteroid cream postoperatively, the tissue gradually returned to normal without treatment.

Cases of acquired phimosis and balanitis may be caused by lichen sclerosus. In boys, the perianal area and scrotum are not affected. The diagnosis is often made through histologic examination following circumcision for phimosis.

6.8

Priapism

Priapism (sustained erection of the penis without sexual arousal) in a 6-year-old boy. Findings included painful penile erection that persisted for 72 hours. No obstruction to urinary flow was noted. Since conservative measures proved unsuccessful, a shunt operation was performed (creation of a surgical shunt between the corpora cavernosa and corpus spongiosum). The postoperative period was free of complications. The cause in this case was not determined.

During childhood, priapism is observed in conjunction with leukemia, sickle cell anemia, and trauma to the perineal area. The treatment for priapism may be disease specific; with leukemia, chemotherapy combined with radiation may be of some help; with sickle cell disease, transfusion of packed red blood cells may be the treatment of choice. Persistent posttraumatic priapism often requires surgical correction.

6.9

Balanitis

Balanitis (inflammation of the glans penis and foreskin) in a 10-year-old boy. The penis was swollen, reddened and partially ulcerated. The foreskin had similar inflammatory changes and was very painful. Lymphadenopathy was noted in the right groin area. The condition responded to antimicrobial therapy.

In uncircumcised boys, retention of smegma (due to poor hygiene) is often the cause of acute infections with erythema, edema, and purulent drainage. Anaerobic and intestinal bacteria can frequently cause ulcerations. Trichomonas, with or without accompanying urethritis, may also cause balanitis. Primary herpes simplex balanitis may be particularly painful and cause blistering edema and regional lymphadenopathy. Herpes simplex may also cause urethritis and severe dysuria without any visible skin changes.

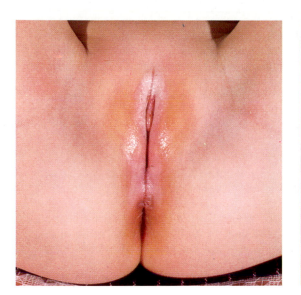

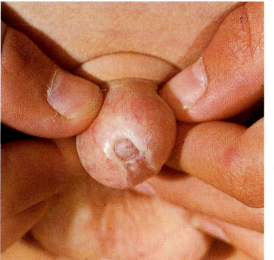

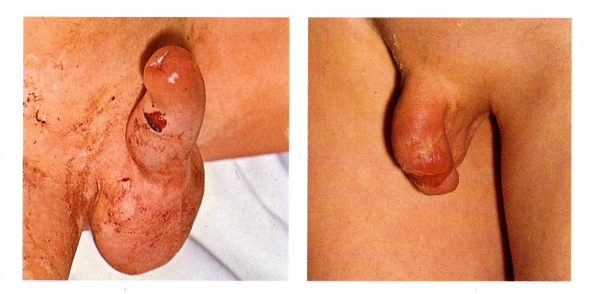

6.10
Vulvovaginitis

Vulvovaginitis in a 5-year-old girl. Erythema, swelling, and purulent drainage were noted in and around the vulva. The infection was caused by *Neisseria gonorrhoeae* (proven by microscopic examination and culture). Cases of sexually transmitted diseases in the preadolescent must be approached with the diagnosis of sexual abuse in mind. The child was successfully treated with penicillin.

Vulvovaginitis in childhood must be differentiated from other forms of vulvovaginitis, which may be caused by Group A or Group B streptococci, staphylococci, *Haemophilus*, *Enterobacter*, *Trichomonas vaginalis*, *Candida albicans*, and herpes simplex virus. Foreign bodies, which may be introduced into the vagina, must be ruled out when dealing with children.

6.11
Molluscum Contagiosum

Molluscum contagiosum in a 4-year-old boy. Several pearl-shaped papules, 2–3 mm in diameter with central umbilication were noted on the skin of the penis. A caseous material could be expressed from these lesions. This cutaneous infection was apparently caused by autoinoculation from lesions originally found on the face of the child.

Skin lesions in molluscum contagiosum can vary widely in size, from the size of a pinhead to pea-sized lesions. Central dimpling or umbilication is usually noted. Microscopic analysis of the caseous material reveals many intracellular inclusion bodies. Eczematous or impetiginous changes are frequent. Molluscum contagiosum has a predilection for the axillae or the anogenital area, but may also be found on the face, the head, and in the mouth. Opinion regarding treatment varies. Without treatment, the lesions of molluscum contagiosum may resolve within 6 to 9 months; however, some cases take years to resolve.

Differential Diagnosis—Similar discrete pearly papular lesions may be seen with warts and milia (page 208).

6.12
Condylomata Acuminata

Condylomata acuminata (genital or venereal warts) in a 4-year-old boy. White, moist, papillomatous growths of warty tissue (identified histologically as genital warts) were noted in the perianal area. Condylomata acuminata is an example of papovavirus infection which may be transmitted either by sexual intercourse or by direct contact. In girls, condylomata acuminata are usually located in the introitus, the labia minora, the labia majora, the perineum, the anus, the clitoris, or the urethra.

Differential Diagnosis—Differential diagnosis includes condylomata lata (secondary syphilis) and carcinoma (in adult patients).

6.13
Condylomata Acuminata

Condylomata acuminata (genital warts) in a 4-year-old boy. Cauliflowerlike, hyperplastic warts were noted on the penis and the glans. Genital warts may be skin colored or reddened papules with a raw appearing surface. They are frequently found on the foreskin, the meatus, the shaft of the penis, the anus, and the scrotum. They can last for a few weeks or up to a year.

Differential Diagnosis—Differential diagnosis includes molluscum contagiosum, milia, and condylomata lata.

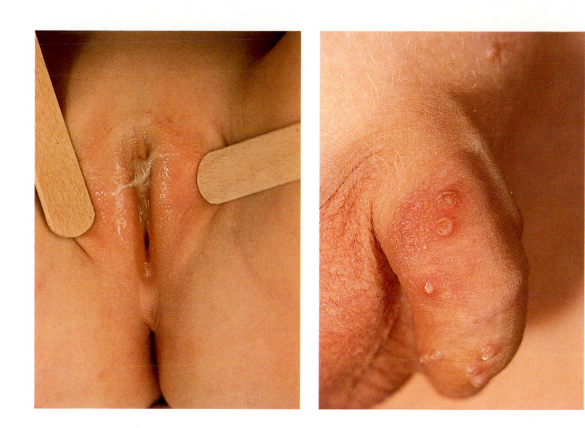

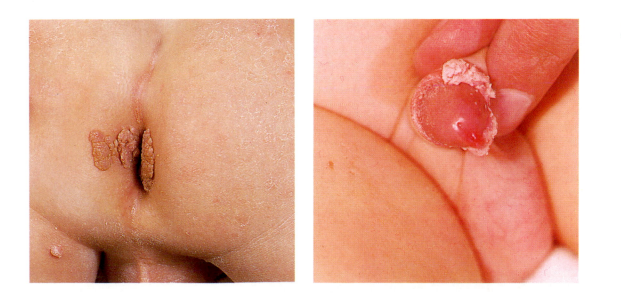

6.14
Indirect Hernia

Indirect hernia in a 3-month-old boy. Of note was the swelling of the right groin near the pubic symphysis. The swelling extended into the scrotum. When the child cried, the swelling increased. The hernia was easily reducible.

Differential Diagnosis—Hydrocele of the spermatic cord or testes must be differentiated from an indirect hernia. Unlike an indirect hernia, a hydrocele will transilluminate.

6.15
Hydrocele

Bilateral hydrocele of the testes and spermatic cord in a 5-month-old boy. Hydroceles occur due to failure of obliteration of the tunica vaginalis. The abnormal collection of fluid inside the tunica vaginalis caused both the left and right scrotum to be taut and painfully swollen. Since there was also hydrocele of the spermatic cord, the swelling was also noted in the area of the groin. The fluid collection could be easily transilluminated. In cases of indirect hernia, transillumination is negative. Presence of hydrocele was confirmed at the time of surgical repair. Hydrocele of the testes or the spermatic cord is usually associated with an indirect hernia.

6.16
Hypospadias

Hypospadias in a 2-year-old boy. The narrowed urethral opening was on the ventral surface of the penis, close to where the penis joined the scrotum. The penis was bent ventrally due to a fibrous band or chordee, and urine passed in a very thin stream. Intravenous pyelogram and voiding cystourethrogram demonstrated no distention of the bladder, ureter, or renal pelvis. Both testes were descended and no hernia was detected. Surgical repair was recommended before the child reached school age.

6.17
Exstrophy of the Bladder

Exstrophy of the bladder with epispadias in a 1-day-old newborn. Exstrophy of the bladder is a developmental defect in which there is abnormal midline fusion of the endoderm and ectoderm. The defect may involve the anterior abdominal wall, the bladder, and the urethra. In this case, the bladder was everted, and the opening to the ureter could be seen on the posterior wall of the bladder. The ureter and renal pelvis were not distended. The urethra opened on the dorsal side of an abnormally short penis (epispadias). The child was treated with antibiotics to prevent infection. At one year of age, rectal prolapse developed, which required operative correction. Corrective surgery for exstrophy of the bladder (cystectomy and ureteral diversion into a sigmoid conduit) was planned at a later date.

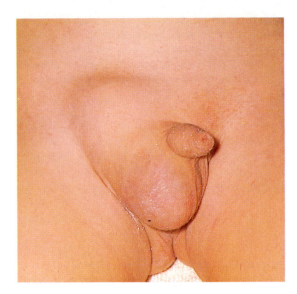

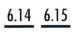

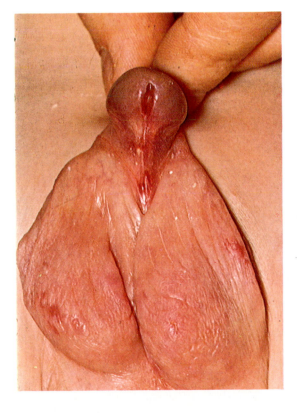

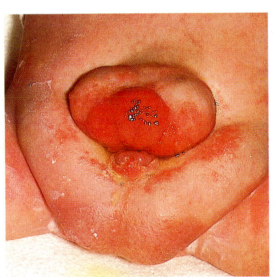

6.18

Imperforate Hymen

Imperforate hymen in a 2-week-old girl. The imperforate hymen protruded from the vaginal orifice as a result of accumulation of secretions in the estrogenized vagina. After incision of the hymen, the mass disappeared. The girl had no associated problems with urination.

In vaginal atresia, the lower part of the vagina directly behind the hymen is closed. Examination of the vaginal orifice reveals a protruding membrane. Endoscopic drainage from below is necessary due to the risk of developing hydrometrocolpos, which can lead to urinary or intestinal obstruction.

6.19

Incomplete Testicular Feminization

Incomplete testicular feminization in a 4-day-old child. Physical findings included normal appearing external female genitalia except for clitoral hypertrophy and a sinus urogenitalis. Because of the swelling of both labia majora, an inguinal hernia was suspected. At the time of surgery, the hernial sac was found to include both testes. The testes were removed. A uterus was not present. Karyotype revealed the infant to be a normal male (XY). The child will be started on estrogen treatment at the onset of puberty.

6.20

Complete Testicular Feminization

Complete testicular feminization in a 16-year-old girl. The patient presented for evaluation with primary amenorrhea. She demonstrated early breast development, but pubic and axillary hair growth was not noted. Physical examination demonstrated a short vagina without obvious cervical opening. At laparotomy, neither ovaries nor uterus was found. At the time of surgery, intraabdominal testes were removed. Chromosomes revealed a normal male karyotype (XY). Psychologically the patient identified with the female gender. Regular treatment with estrogen was begun in order for the girl to develop secondary sexual characteristics.

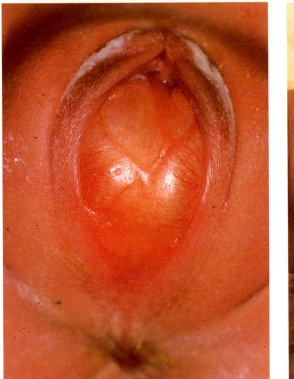

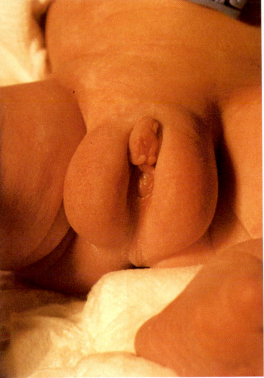

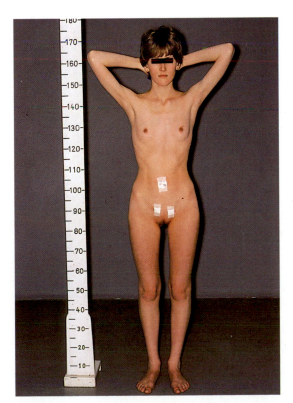

7.1

Asymmetric Tonic Neck Reflex

Asymmetric tonic neck reflex is elicited by rapidly turning the head of the supine infant to one side. This maneuver will lead to extension of the arm and leg on the side to which the face is turned. The opposite side will adopt a flexion posture; the so-called "fencing position." The reflex may be normal during the first 2 to 4 months of life.

7.2

Galant Spinal Reflex

Stroking the back along the paravertebral spine causes sideward bending of the spinal column, with the concave side toward the side being stimulated.

7.3

Foot Grasp Reflex

Light pressing on the soles of the feet causes the toes to curl.

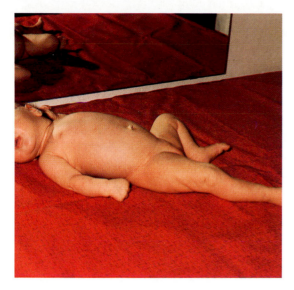
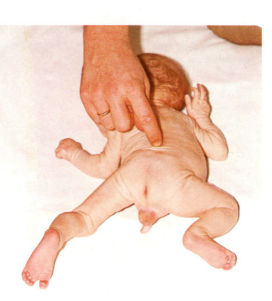

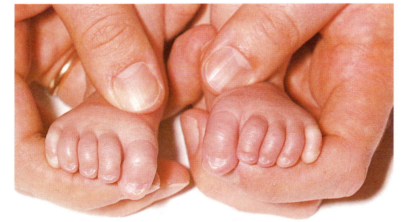

7.4

Palmar Grasp

Palmar grasp reflex in a healthy 2-week-old child. This primitive reflex involves the grasping of a finger laid on the inner surface of the child's hand.

7.5

Rooting Reflex

Rooting reflex in a healthy 2-week-old child. The mouth is open and the head turns toward the finger that gently strokes the mouth.

7.6

Stepping Reflex

Stepping reflex (automatic walking) in a healthy 2-week-old child. Walking movements are elicited when the child is held upright, inclined forward, and the soles of the feet are gently touched to a flat surface.

7.7

Placing Reflex

Placing reflex (climb reflex) in a healthy 2-week-old child. After touching the edge of the table with the dorsum of the foot, the child will lift the leg and set the foot flatly on the table.

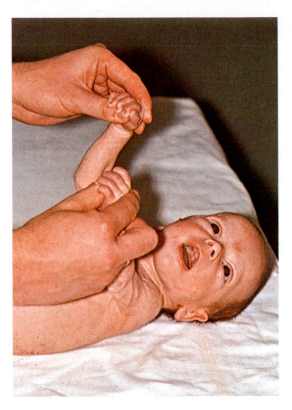

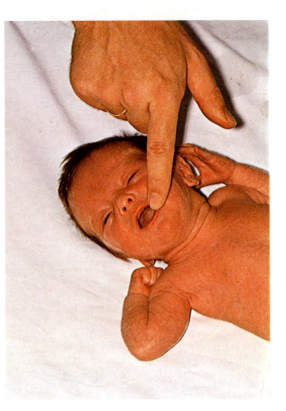

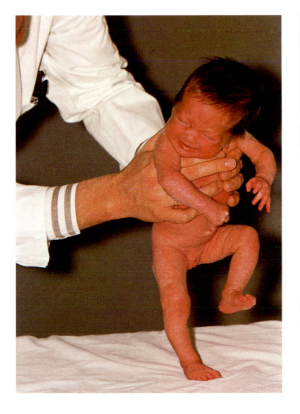

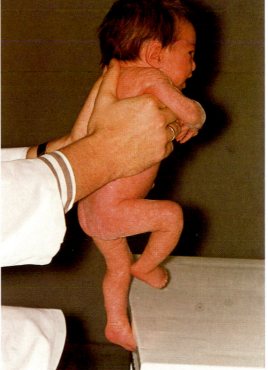

7.8

Moro Reflex

Moro reflex in a healthy 2-week-old child. The Moro reflex is elicited when the child is placed supine and the infant is either gently shaken or support is suddenly withdrawn. The reflex has two phases. The infant will first demonstrate exten- sion and abduction of the arms, followed by flexion and adduction of the arms and splaying of the fingers. The Moro reflex is a primitive reflex that usually disappears by 3 months of age.

7.9

Asymmetric Moro Reflex

Asymmetric response to an attempt at eliciting the Moro reflex in a 3-week-old child. The left arm extended and abducted appropriately, but the right arm did not change position. The cause of this asymmetric response is severe birth trauma that led to right-sided hemiplegia.

7.10

Parachute Reflex

The Parachute reflex is elicited by the rapid tilting forward of a 7-month-old child who had previously been held upright. The child protects herself by extending her arms and splaying her fingers.

7.11

Parachute Reflex

Attempts to elicit parachute reflex in a 1-year-old boy with cerebral palsy. When the child is held upright and tilted forward, the arms and fingers remained flexed (abnormal response). The child had cerebral palsy due to intrauterine asphyxia. After birth, there was evidence of asphyxia and the child required support with mechanical ventilation for several days. The long-term effects of this intrauterine as- phyxia included cerebral palsy, seizure disorder, and devel- opmental delay.

Children with cerebral palsy may present with the follow- ing characteristics:

1. Persistence of primitive reflexes (such as atonic neck reflex)
2. Absence of complex reflexes (such as the parachute reflex, support reflex, placement reflex, and balance re- actions)
3. Occurrence of pathologic reflexes (such as extension reflex)
4. Abnormal muscle tone (such as spastic dyplegia)
5. Inability to learn motor skills such as grasping, sitting, standing, walking, and crawling
6. Asymmetric posture and disturbances of spontane- ous movement

7.12

Automatic Reaction

Automatic reaction in a healthy 10-day-old child. When placed on his stomach, the child immediately turns his head to the side to maintain his airway.

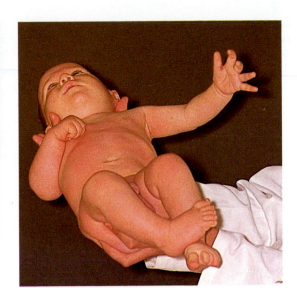

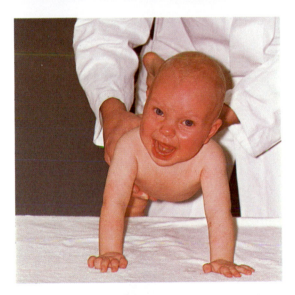

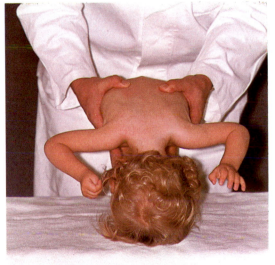

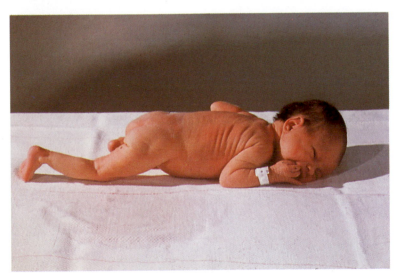

7.13

Sideways Parachute Reflex

Sideways parachute reflex (support reaction) in a healthy 8-month-old boy. When pushed to one side, a positive righting reaction of the torso and head occurs, along with shortening of the unweighted left side of the torso and support from the open hand of the extended right arm. A positive sideways parachute reflex generally begins at the age of 7 months.

7.14

Sideways Parachute Reflex

Sideways parachute reflex (support reaction) in an 8-month-old boy with cerebral palsy. When pushed to one side, there is a negative righting reaction of the head and torso with no support from the right arm. The hand remains rolled in a fist.

7.15

Positive Standing with Support

Standing with support (readiness to stand) is demonstrated in a healthy 8-month-old boy. The posture is symmetric, the trunk is held slightly forward, the hips are extended, and the legs rotated slightly outward and abducted. At age 10 months, a normal child will begin to stand, while holding on to support, and lift himself to stand.

7.16

Negative Standing with Support

Negative standing with support (readiness to stand) is demonstrated in a 1-year-old girl with cerebral palsy. The arms are in a jug-handle position. Hands are closed in a fist, the thumbs are tucked in, the hips are slightly bent, and the legs rotated inward and crossed.

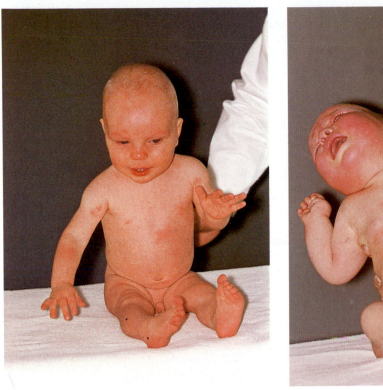 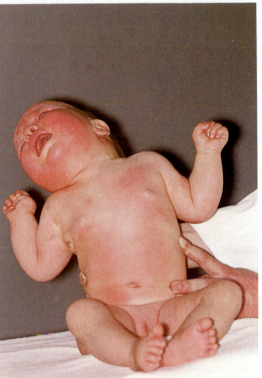

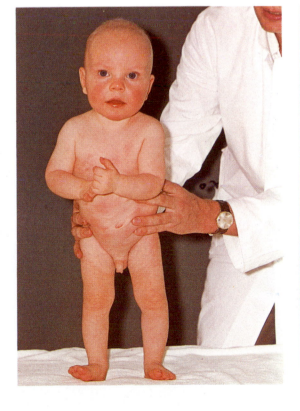 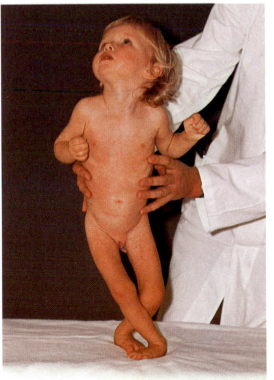

7.17

Positive Body Righting Reflex

Positive body righting reflex in a healthy 8-month-old child. When the trunk is bent sideways, the head is held vertically. The upper torso is contracted and the unweighted leg is abducted and flexed.

7.18

Positive Landau Reflex

Positive Landau reflex in a healthy 8-month-old boy. When suspended in the horizontal position, with a hand supporting the child beneath the abdomen, the normal response is to maintain the head, trunk, hips, and legs in extension. Passive bending of the neck is followed by flexion of the trunk and hips. The Landau reflex may be seen as early as 4 months of age.

7.19

Negative Body Righting Reflex

Negative body righting reflex in a 1-year-old girl with cerebral palsy. When the torso is bent sideways, the head remains in the same axis as the torso. The upper body is contracted and the legs are adducted and extended (scissoring).

7.20

Negative Landau Reflex

Negative Landau reflex in a 1-year-old girl with cerebral palsy. The head is not lifted, the arms are bent, and neither the back nor the legs are extended.

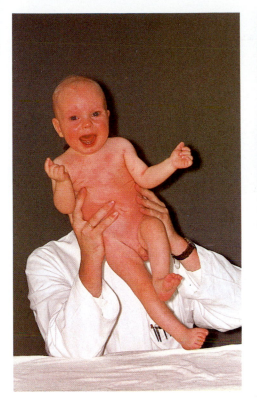

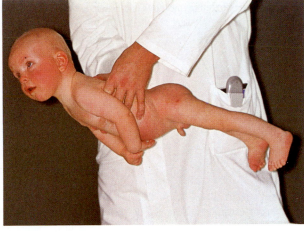

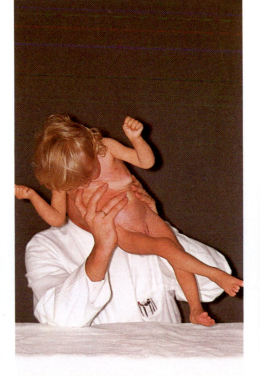

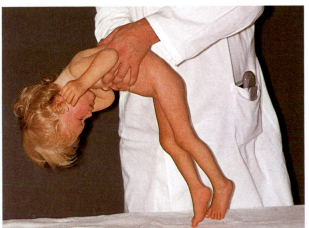

7.21

Traction Attempt

Traction attempt (pull to sitting position) in a 3-month-old boy. The arms remain slightly bent and the head is brought up in the process of sitting.

7.22

Traction Attempt

Attempts to pull to a sitting position in a 4-month-old girl with cerebral palsy. The arms were extended during the maneuver, and the head was noted to fall back.

7.23

Obligatory Neck Reflex

Obligatory neck reflex in a 4-year-old boy with cerebral palsy. Obligatory extension and turning of the head were noted. Other signs of abnormal neurologic development in this child include hyperextension of the legs (scissoring), plantar flexion of the feet, extension and pronation of the arms, and arching of the back.

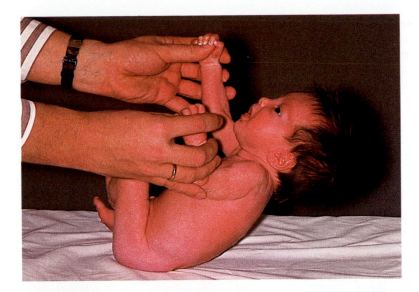

7.21

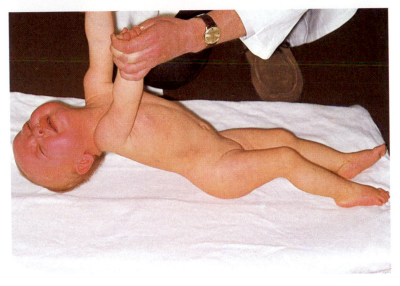

7.22

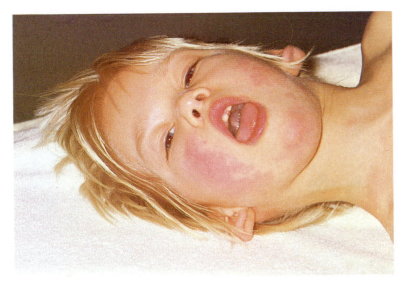

7.23

7.24

Spastic Hemiplegia

Spastic hemiplegia of the right side in a 3-month-old boy with cerebral palsy. The right arm is always flexed, adducted, and pronated. The fist is closed with the thumb tucked in. The right leg is rotated inward and adducted; the left leg is rotated outward. The right foot is maintained in a slightly equinovarus position. Muscle tone of the right arm and leg is increased. Achilles tendon reflexes are greater on the right and the grasp reflex on the right is strongly positive. A left convex scoliosis of the spine was also noted. The cause of the hemiplegia was uncertain. The child became involved in intensive physical therapy with some improvement.

7.25

Decorticate Posture

Decorticate posture noted after drowning in a 4-year-old boy. The arms are flexed, the hands tightly fisted, and the legs extended. Bilateral contactures were noted. The child maintained an opisthotonic posture. The child remained in a comatose state, apparently awake but with no response to external stimula (coma vigil).

7.26a 7.26b

Infantile Spinal Muscular Atrophy (Werdnig-Hoffmann Disease)

(Sever) Intermediate

Werdnig-Hoffman disease in an 11-year-old boy. Findings included widespread muscular atrophy leading to weakness, hypotonia and areflexia. The child was unable to sit or stand, but had contractures of the hands and feet. Other findings included paradoxical respiration (due to weakness of the intercostal muscles but otherwise normal diaphragmatic function) and fasciculation of the tongue. The disease became manifest at 1 year of age presenting with muscle weakness.

Werdnig-Hoffman disease is caused by atrophy of the anterior horn cells of the spinal cord as well as atrophy of the motor nuclei in the brainstem. Nerve atrophy leads to secondary muscular atrophy. The disease is frequently complicated by bronchopneumonia. The diagnosis may be confirmed through electromyography (demonstrating denervation) and muscle biopsy (demonstrating degeneration).

7.27

Friedreich's Ataxia

Hereditary Friedreich's ataxia in an 11-year-old boy. Muscular atrophy of the lower extremities and pes cavus (high arched feet) have been present since the age of 1 year. This neurologic disorder may present with ataxic gait, muscle weakness (due to peripheral neuropathy), sensory loss (especially in the feet), intention tremor, dysarthria, and loss of reflexes. Friedreich's ataxia is a loss of progressive cerebellar and spinal cord dysfunction caused by the degeneration of the spinal, cerebellar, and corticospinal tract. Nerve conduction studies demonstrate decreased velocity.

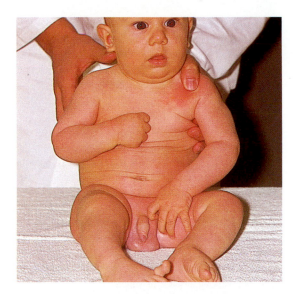

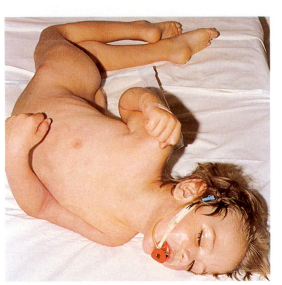

7.24 7.25

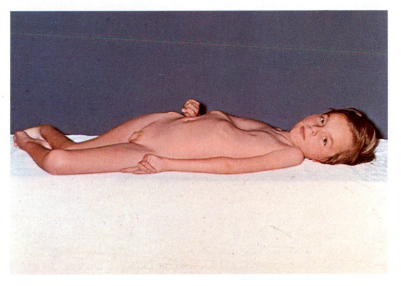

7.26a

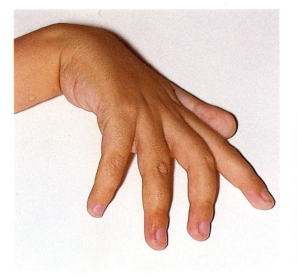

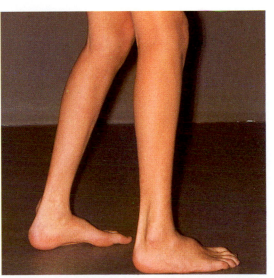

7.26b 7.27

7.28

Hydrocephalus

Hydrocephalus in a 14-month-old girl resulting from intra-uterine toxoplasmosis. Enlargement of the head had been noted since birth, along with thinning of the cranial bones, dilatation of the scalp veins, and downward deviation of the eyes (sunset phenomenon). Fundoscopic examination of the eyes revealed chorioretinitis, a finding typical for toxoplasmosis. The protein content of the cerebrospinal fluid was elevated. Skull radiographs demonstrated intracranial calcifications. Serum IgM specific for *Toxoplasma* was detected using indirect fluorescent antibody technique.

7.29

Progressive Hydrocephalus

Progressive hydrocephalus in a 4-week-old boy. The findings included increased head circumference, large bulging anterior fontanel, and "sunset phenomenon" of the eyes (downward displacement of the eyes with retraction of the upper eyelid). The etiology of this communicating hydrocephalus was unclear. To control the symptoms of progressive hydrocephalus, a shunt procedure was performed.

Differential Diagnosis—Abnormal enlargement of the head within the first year of life may be due to chronic subdural effusion. In this case, the parietal region protruded more than the frontal area (opposite of the findings in hydrocephalus). In cases of familial macrocephaly (see Figure 7.31), no symptoms of illness are noted. Enlargement of the head due to excessive brain growth (megalocephaly) appears in storage diseases such as Hurler's disease, Tay-Sachs disease, and metachromatic leukodystrophy. With hydranencephaly (absence of cerebral hemispheres), only the cerebellum and brainstem are present. The cerebrum is replaced by a fluid-filled cavity. The head circumference is normal or only slightly enlarged and the shape of the head may be normal. When transilluminated, the skull lights up brightly. There is a striking absence of voluntary motor movements in hydranencephalic children.

7.30

Congenital Hydrocephalus

Congenital hydrocephalus in a 1-day-old premature infant. The infant was born 4 weeks before the expected due date and weighted 4,800 g. The child had a greatly enlarged head (head circumference 54 cm) with widely opened cranial sutures, large bulging fontanel, low-set ears, large forehead, and a relatively small face.

Prenatal infection was not suspected due to the lack of other deformities or symptoms. Death resulted from respiratory failure at 5 weeks of age. The autopsy revealed the cause of hydrocephalus as congenital aqueductal stenosis. Congenital aqueductal stenosis may lead to obstructive hydrocephalus with extreme enlargement of the lateral and third ventricles.

7.31

Familial Macrocephaly

Familial macrocephaly in a 4-month-old boy. At birth, the head circumference was 37.5 cm. The head is enlarged, but of normal configuration. The fontanel is normal in size, the cranial sutures are not widenened, and the face appears relatively normal. Psychomotor development is appropriate for age. Computed tomography revealed no signs of hydrocephalus, subdural effusion, or tumor. Both the father and the 5-year-old brother are macrocephalic as well.

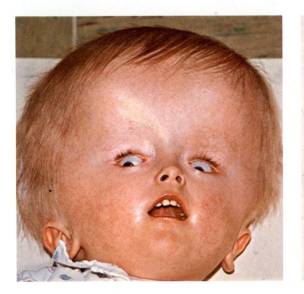
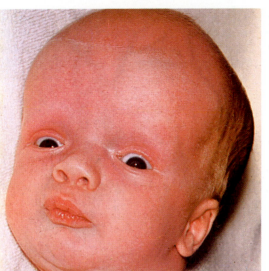

7.28 7.29

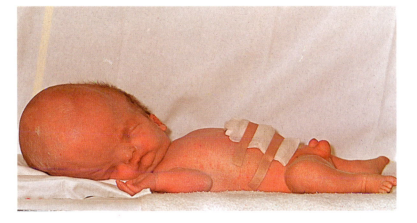

7.30

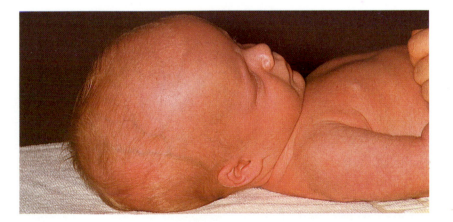

7.31

7.32 7.33

Hydrocephalus

These figures demonstrate the findings in a 3½-month-old girl after placement of a ventriculoatrial shunt for hydrocephalus. The child was born prematurely at 30 weeks gestation and developed progressive hydrocephalus. After the operation, the head circumference decreased from 42 cm to 39.5 cm. The large fontanel and widely spread cranial sutures were no longer seen. After the operation, the parietal and occipital bones overlapped. The cause of hydrocephalus was uncertain but probably was related to intraventricular hemorrhage and posthemorrhagic hydrocephalus.

7.34

Dandy-Walker Syndrome

Dandy-Walker syndrome in a 1-day-old girl. Dolichocephaly, bulging anterior and posterior fontanels, and widely spread cranial sutures were noted. Occipital transillumination of the cranium revealed enlargement of the fourth ventricle. Computed tomography demonstrated not only enlargement of the ventricles (due to congenital obstruction of the foramen of Luschka and foramen of Magendie), but also shifting of the cerebellar hemispheres.

7.35

Oxycephaly

Oxycephaly in a 2-week-old boy. The "towerlike" cranium is caused by cranial synostosis involving the coronal sutures. The high forehead and exophthalmos are a result of the depression of the roof of the orbits. Papilledema and optic atrophy may develop later. Other malformations occur with oxycephaly such as syndactyly, cardiac defects, and choanal atresia. Oxycephaly is one of the main findings in Apert syndrome, Carpenter syndrome, and Crouzon syndrome (pages 30 and 32).

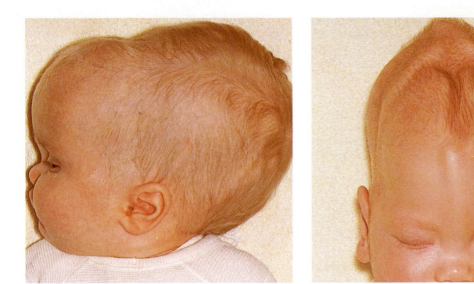

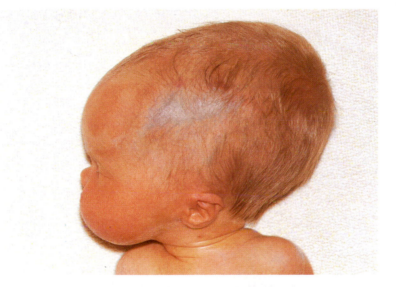

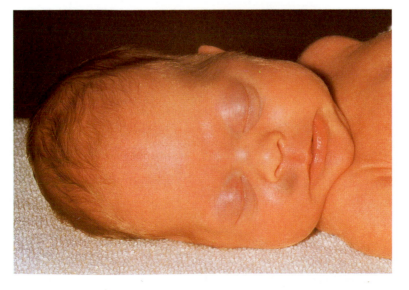

7.36

Meningocele

An apple-sized sacral meningocele in a 4-day-old newborn. The infant was without symptoms of hydrocephalus or other neurologic disease. The diagnosis of meningocele with spinal bifida was confirmed radiologically and at the time of operative repair.

Spina bifida with meningocele (or meningomyelocele) may present as a midline defect usually in the lumbosacral area. The defect is covered by a thin membrane of meninges. Spinal bifida is associated with Arnold-Chiari malformation and aqueductal stenosis.

7.37

Meningomyelocele

Closed lumbosacral meningomyelocele causing partial paralysis of the legs and incontinence of urine and stool. The lesion was repaired on the first day of life. The infant did not develop subsequent hydrocephalus.

7.38

Meningomyelocele

Open thoracolumbar meningomyelocele in a newborn infant. The child was completely paralyzed below the level of the lesion. Surgery to close the spinal defect was performed on the second day of life. A shunt procedure was performed during the fourth day of life due to progressive hydrocephalus.

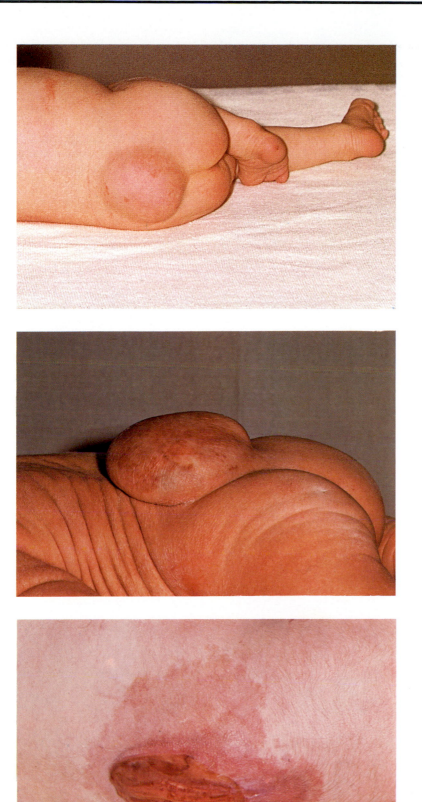

7.39

Diastematomyelia

Diastematomyelia (congenital midline cleft of the spinal cord) in an 11-year-old boy. Physical findings included localized hypertrichosis (tufts of hair) in the area of the mid to lower thoracic spine. Diastematomyelia of the third to twelfth thoracic vertebrae was detected with magnetic resonance imaging. No other neurologic deficits were noted.

7.40   7.41

Encephalocele

Frontal encephalocele before and after operative repair in infancy. Physical findings demonstrated a 4 × 5 cm large, dark red sac protruding from the forehead and covering the nose and right eye. The encephalocele developed through a 5-mm defect in the skull. The encephalocele was surgically removed. At the age 3 months, a ventricular shunt was placed due to progressive hydrocephalus.

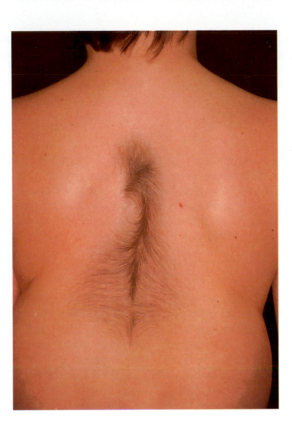

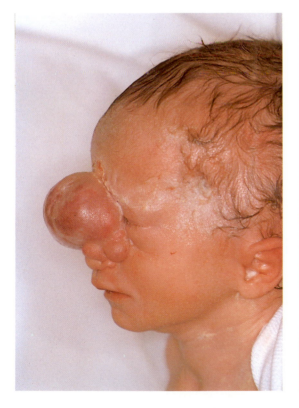

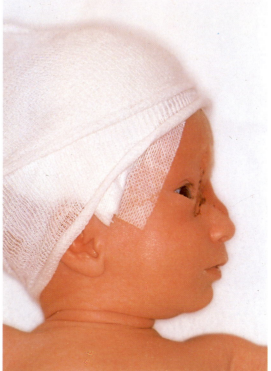

7.42

Cranial Meningocele

Cranial meningocele in a 3-day-old newborn. In cranial meningocele, there is herniation of meninges through a skull defect. The fluid-filled mass transilluminated in a uniform fashion. Surgical correction was undertaken, and there were no neurologic sequelae.

Cranial meningocele (and meningoencephaloceles) associated with cranial defects usually occur in the occipital area. They are frequently associated with underlying problems of the ventricular system such as hydrocephalus.

7.43

Meningoencephalocele

Occipital meningoencephalocele in a newborn infant. The infant had a large cranial defect in the occipital area and multiple other anomalies (ventriculoseptal defect, coarctation of the aorta, hydronephrosis). No operation was attempted, and the child died at 24 days of age due to increased intracranial pressure. In addition to the large meningoenceph-

alocele, postmortem examination revealed obstructive hydrocephalus, cerebellar aplasia, microgyri, and gliosis.

An encephalocele involves herniation of the brain through a skull defect and may be accompanied by other cerebral malformations or hydrocephalus.

7.44

Teratocarcinoma

Malignant teratocarcinoma in a 6-month-old girl. At birth, a plum-sized, doughy tumor at the upper end of the anal cleft was noted. There were no neurologic symptoms. On palpation of the abdomen, no masses were appreciated. At surgery, a cystic teratocarcinoma that extended to the spinal column and into the abdominal cavity was removed. Although there were no immediate postoperative complications, 1 month after the operation, a grapefruit-sized tumor was discovered in the child's pelvis. The mass could be palpated in the lower abdomen. It displaced both ureters laterally and shifted the rectosigmoid colon forward. Laparotomy revealed that this was part of the original teratocarci-

noma, which had penetrated the pelvis. After the second operation, radiation therapy and chemotherapy were given.

Germ cell tumors, such as teratocarcinoma, can occur in the gonads, central nervous system, sacrococcygeal area, retroperitoneum, and mediastinum. The mass may cause obstruction of either the genitourinary or the gastrointestinal system.

Differential Diagnosis—Similar sacrococcygeal masses may occur in cases of lipoma or meningomyelocele. Hemangiomas and neurogenic tumors must also be considered.

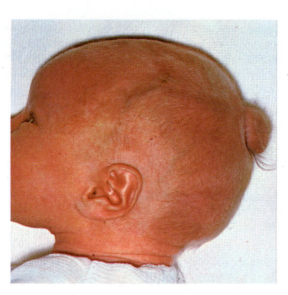

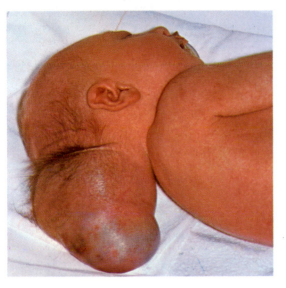

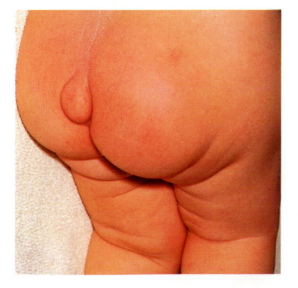

7.45

Gingival Hypertrophy

A 12-year-old girl with gingival hypertrophy caused by taking diphenylhydantoin for a seizure disorder. Hypertrophy may be so severe as to cover the crowns of the teeth. Because of gingival hypertrophy, the mouth is more susceptible to trauma, and poor oral hygiene may lead to increased inflammation.

Differential Diagnosis—Idiopathic gingival hyperplasia may occur and can lead to thickening of the lips and anomalies of tooth placement. Patients with idiopathic gingival hyperplasia may also suffer from mental deficiency and hypertrichosis.

7.46

Acrodynia

Acrodynia (Feer's disease) in a 3-year-old girl. Findings included redness and swelling of the gums with increased salivation. The red tips of the fingers and toes, extreme pruritis, and pain in the hands and feet are characteristic of acrodynia. Detailed medical history revealed the presence of chronic mercury poisoning.

7.47

Hypertrichosis

Hypertrichosis in a 12-year-old boy who had been treated with diphenylhydantoin for a seizure disorder. An excess of body hair was first noted on the extensor surface of the arms and later noted on the torso and face. Therapy with diphenylhydantoin is also associated with gingival hypertrophy.

Hypertrichosis is caused by many medications, including prolonged therapy with corticosteroids, diazoxides, androgens, and other anabolic agents. While hypertrichosis caused by many medications may disappear 6 to 12 months after cessation of therapy, the hirsutism seen with androgens or anabolic steroids is usually irreversible. Specific syndromes may also be associated with hypertrichosis, including Brachman-de Lange syndrome, craniofacial dysostosis, trisomy 18, and Bloom syndrome.

7.48

Cushing Syndrome

Cushing syndrome in a 1½-year-old boy who had been treated with dexamethasone for infantile myoclonic seizures. Findings included "full moon" face, obesity, and hypertrichosis. Glucose intolerance also occurred due to steroid treatment. Later, use of clonazepam (Clonopin) for control of the seizures proved effective and Cushing syndrome disappeared with the cessation of dexamethasone therapy.

7.45

7.46

7.47   7.48

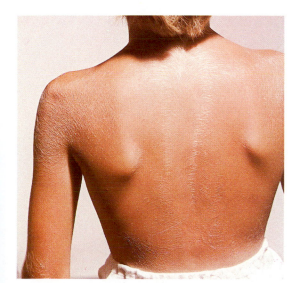

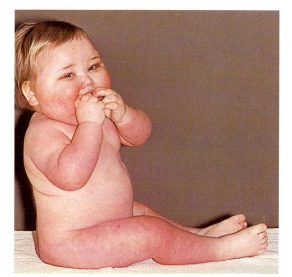

7.49

Kearns-Sayre Syndrome

Kearns-Sayre syndrome in a 16-year-old girl. The physical findings included ptosis and bilateral ophthalmoplegia. The disorder started 2 years earlier and increased steadily in severity. The mother and older sister had similar symptoms. The girl also had atypical pigmentary degeneration of the retina and a cardiac conduction disorder (right bundle branch block). The symptoms were due to a primary progressive degenerative dystrophy of the extraocular muscles. The etiology and pathogenesis of this disorder is unclear. It has been postulated that this may be due to a disorder of mitochondrial DNA.

7.50

Central Facial Nerve Palsy

Central facial nerve palsy in an 11-year-old boy. The nasolabial fold on the paralyzed right side was flattened. The boy could not whistle. Both eyes could be closed tight and the forehead was smooth on both sides. Possible causes for central facial nerve palsy include brain tumors, brain trauma, encephalitis, Guillaume-Barre syndrome, and mastoiditis. Idiopathic facial nerve palsy is known as Bell's palsy.

7.51

Möbius Syndrome

Möbius syndrome in a 2-month-old boy. When the child looked to the right, the right eye could not be abducted (abducens paralysis). The child displayed little facial movement associated with crying and was noted to have ptosis of the right eye (facial paralysis). The disorder was present since birth.

Möbius syndrome is a congenital, nonprogressive failure of several cranial nerves, especially the sixth (abducens) and seventh (facial) cranial nerves. The syndrome is due to agenesis or early atrophy of the cranial nerve nuclei and their nerves. The oculomotor, glossopharyngeal, hypoglossal, and accessory nerves may also be involved.

7.52

Strabismus

Strabismus in a 3-year-old boy. The squint angle is about 15 degrees in relation to the cornea. The impression of strabismus was accentuated by the low nasal bridge and wide separation of the eyes. The right eye was used exclusively for fixation, leaving the left eye likely to develop amblyopia.

7.53a and 7.53b

Congenital Palsy of the Superior Oblique Muscle

Congenital palsy of the superior oblique muscle in a 3-year-old girl. Findings included the typical compensatory head tilt (the head inclined toward the right shoulder and the child avoided looking downward and toward the right) (Figure 7.53a). In the Bielschowsky head tilting test, the affected eye looked upward (Figure 7.53b).

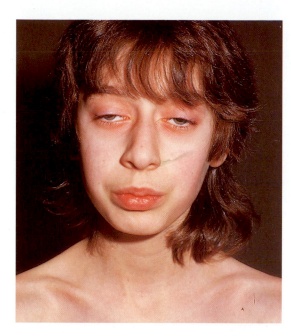
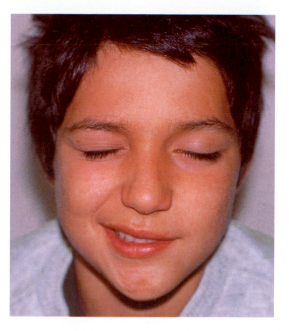

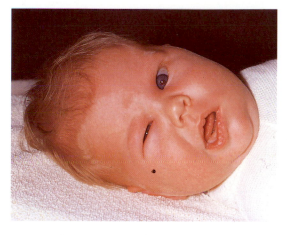
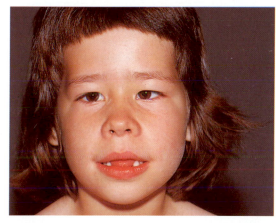

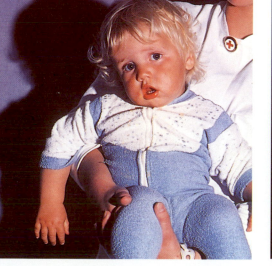
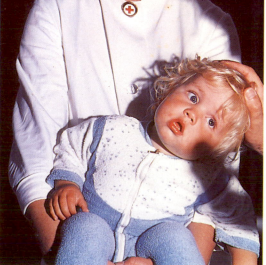

7.54

Progressive Spinal Muscle Atrophy

Progressive spinal muscle atrophy (Werdnig-Hoffman disease) in a 4-month-old girl. In an attempt to pull to sitting position (traction attempt), the arms were fully extended and the head immediately fell backward. The child had had severe muscular hypotonia and respiratory difficulty since birth. The diagnosis was confirmed by muscle biopsy. The disease progressed rapidly, and the child died at 11 months of age.

7.55

Progressive Neuropathic Muscular Atrophy

Progressive neuropathic muscular atrophy in a 15-year-old girl. The findings included high arched feet (pes cavus) with hammer toes due to symmetrical atrophy of the extensor and abductor muscles of the feet. Atrophy of the muscles below the middle third of the thigh was also noted, giving the patient a "stork leg" appearance. Typical steppage gait was noted. Achilles tendon reflex and patellar tendon reflex could not be elicited. Motor and sensory nerve conduction velocity of the peroneal nerve was decreased. Electromyogram and muscle biopsy were typical for neurogenic atrophy. The disorder has a dominant pattern of inheritance; both the mother and maternal grandfather were affected.

Differential Diagnosis—The differential diagnosis of concave foot with hammer toes includes hereditary Friedreich's ataxia (progressive cerebellar and spinal cord dysfunction) in which a combination of ataxia, corticospinal tract dysfunction (with a positive Babinski sign), and absent deep tendon reflexes are noted. Other neurogenic myopathies such as Roussy-Levy syndrome can also lead to pes cavus. Pes cavus is usually a manifestation of underlying neuromuscular disease.

7.56

Rett Syndrome

Rett syndrome in a 16-year-old girl who demonstrates characteristic handwashing motions. The neurologic symptoms began during the second year of life including delay in psychomotor development, dementia with autistic behavior, ataxia, loss of purposeful hand motions, and bizarre, stereotypic movements with rhythmic kneading and pressing of the fingers. The girl demonstrated periods of hyperventilation with expiratory moans and grimacing typical of Rett syndrome.

7.54

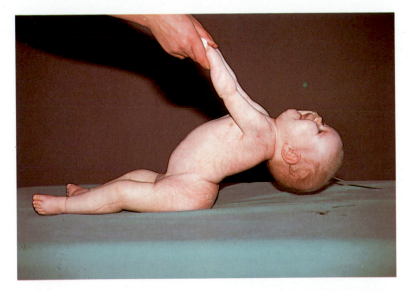

7.55

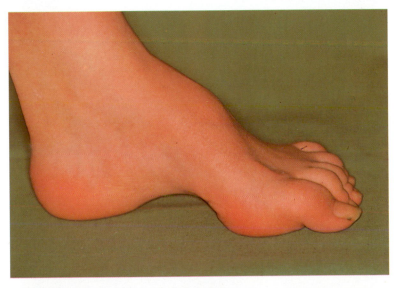

7.56

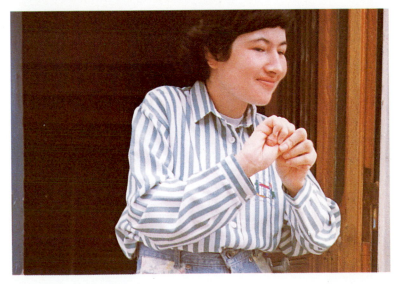

8.1—8.3

Dermatomyositis

A 9-year-old girl with dermatomyositis. The symptoms included skin findings and muscular pain and weakness. The face had a butterfly-shaped erythema over the malar area and a lilac coloring of the upper eyelids. Gingival and nasal mucous membranes were also reddened. Over the arms and legs there was thickening of the skin resembling scleroderma, nonpitting edema, and a maculopapular rash. Scaly erythematous areas with atrophy were noted over the extensor surfaces of the knee, elbow, and finger joints; later, these areas were noted to be hyperpigmented. Extension at both elbow joints was restricted. Evidence of myositis was seen in the painful response to palpation of the muscles, diminished strength (making standing impossible), areflexia, and typical findings on electromyography. Laboratory investigation revealed elevated serum levels of creatine kinase, transaminase, and aldolase. A dermal muscle biopsy confirmed the diagnosis of dermatomyositis. The child rapidly improved after starting prednisone therapy, but recovery (disappearance of muscle weakness and skin changes) occurred only after several months of treatment.

Differential Diagnosis—During the chronic stage, with the absence of any visible skin findings, dermatomyositis may be difficult to distinguish from other muscular diseases (poliomyelitis, viral myositis, muscular dystrophy, myasthenia gravis). Differentiation can be made through electromyography, enzyme analysis, muscle biopsy, or the presence or absence of specific neurologic symptoms.

Since arthritis or arthralgia may be associated with dermatomyositis, dermatomyositis must be differentiated from juvenile rheumatoid arthritis and mixed connective tissue disease. The butterfly-shaped erythema of the face is also seen in systemic lupus erythematosus. Hardening of the skin and structures under the skin may occur in scleroderma.

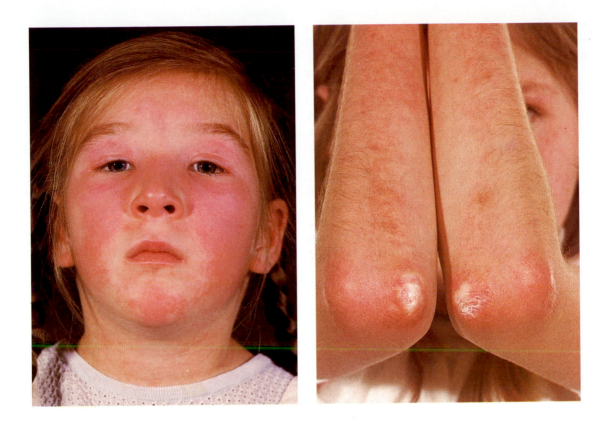

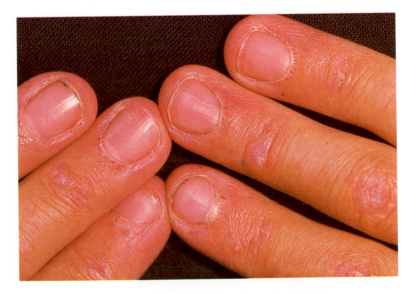

8.4
Juvenile Rheumatoid Arthritis

Juvenile rheumatoid arthritis (polyarticular form) in a 9-year-old girl. Findings included painful swelling with restricted movement of the metacarpal phalangeal joints and the metatarsal phalangeal joints. The right knee joint was also involved. Despite treatment with acetylsalicylic acid (aspirin) there was chronic progression of the disease with bouts of fever, leukocytosis, and worsening arthritis. Treatment with indomethacin, prednisone, and chloroquine was required. Aggressive treatment was able to control the symptoms. There was no other organ involvement (as there is in Still's disease) and no iridocyclitis was noted. There are several clinical subgroups of juvenile rheumatoid arthritis. This girl apparently suffered from polyarticular disease, in which there is multiple joint involvement. The onset of polyarticular juvenile rheumatoid arthritis is frequently late in childhood. Serum rheumatoid factor and antinuclear antobidies are frequently positive. Polyarticular juvenile rheumatoid arthritis is associated with HLA type DR4. The long-term outcome of children with polyarticular disease is poor (with severe arthritic disease).

Differential Diagnosis—The early stages of rheumatoid arthritis must be distinguished from other causes of acute arthritis, including osteomyelitis, vital infection, sepsis, and gonorrhea. Tuberculous joint disease, gout, leukemia, trauma, and aseptic necrosis must all be considered. In rheumatic fever, the arthralgia and arthritis may be migratory, and endocarditis may occur. Systemic lupus erythematosus may exhibit very similar arthritic symptoms and must be differentiated by means of other clinical findings. Ankylosing spondylitis is rare in childhood, but can follow juvenile rheumatoid arthritis of the pauciarticular type. Patients with ankylosing spondylitis have more frequently type HLA-tB27 (noted in 90% of patients with ankylosing spondylitis, but in only 5% to 7% of the general population).

8.5
Juvenile Rheumatoid Arthritis

Juvenile rheumatoid arthritis (polyarticular form) in a 16-year-old girl. The interphalangeal joints of both hands were thickened. Finger movement was painful and greatly restricted. No erythema was noted. Pain and stiffness were present in both hip joints. Symptoms were first noted at the age of 12 years and gradually progressed. Rheumatoid factor and antinuclear antibodies were positive. Radiographs demonstrated periosteal bone degeneration in the phalanges. There was no iridocyclitis or involvement of other organ systems. Symptomatic treatment led to improvement, but recurrence was frequent.

Children with rheumatoid factor-negative polyarticular juvenile rheumatoid arthritis appear to have a less severe course when compared to rheumatoid factor-positive children.

8.6   8.7
Osteomyelitis

Acute hematogenic osteomyelitis in a 6-week-old infant. The findings included swelling and restricted movement in the area of the left shoulder joint and both knee joints. The left leg was maintained in an adducted position. The infant was febrile and had hepatosplenomegaly. Cultures from both the blood and joint aspirate revealed *Staphylococcus aureus*. Characteristic radiographic findings of osteomyelitis (periosteal elevation in the metaphyseal area) were seen in the left proximal femur, in both distal femurs, and in the left proximal humerus. The child was successfully treated with antibiotic therapy.

Differential Diagnosis—In older children, the differential diagnosis of joint swelling includes rheumatic fever (pain and swelling in several joints, carditis), leukemia, Ewing sarcoma, metastatic tumors (such as neuroblastoma), and scurvy. With chronic osteomyelitis of uncertain etiology, tuberculosis, syphilis, brucellosis, actinomycosis, and other systemic mycoses must be considered.

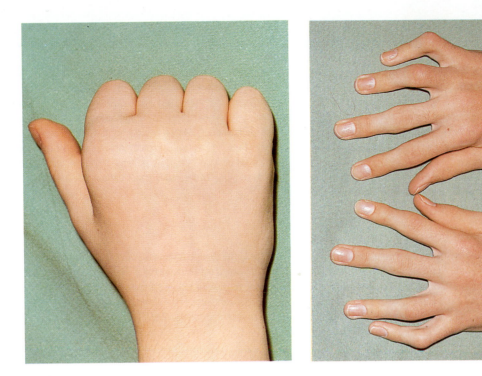

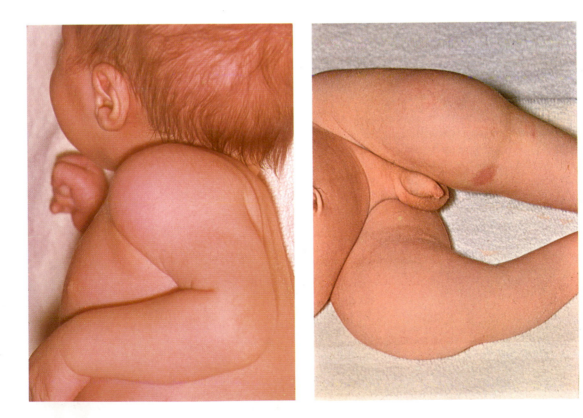

8.8 Juvenile Rheumatoid Arthritis

Arthritic involvement of the right knee in a 10-year-old girl. Of note was the painful, nonerythematous swelling of the right knee with restricted movement. Initially, a high fever lasted for 1 week. The probable diagnosis was juvenile rheumatoid arthritis (pauciarticular form). Pauciarticular juvenile rheumatoid arthritis usually affects one or more of the larger joints. Antinuclear antibodies are positive in most of these cases. Rheumatoid factor is usually negative. The diagnosis was confirmed by aspiration of joint fluid and synovial biopsy during an acute episode.

Differential Diagnosis—Acute septic monoarthritis must be considered. Causative agents include *Haemophilus in-fluenzae, Neisseria gonorrhoeae, Salmonella,* and *Brucella.* Other causes of more persistent monoarthritis of infectious etiology may include tuberculosis or congenital syphilis. Noninfectious causes for swelling of the knee include synovial chondromatosis and pigmented villonodular synovitis. Characteristic of pigmented villonodular synovitis is proliferation of the synovial membrane and hemosiderin impregnation. Joint aspirate usually reveals pigmented or serosanguinous fluid. Fibromas, hemangiomas, xanthomas, and sarcomas may also originate in the synovial membrane and cause swelling of the joints under certain circumstances.

8.9 Juvenile Rheumatoid Arthritis

Juvenile rheumatoid arthritis (systemic onset or Still's disease) in a 5-year-old boy. Systemic juvenile rheumatoid arthritis may have prominent extraarticular manifestations. The findings included a red evanescent macular rash on the face, torso, and extremities. The child had frequent bouts of fever and arthralgia (especially of the hands, fingers, and knees) without arthritis or lymphadenopathy. The child had pleuritis but no symptoms of pericarditis. Initially, the acute febrile episode responded well to prednisone therapy; however, due to several relapses over a 12-year period, the child was also treated with D-penicillamine.

8.10 Erythema Marginatum

A 12-year-old boy with rheumatic fever (presenting with chorea and rheumatic carditis). Erythema marginatum, the characteristic skin rash of rheumatic fever, was noted. The typical numerous bright red macules (rings or stripes) were seen over the back and abdomen. The appearance of the rash varied day by day, and after 2 days the rash was no longer detected. Gradual improvement of the chorea and carditis followed treatment with acetylsalicylic acid (aspirin) and prednisone.

Erythema marginatum may occur in 5% to 10% of children with rheumatic fever (especially when there are cardiac findings). It is not pathognomonic. The rash is evanescent and may come and go during the several weeks the child is affected.

Differential Diagnosis—See erythema annulare centrifigum (page 170 and 266).

8.11 Arthrogryposis

A 3-month-old boy with arthrogryposis. Congenital joint contractures were noted at birth, involving both the large and small joints. Other findings included muscular hypoplasia, generalized thickening and dimpling of the skin, hip subluxation, bilateral talipes equinovarus, opisthotonic posture, and scoliosis of the spine. Treatment included physical therapy, casting, and orthopedic surgery.

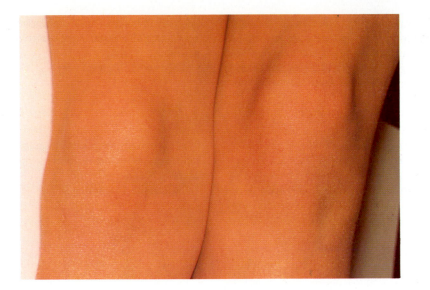

8.8

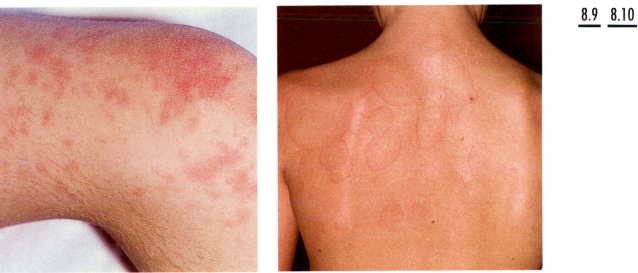

8.9 8.10

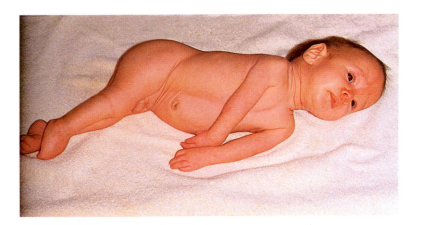

8.11

8.12

Systemic Lupus Erythematosus

Systemic lupus erythematosus in a 6-year-old boy. Findings included a butterfly-shaped, nonpruritic, scaly, erythematous rash involving the cheeks and the bridge of the nose. Hypersensitivity to sunlight which can lead to blistering occurs in approximately one-third of the cases. Cutaneous facial symptoms of systemic lupus erythematosus include discoid lupus, nonpruritic urticaria, and changes similar to erythema multi forme.

Differential Diagnosis—See pages 154, 170, 272.

8.13

Systemic Lupus Erythematosus

Systemic lupus erythematosus in a 7-year-old girl. Findings included several irregular ulcerations of the mucous membranes that were covered with a white pseudomembrane. Other cutaneous symptoms and evidence of systemic disease led to the diagnosis. About 25% of all patients with systemic lupus erythematosus experience changes in the mucous membranes (especially the palate, inner cheek, or gum). In the early stages, erythematous lesions may evolve into painful ulcers.

Differential Diagnosis—Similar findings may be seen in ulcerative stomatitis (page 246).

8.14

Erythema Nodosum

Erythema nodosum in a 10-year-old boy. Findings included painful indurated nodules over both legs and arthritis of the knee. Numerous round and elliptical nodules of varying sizes were found over the shins of both legs. These nodules were raised above the skin surface and felt hot and painful when touched. The overlying skin was taut and glistening. At first, the skin overlying the nodules was a bright red; later, the skin developed a blue-red discoloration. The underlying cause of erythema nodosum was an infection with *Yersinia pseudotuberculosis* (serum antibody titer: 1:5,000). Within 3 weeks of appropriate antibiotic therapy, the lesions resolved without scar formation, leaving behind a brown discoloration. Erythema nodosum may also be seen in rheumatoid arthritis, sarcoidosis, ulcerative colitis, systemic lupus erythematosus, and allergic drug reactions.

Differential Diagnosis—Erythema nodosum must be differentiated from erythema induratum, polyarteritis nodosa, Weber-Christian syndrome (nodular paniculitis), subcutaneous fat necrosis, thrombophlebitis, and fungal infection.

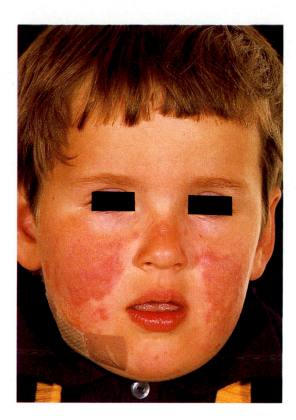

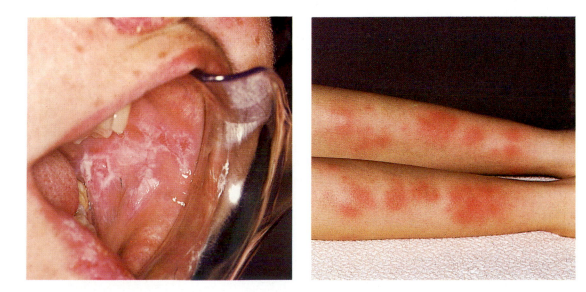

8.15

Scheuermann's Disease

Scheuermann's disease (juvenile kyphoscoliosis) in a 14-year-old boy. Findings included excessive, uncompensated deep kyphosis of the thoracic spine and compensated excessive lordosis of the lumbar spine. The boy complained of dull back pain after exertion. In the area of the thoracic spine, radiographs revealed irregularities of the endplates, wedge-shaped vertebral formation, Schmorl nodes (recesses in the vertebral body), and separation of the epiphyseal areas from the anterior vertebral margin. The boy improved after physical therapy and swimming.

8.16

Scoliosis

Scoliosis (persistent lateral curvature of the spine) in a 15-year-old girl with excessive fixed lateral bending of the spine (thoracic right convex). The trunk projected to the right. On the left side, the triangle formed by the contour of the chest, pelvis, and hanging arm, was lower than that on the right. There was a thoracolumbar bulge in the dorsal profile due to contorsion of the vertebral bodies.

Milder scoliosis is usually discovered during the prepubertal accelerated growth phase. Numerous causes are possible including neuromuscular disease, connective tissue disorders, injury, inflammation, and tumor. Milder scoliosis may be treated with physical therapy; severe scoliosis requires surgery.

8.17

Genu Valgum

Genu valgum (knock-knees) in a 6-year-old boy. Both legs were angulated outward (with a reduced external angle between the thigh and lower leg) and bilateral talipes valgus was noted. The inner malleolar distance was 12 cm. Both knee joints were hyperextended.

Genu valgum noted at 2 to 6 years of age is frequently physiologic. However, unilateral genu valgum is always pathologic (e.g., result of an injury). Bilateral genu valgum can occur in systemic diseases affecting the skeleton, in endocrine disorders, and as a congenital malformation. A familial pattern of inheritance has been noted.

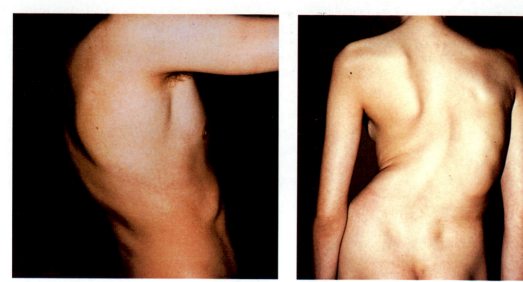

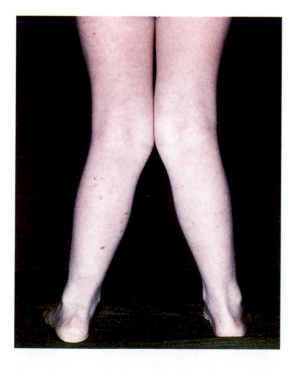

8.18

Patellar Subluxation

Patellar subluxation in a 12-year-old girl. Lateral dislocation of the left patella was noted. Extension of the knee joint was greatly restricted. Subluxations occur at the start of flexion from the extended position. Spontaneous repositioning of the patella is possible. If the dislocation persists, fixation of the knee joints in a slightly flexed or knock-knee position is typical. Knee-joint effusion is common. Recurrent subluxation of the patella (slipping patella) occurs due to weak ligaments, paralysis, or flattening of the condyles; traumatic patellar subluxation arises through direct trauma.

8.19

Cleft Foot

Cleft foot before and after surgical correction (at the age of 1 to 1½ years). The cleft formed due to inadequate development of the middle digital rays with partial fusion of the lateral digital rays. Radiographs demonstrated displacement of the metatarsal and tarsal bones in addition to absence of the central ray portions. Walking and standing were not affected. A normal shoe could be worn after surgical correction.

8.20

Flatfoot

Flatfoot (pes planus) in a 9-year-old boy with cerebral palsy. Findings included total absence of the longitudinal vault of the foot, step position of the talus, heel in valgus, and abduction of the forefoot. The talus head was palpable under the protruding plantar skin, adhered firmly to the subcutaneous tissue and was covered with callus.

Flatfoot occurs in isolation or is associated with arthrogryposis, cerebral palsy, neurofibromatosis, trisomy 13 or 18 (rockerbottom feet). Flexible flatfeet may be surgically corrected; in severe cases the defective position is not correctable.

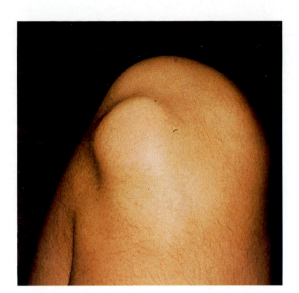

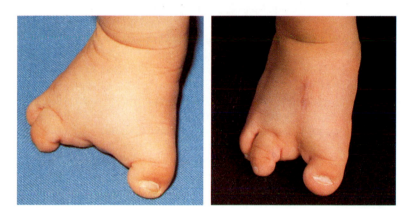

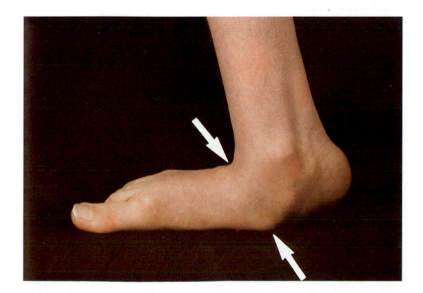

9.1

Scleroderma

Morphea (localized scleroderma) in an 8-year-old girl. The skin was first noted to have indurated, erythematous lesions on the flexor surface of the right leg and on the back. These foci later faded centrally and appeared violet in color at the margins. After several weeks, the lesions became indurated and waxy in appearance. Scarring and fibrosis occurred, causing the lesions to be firmly adhered to the underlying tissue. The lesions gradually resolved over an eight month period without therapy.

Scleroderma is chronic inflammatory disturbance of the connective tissue. Isolated cutaneous involvement, as seen in this case, is referred to as morphea.

Differential Diagnosis—Skin changes resembling scleroderma frequently occur after bone marrow transplant (chronic graft-versus-host disease). Atrophic plaques resembling morphea can also be seen following injections of corticosteroids. In cases of scleredema adultorum, localized nonerythematous, nonpitting induration of the skin occurs, which may limit mobility. Scleredema adultorum, which is rare in childhood, develops suddenly 1 to 6 weeks after an acute streptococcal infection. The lesions appear on the face, neck, back, and later on the arms and thorax. The condition is self-limited and resolves within months or years. No effective treatment is known.

9.2

Scleroderma

Morphea (frontoparietal scleroderma, *en coup de sabre*) on the left side of the forehead of a 17-year-old girl. The lesion was an elongated, indurated, hyperpigmented area of skin 1–2 cm wide which extended from the forehead to the parietal area. Where the scalp was affected, there was alopecia. There were no other lesions. Hemiatrophy of the face, which

frequently occurs, was absent in this case. The ESR was normal. In other cases of morphea, similar frontoparietal lesions with an ivory colored, hardened plaque and hyperpigmented borders may occur. Usually, there are no other lesions. Treatment is difficult; however, spontaneous regression of scleroderma is possible.

9.3

Scleroderma

Progressive scleroderma in a 16-year-old girl. For 3 years, she experienced increasing pain and swelling of the fingers. When her hand was closed in a fist, the skin over the swollen fingers was taut and shiny. In addition, the skin over the hands and the knees was hardened, causing restricted movement. A 2-cm-long hardened area of skin was noted on the left side of the neck. The girl complained of coldness, paresthesia, and acrocyanosis of the hands (Raynaud's phenomenon). No involvement of the gastrointestinal tract, the heart, the lungs,

or the kidneys was noted. As is typical in scleroderma, the ESR was only slightly elevated, and the serum rheumatoid factor was positive. Antinuclear antibodies could not be detected.

Differential Diagnosis—Scleroderma must be differentiated from disseminated morphea (which does not affect the internal organs). Scleroderma may be differentiated from dermatomyositis by the lack of muscle involvement.

9.4

Raynaud's Disease

Raynaud's disease in an 11-year-old girl. Findings included episodic symmetrical blanching, cyanosis, and reddening of the fingers and toes associated with paresthesia and pain. The symptoms disappeared after a short time but recurred frequently. Peripheral pulses were palpable. Doppler sonog-

raphy demonstrated poor perfusion of the hands and feet which decreased further with cooling. Diseases associated with Raynaud's disease (systemic lupus erythematosus, rheumatoid arthritis, scleroderma, diabetes mellitus) were excluded.

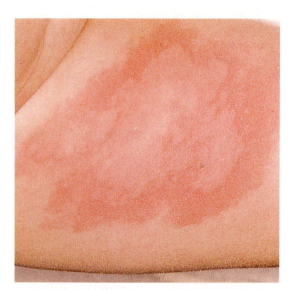

9.1

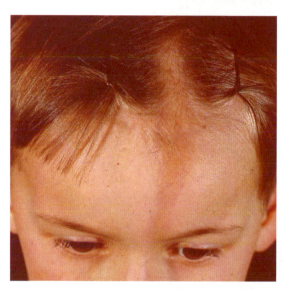
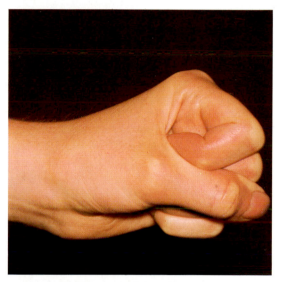

9.2 9.3

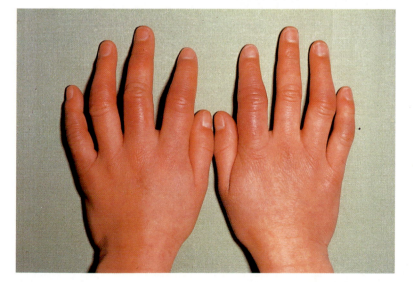

9.4

9.5

Erythema Multiforme

Erythema multiforme (Stevens-Johnson syndrome) in a 12-year-old boy. Two weeks after antibiotic treatment for bronchopneumonia, the child developed a nonpruritic generalized exanthem. The rash was characterized by circular lesions, 1–2 cm in diameter on the arms and legs; the lesions had a sunken, blue discolored center with a bright red raised border. Some of the lesions developed central vesiculation. The rash rapidly responded to 4 days of prednisone treatment. As is the case with the majority of children with erythema multiforme, the underlying cause was not determined. Erythema multiforme is associated with viral infections (herpes simplex), bacterial infections (*Mycoplasma*), and certain medications (sulfonamide, anticonvulsants, penicillin, barbiturates). In approximately 40% of the cases, the oral mucous membranes are affected (Stevens-Johnson syndrome, page 172). The characteristic skin rash usually presents no difficulty regarding differential diagnosis.

9.6

Scarlatiniform Exanthem

Scarlatiniform exanthem in a 12-year-old boy. The child was treated with carbamazepine (Tegretol) for a seizure disorder. Three weeks after therapy was initiated, the child became febrile, and a generalized skin rash was noted. The rash was slightly pruritic and consisted of dense red papules the size of a pinhead. The mucous membranes were not affected. There was no arthritis, lymphadenopathy, or hepatosplenomegaly. After discontinuing the anticonvulsant medication, the exanthem disappeared, and the child's fever abated.

Other known allergic side effects of carbamazepine include maculopapular and urticarial exanthem, edema, and agranulocytosis.

9.7

Urticaria

Urticaria in a 3-year-old boy. The rash is characterized by pruritic, erythematous, raised skin lesions (approximately the size of a penny) that appeared suddenly over the entire body. The rash may be accompanied by facial edema. Fever is not associated with the rash.

The cause of urticaria is frequently unknown. Individual lesions may resolve quickly (within two days) but new lesions may appear later. The diagnosis of urticaria is generally simple; however, sometimes it is difficult to differentiate urticarial lesions from erythema multiforme or anaphylactoid purpura.

9.8 9.9

Urticaria

Generalized urticaria in a 5-year-old boy. The rash appeared every time the child ate fish. The rash was characterized by pruritic wheals with a white, edematous center surrounded by an erythematous base. Lesions were found on the face and over the body. Some of the lesions formed ring- and garland-shaped patterns. Along with the urticarial rash, the child developed subglottic edema, which responded rapidly to intravenous corticosteroids.

There are many forms of urticaria in childhood. Papular urticaria appear in small children at the site of insect bites. The lesions have a papular center on an urticarial base, often with a small blister in the center. These pruritic lesions are arranged in groups and are usually located on the exposed parts of the extremities. Other forms of urticaria included cholinergic urticaria. Cholinergic urticaria are brought on by exertion, heat, and emotional stress. The rash is characterized by small wheals or papules, 2–3 mm in diameter, surrounded by a 2- to 3-mm-wide erythematous base. The lesions are nonpruritic and develop on the torso, upper arms, and upper legs. They may disappear in minutes or after 1–2 hours. Severe outbreaks of cholanergic urticaria may be accompanied by systemic cholinergic symptoms (sweating, salivation, abdominal pain, diarrhea).

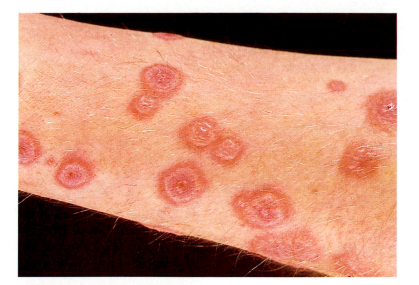

9.5

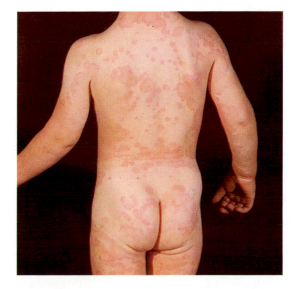

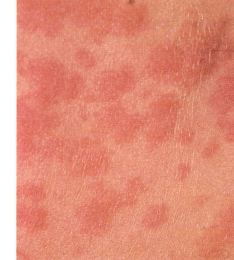

9.6   9.7

9.8   9.9

9.10

Erythema Multiforme

Erythema multiforme in an 8-year-old boy. The findings included dark erythematous nonpruritic papules on the face and torso, which became partially confluent. Characteristic central clearing (iris or target lesions) may occur. Mucosal involvement is common.

The term "multiforme" is used to describe these skin lesions because the rash may manifest in various ways (either as erythematous macules or papules) or as vesiculobullous lesions). In contrast to urticaria, there is no itching, the course of the disease is longer, and relapses may occur more frequently.

9.11

Erythema Annulare Centrifugum (Darier)

Erythema annulare centrifugum on the chest of a 1-year-old boy. Numerous nonpruritic erythematous garland-shaped lesions were noted on the torso and extremities. The center of the lesions may be a pale red with an erythematous border. The lesions may spread centrifugally and remain for several weeks. The exact cause is unknown.

Characteristic of erythema annulare centrifugum is the chronic progressive nature of the rash and the development of ring-shaped lesions from the small red papules. The edge of the lesions may be flat or slightly raised and may be slightly scaly.

Differential Diagnosis—Differential diagnosis of erythema annularre centrifugum includes tineal infections, granuloma annulare, and systemic lupus erythematosus.

9.12 9.13

Erythema Multiforme

Erythema multiforme on the arm of a 6-year-old boy. The multiple erythematous lesions coalesced giving the rash a garland-shaped appearance. Characteristic target lesions were seen on the arms and legs (erythematous macules with a light red border and sunken dusky center). The rash was symmetrically arranged in a garland-shaped pattern on the extensor surfaces of the extremities. At the time the rash appeared the child was febrile. Pneumonia was detected by chest radiograph. The rash appeared in bursts over several days and disappeared after 2 weeks.

Differential Diagnosis—Erythema multiforme must be differentiated from other erythematous rashes including the rashes associated with porphyria, systemic lupus erythematosus, and Kawasaki disease (page 174).

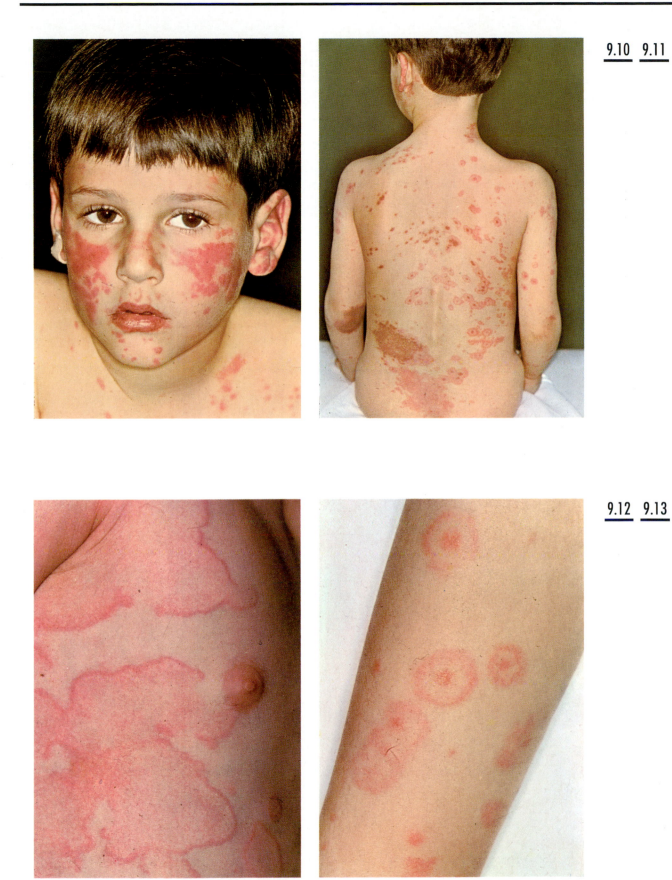

9.14

Stevens-Johnson Syndrome

Butterfly-shaped, erythematous malar rash with hemorrhagic exudative vesicular inflammation of the oral mucosa, nasal mucosa, and conjunctiva in a 9-year-old boy. Stomatitis was present and led to an inability to feed. A generalized maculopapular and bullous rash was noted over the body. Due to the stomatitis, the child had to be fed parenterally. Systemic corticosteroid treatment and local treatment of the mucous membrane lesions were successful in treating this illness. The rash resolved after 1 week with no evidence of scarring.

9.15

Stevens-Johnson Syndrome

Stevens-Johnson syndrome in a 3-year-old boy. Findings included inflammation of the urethra and the foreskin, with swelling and purulent drainage. The child had pain on urination. In addition, the child had a high fever and developed a rash compatible with erythema multiforme exudativum (maculopapular lesions with partial vesiculation and hemorrhage). A bullous eruption was noted over the mouth, anus, and the eyes. Stevens-Johnson syndrome was secondary to the administration of barbiturates 10 days previously. The child recovered after 2 weeks.

9.16

Stevens-Johnson Syndrome

Stevens-Johnson syndrome in a 3½-year-old boy. Findings included redness and swelling of the skin around the anus without vesicle formation. By contrast, large vesicles, which ulcerated and were covered with a hemorrhagic crust, were found around the mouth. Other mucous membrane and skin changes were characteristic of Stevens-Johnson syndrome. The patient responded to oral prednisone and symptomatic therapy.

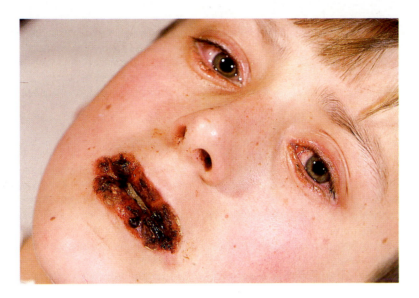

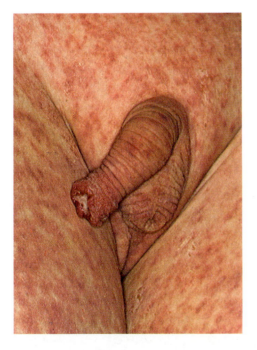

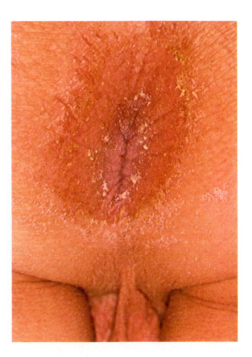

9.17

Acrodynia

Acrodynia (Feer's disease) in a 3½-year-old girl. The child had absorbed abnormally high levels of mercury because of exposure to a topical ointment containing mercury. Symptoms included redness and swelling of the hands (pink disease), and scaling of the fingers associated with acute pain (acrodynia). Similar skin changes were noted on the feet. Muscular hypotonia (with diminished Achilles and patellar tendon reflexes), tachycardia, elevated blood pressure, increased perspiration, anorexia, behavioral changes (irritability), and insomnia were also noted. After the exclusion of other causes, mercury intoxication was diagnosed. The child was removed from the source of mercury poisoning and gradually improved with symptomatic treatment.

9.18–9.20a

Kawasaki Disease

Kawasaki disease (mucocutaneous lymph node syndrome) in a 9-year-old boy. The child developed high fever and signs of a systemic illness. Symptoms included a nonpurulent conjunctivitis, stomatitis (Figure 9.18), cherry-red lips, and painful cervical lymphadenopathy. The hands were edematous and swollen, and the fingertips were reddened and painful (Figure 9.19). After some improvement, desquamation, especially at the fingertips (Figure 9.20a) was noted. In addition, palmar erythema and uveitis (which occurs in 80% of all patients) were noted. The patient was treated with acetylsalicylic acid and intravenous gammaglobulin to prevent future development of coronary artery disease.

Differential Diagnosis—Strawberry tongue, erythematous exanthem, and desquamation are also found in scarlet fever. In toxic shock syndrome (due to toxin-producing strains of *Staphylococcus*) a generalized erythematous macular exanthem is typically followed by desquamation 1 to 2 weeks later (especially on the hands and feet). Stomatitis and many of the cutaneous findings seen in Kawasaki disease, may also be seen in Stevens-Johnson syndrome.

9.20b

Kawasaki Disease

Kawasaki disease in a 1½-year-old boy with cherry-red lips (cheilitis). The other symptoms and the characteristic clinical course supported the diagnosis of Kawasaki disease.

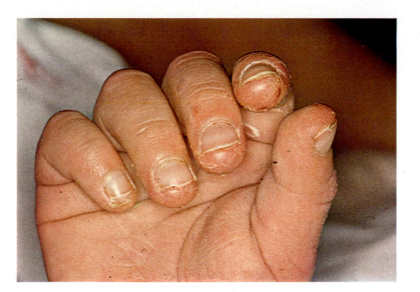

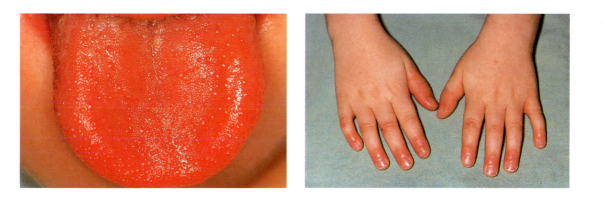

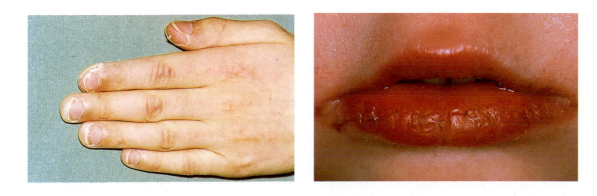

9.21

Granuloma Annulare

Granuloma annulare in a 16-year-old boy. Of note was an erythematous, firm, painless nodule, 1×2 cm in size, over the metacarpal phalangeal joint of the right hand. The characteristic features of granuloma annulare were demonstrated histologically (granuloma with central necrosis, mucin deposition, and peripheral infiltration of lymphocytes, histiocytes, and giant cells). In granuloma annulare, there is typically a ring of dense, small, firm, natural skin-colored, and light red papules found primarily on the extensor surface of the fingers, hands, arms, legs, and feet.

Differential Diagnosis—Granuloma annulare must be differentiated from necrobiosis lipoidica (frequently localized on the legs), rheumatoid nodules (often near joints) and sarcoidosis.

9.22

Granuloma Annulare

Granulaoma annulare in a 15-year-old boy. The rash has a ringlike appearance with a raised reddened border. In contrast to tinea corporis, there is no desquamation. After persistence for several months, the rash healed after local and systemic corticosteroid treatment.

9.23

Granuloma Annulare

Granuloma annulare in a 14-year-old girl. A large erythematous area of skin with a slightly atrophic center was noted on the dorsum of the foot. More typical of this lesion is a ring of erythematous papules around a sunken center. The cause of granuloma annulare is uncertain; its occurrence is relatively frequent, primarily in children. Generally, granuloma annulare causes no discomfort and disappears spontaneously after months or years without associated scarring.

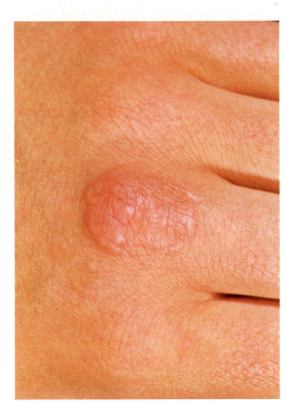

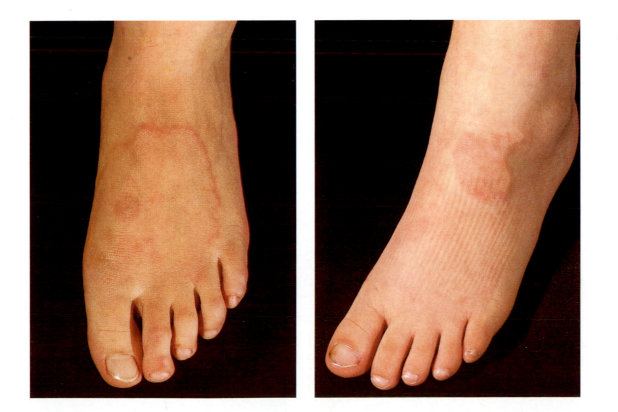

9.24 9.25

Seborrheic Dermatitis

Seborrheic dermatitis in a 3-month-old boy. Generalized scaling and yellow crusting of the scalp was noted. Round erythematous lesions converged to form larger honeycomb-like areas over the torso and extremities. The lesions on the trunk and extremities were scaly and erythematous. Seborrheic dermatitis is frequently found in the scalp, in the flexor surface of the joints, and in the anogenital area. The rash was nonpruritic. The rash began in the child's sixth week of life and resolved in the seventh month of life after various trials of symptomatic therapy.

Differential Diagnosis—Seborrheic dermatitis must be differentiated from a variety of other dermatologic conditions, including atopic dermatitis (page 182), contact dermatitis, diaper dermatitis (page 180), psoriasis (page 218), tinea versicolor (page 254), tinea capitus (page 254), tinea corporis (page 250), and pityriasis rosea (page 216).

9.26 9.27

Leiner's Disease

Leiner's disease in a 3-month-old boy. Of note is the generalized erythema and scaling of the skin. Children with Leiner's disease may have a disorder of the complement system. Complications include anemia, hyperproteinemia, persistent diarrhea, failure to thrive, and secondary bacterial infection. The dermatitis improved after 4 weeks of treatment.

Differential Diagnosis—The differential diagnosis includes other scaling dermatoses (seborrhea, ichthyosiform erythroderma, and *Candida* dermatitis).

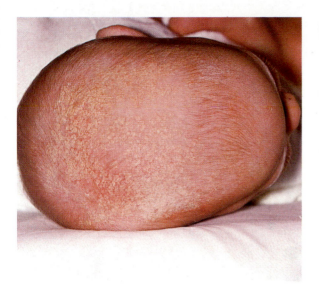

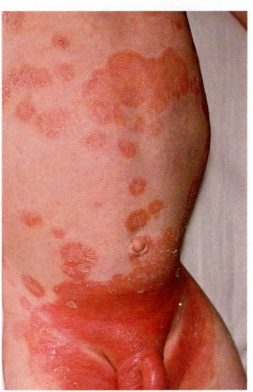

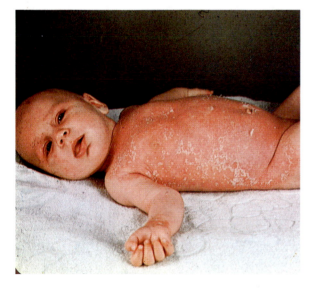

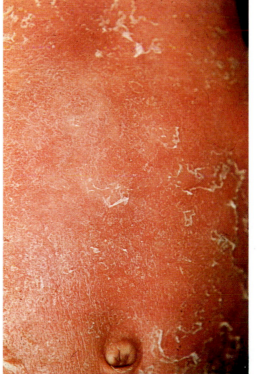

9.28

Candida Dermatitis

Candida dermatitis in an 8-year-old girl. The skin around the anogenital area (including the labia majora) was reddened, swollen, and slightly scaly. A potassium hydroxide (KOH) preparation revealed numerous microscopic *Candida* hyphae. Fungal cultures were also positive for *Candida albicans*.

Candida dermatitis has a predilection for the folds of the skin, the diaper area, the areas near orifices and the fingers (due to contact with saliva). The lesions have bright erythematous centers and irregular scaling edges. Satellite lesions may be found nearby.

9.29

Candida Dermatitis

Candida dermatitis in a 4-month-old boy. The skin of the anogenital area (including the foreskin) was erythematous and scaly with sharply defined erythematous borders. *Candida albicans* was identified in culture. The child originally had a seborrheic dermatitis that became secondarily infected with *Candida*. Treatment with nystatin-containing prepara-tions produced rapid improvement, but there were repeated occurrences. The rash completely resolved by 11 months of age. During one relapse, vesiculopustular lesions on an erythematous base were noted, which were also caused by *Candida albicans*.

9.30

"Pomatum" Crust

So-called "pomatum" crust (caused by the residue of oint-ment) on both sides of the groin in a 3-month-old girl.

9.31

Diaper Dermatitis

Diaper dermatitis in a 4-month-old boy. A well-defined, intensely red rash with fine scaling was found over the entire diaper area. Papules and vesicles on erythematous bases were initially present. The rash was chronic and progressive in nature. The cause of the dermatitis was maceration of the skin due to contact with urine and feces in the diaper. The rash responded well to topical treatment.

Seborrheic or atopic dermatitis may predispose to diaper dermatitis. Frequently, candidal or bacterial infections may occur as a secondary complication.

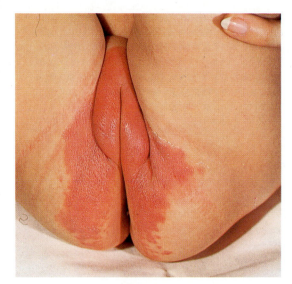
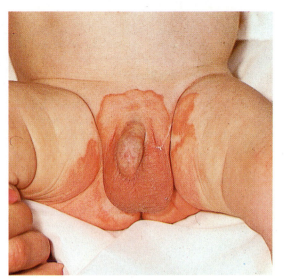

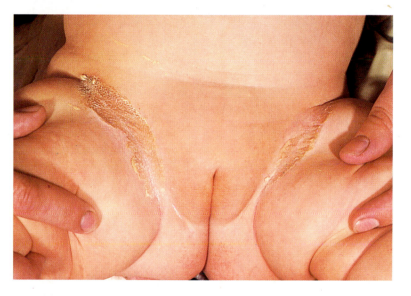

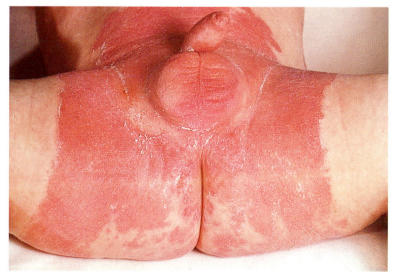

9.32

Atopic Dermatitis

Atopic dermatitis in a 12-year-old boy. Findings included lichenified dried skin with excoriations over the hands and arms (evidence of long-standing disease). During the first year, the skin changes were localized to the face and the extensor surfaces of the extremities and consisted of raised, confluent, pruritic, edematous papules that later formed crusted blisters. The course of the condition was chronic and progressive in nature with intermittent spontaneous remissions. The lichenified areas were treated with topical corticosteroid cream.

Atopic dermatitis during the first year of life frequently appears on the face, but may involve other areas as well. Later in childhood, atopic dermatitis may involve the extensor and flexor surfaces of the extremities. During the first year of life, edematous, erythematous papules which may be single or confluent predominate; later in childhood, thickening and lichenification is more common.

9.33

Atopic Dermatitis

Atopic dermatitis in a 13-year-old girl. Findings included numerous isolated or confluent papules on the face with excoriations due to scratching. Hypopigmented facial patches (pityriasis alba) were also noted. Similar areas of atopic dermatitis (some with lichenification and scaling) were present on the neck.

9.34

Atopic Dermatitis

Atopic dermatitis in a 10-year-old boy. Findings included lichenification of the skin and excoriation due to scratching. The prognosis for atopic dermatitis is relatively good.

Marked improvement occurs in half the patients by 14 years of age. Rarely does the disease extend beyond the age of 30. Family history is positive in 70% of the cases.

9.35

Atopic Dermatitis

Impetiginized atopic dermatitis in a 6-month-old boy. Findings include pruritic papules and blisters on the dorsal side of the hands and fingers, which were excoriated and became infected with staphylococci. Erythematous pruritic lesions with partial scaling and vesicle formation were also found on the arms, the scalp, and the torso. The child had other allergic manifestations including hayfever and bronchial asthma (seen in 30–50% of all patients).

9.32

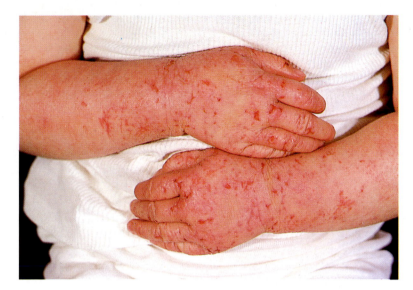

9.33

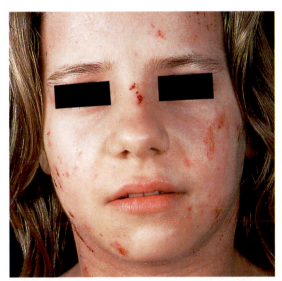

9.34   9.35

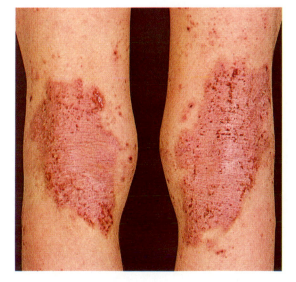

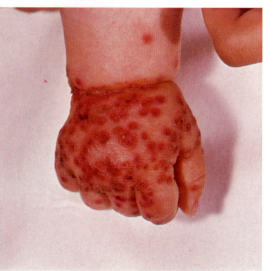

9.36

Polymorphous Light Eruption

Polymorphous light eruption in a 5-year-old boy. Red, partially scaling papules on the lower half of the face appeared several hours after prolonged exposure to sunlight. These lesions formed plaques and were somewhat pruritic. The upper half of the face was spared because it was shielded from sun exposure by a cap. Papular lesions were also found on other light-exposed sites (arms, legs). The lesions resolved after 5 days.

The delayed appearance after exposure to sunlight, the typical skin lesions on exposed parts of the body, the resolution in 7 to 10 days (with avoidance of further exposure to sunlight) are characteristic of polymorphous light eruption.

9.37

Contact Dermatitis

Allergic contact dermatitis ("contact eczema") in an 8-year-old girl with an extensive red, papular, scaly rash on her face. The lesions appeared 10 days after the use of a facial ointment for dry skin. The patch test (allergy test)—using the same ointment—produced a delayed erythema with papules.

9.38

Darier's Disease

Darier's disease (keratosis follicularis) in a 14-year-old girl. The rash began as many small, closely grouped firm papules on the face, neck, trunk, and flexor surfaces (systemic distribution). The lesions evolved to form extensive gray-brown plaques with scaling. The rash was first noted at 10 years of age. Darier's disease is an autosomal dominant trait. Characteristic histologic changes of intradermal vesiculation and hyperkeratosis were noted.

9.39

Photodermatitis

Photodermatitis in a 16-year-old girl. Findings included extensive brown skin pigmentation with no erythema or vesiculation after use of a perfume that contained oil of bergamot and subsequent exposure to sunlight. The strange pigmentation pattern at the contact sites are characteristic of "bergamot" dermatitis. The phototoxic substance in oil of bergamot is 5-methoxypsoralen.

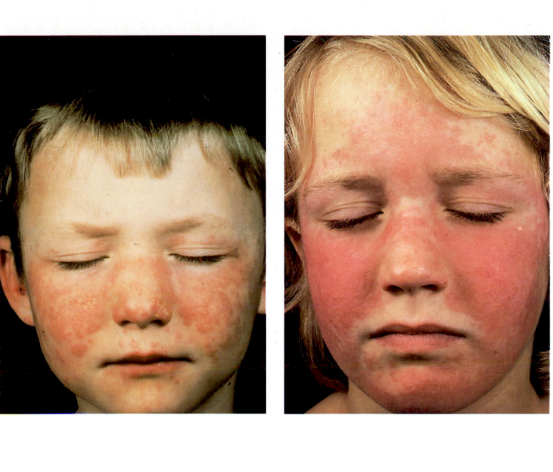

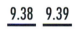

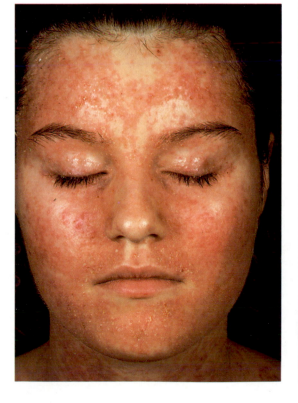

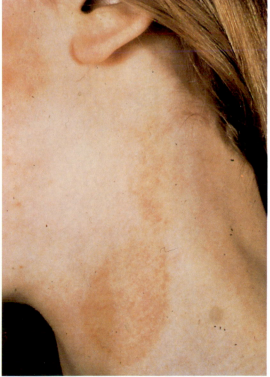

9.40

Infantile Atopic Dermatitis

Infantile atopic dermatitis (infantile eczema) in an 8-month-old girl. Rough, scaly, excoriated lesions were found over the entire body (including flexor surfaces); crusted lesions were also found in the scalp. The cause of infantile eczema is unknown. The child responded to topical treatments with corticosteroid cream and tar-containing preparations. Serum IgE levels were not increased, but this does not rule out the possibility of atopic dermatitis. Increased serum IgE occurs more frequently in patients suffering from bronchial asthma. Delayed hypersensitivity may be compromised in these cases (decreased T lymphocytes and decreased reactivity of T lymphocytes in vitro toward mitogens and specific antigens).

9.41

Atopic Dermatitis

Atopic dermatitis (infantile eczema) in a 3-month-old boy. Scaly, erythematous lesions were noted over the body and scaling crusting lesions were noted in the scalp (cradle cap). At 4 years of age, the child was also noted to have bronchial asthma. The family history was positive for asthma. The only way to distinguish infantile atopic dermatitis from seborrheic dermatitis is to observe the clinical course (seborrheic dermatitis will disappear after several weeks or months and will not recur).

9.42

Atopic Dermatitis

Atopic dermatitis in a 3-year-old boy. Generalized erythema and edema of the skin were noted. The lesions of the face were extremely scaly and the lesions of the neck were exudative and secondarily infected (impetiginization). The pinna of the ear and the external auditory canals were also inflamed. In addition to secondary bacterial infection, complications may include eczema herpeticum (page 240), conjuctivitis, and cataracts. The child died suddenly, with no obvious cause at autopsy.

9.43

Photoallergic Dermatitis

Photoallergic reaction in an 8-year-old boy after treatment with tetracycline. The parts of the body exposed to light (especially the cheeks and nose) were red and swollen. Some areas were blistered and excoriated. The lesions were extremely pruritic. In susceptible individuals, exposure to light may lead to a delayed hypersensitivity reaction. Preventive treatment involves the use of sunscreen or avoidance of specific medications that may cause photoallergic response.

Differential Diagnosis—If the eliciting factor for photosensitivity is unknown, a variety of photodermatoses must be considered:

1. Summer prurigo (pruritic papules with secondary excoriation)
2. Immune disorders, including polymorphous light eruptions (papulovesicular lesions) or urticaria solaris (urticarial lesions)
3. Genetic orders associated with photosensitivity included xeroderma pigmentosum (a wide variety of skin lesions), and Bloom syndrome (photosensitivity and dwarfism)
4. Inborn errors of metabolism, including porphyria (erthematous wheals and blisters) and Hartnup disease
5. Hydroa vacciniforme (vesiculobullous eruption with scarring)
6. Infectious diseases including recurrent herpes simplex infection

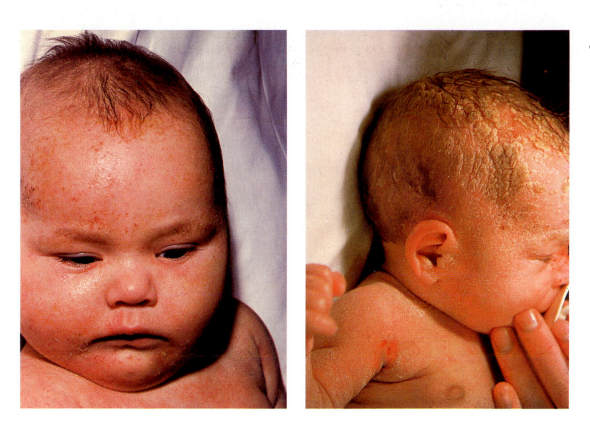

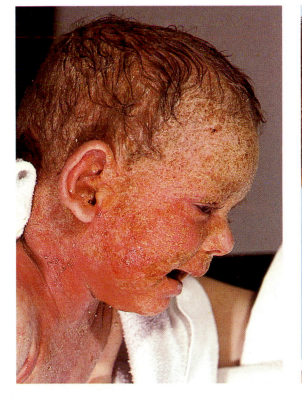
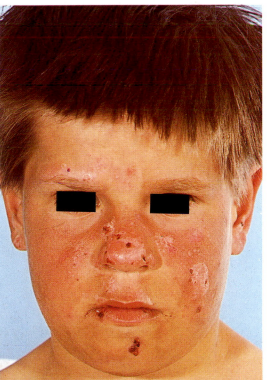

9.44   9.45
Staphylococcal Scalded Skin Syndrome

Staphylococcal scalded skin syndrome (Ritter's disease) in a 6-day-old boy. The skin was erythematous with vesicle formation and widespread wrinkling and loosening of the epidermis. Signs of systemic illness included high fever, irritability, and leukocytosis. Nasopharyngeal cultures grew *Staphylococcus aureus* (group II phage type). Systemic antibiotic treatment led to gradual healing without scar formation. Staphylococcal scalded skin syndrome may be a specific form of toxic epidermal necrolysis (Lyell's disease) in the young infant. Both conditions may be caused by a staphylococcus that produces an exfoliative toxic substance.

9.46
Toxic Epidermal Necrolysis

Toxic epidermal necrolysis (Lyell's disease) in a 4-year-old boy. A painful erythematous rash was noted on the face and chest. Some areas of skin formed flaccid bullae that were filled with a clear liquid. Light rubbing of the skin would lead to formation of bullae and exfoliation (Nikolsky sign). The child had signs of systemic illness, including high fever and malaise. The cause in this case was sulfonamide medication. The child was successfully treated with systemic corticosteroid therapy and local antibacterial treatment to prevent secondary infection.

The skin changes of toxic epidermal necrolysis are often first noted in the axilla and groin. Toxic epidermal necrolysis may more often be fatal than staphylococcal scaled skin syndrome. Toxic epidermal necrolysis is a hypersensitivity phenomenon usually caused by a reaction to medication (sulfanomide, barbiturate).

9.47
Toxic Epidermal Necrolysis

Toxic epidermal necrolysis (Lyell's disease) in a 2-year-old girl. An erythematous rash was noted over the hands with vesicle formation on the palms and fingertips. The cause in this case was unknown. Fluid loss from the denuded skin may lead to dehydration. In addition to the usual skin lesions, conjunctivitis and stomatitis were noted.

Differential Diagnosis—The differential diagnosis of toxic epidermal necrolysis includes staphylococcal scaled skin syndrome (Ritter's disease), burns, and Stevens-Johnson syndrome. In adults, pemphigus vulgaris (flat blisters on nonerythematous skin) should be considered.

9.48
Photoallergic Reaction

Photoallergic reaction in a 10-year-old girl. Vesicles and bullae (partially covered with crusting areas) rapidly appeared over the hands after exposure to sunlight. The lesions were nonpruritic. These lesions healed leaving hyperpigmented areas. The cause in this case was exposure to cologne containing oil of bergamot.

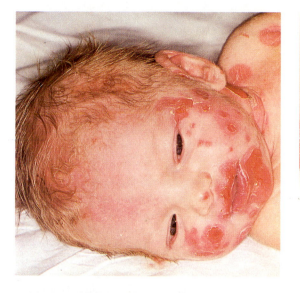

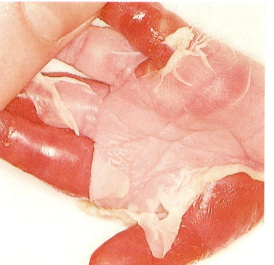

9.44 9.45

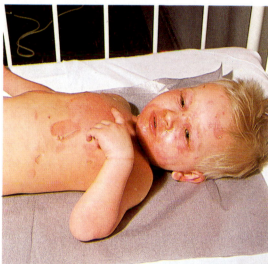

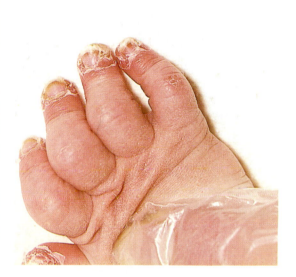

9.46 9.47

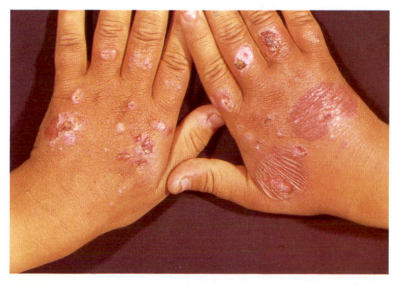

9.48

9.49

Chronic Bullous Dermatosis

Chronic bullous dermatosis of childhood (linear immuno-globulin A [IgA] dermatosis) in a 4-year-old girl. Findings included numerous crust-covered bullae on an erythematous base over the cheeks, perioral area, and on the neck. The bullae appeared suddenly and were initially considered to be bullous impetigo or bullous erythema multiforme. Linear IgA deposition at the dermoepidermal junction was detected in the erythematous skin by immunofluorescence. Chronic bullous dermatosis usually responds well to treatment with sulfapyridine or dapsone.

Differential Diagnosis—Bullous pemphigoid is clinically similar to chronic bullous dermatosis; however, in bullous pemphigoid, linear IgG deposits are found in the basement membrane zone by immunofluorescence. In dermatitis herpetiformis, granular IgA is found in the dermal papillae.

9.50

Bullous Pemphigoid

Bullous pemphigoid in a 15-year-old girl. Findings included numerous taut, fluid-filled blisters, 0.5 cm in diameter, on a nonerythematous base on the left side of the neck. Pictured here after biopsy (with suture) to confirm the diagnosis. The findings were localized to the neck; no mucous membrane involvement was noted. Histologic examination revealed the typical findings of subepidermal blisters with eosinophilic cells, linear IgG and C3 deposition in the basal membrane. There was no inflammatory infiltrate.

Differential Diagnosis—Chronic bullous dermatosis of childhood (linear IgA dermatosis), dermatitis herpetiformis, erythema multiforme, and pemphigous vulgaris.

9.51 9.52

Dermatitis Herpetiformis

Dermatitis herpetiformis (Duhring's disease) in an 11-year-old girl. Numerous small, partially excoriated and encrusted vesicles on an erythematous base were noted on the extensor surface of both thighs (Figure 9.51). These lesions were intensely pruritic. Isolated blisters 1–2 cm in diameter (Figure 9.52) appeared later at other sites (face, shoulders, axilla). The course was lengthy with frequent exacerbations and remissions. The diagnosis was confirmed by biopsy and immunofluorescence test for IgA.

Differential Diagnosis—The papular or vesicular form of dermatitis herpetiformis must be differentiated from scabies, eczema, and insect bites. The bullous form can be confused with bullous erythema multiforme or bullous pemphigoid.

9.53

Scabies

Scabies in a 5-year-old boy with secondary lesions (partially encrusted vesicles and papules) on the skin of the abdomen. The lesions were intensely pruritic. Typical primary lesions (threadlike mite burrows with a tiny vesicle at the end) were found on the fingers and hands. The mites were detected microscopically.

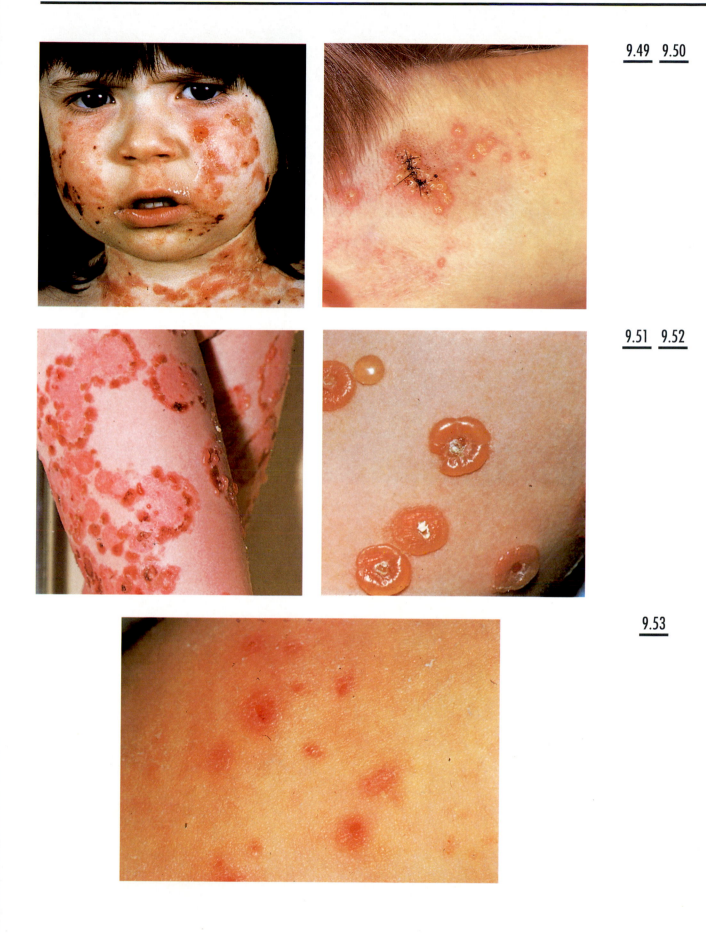

9.54
Infantile Acne

Infantile acne in a 1-year-old boy. Typical skin lesions (comedones) were noted on the face. These lesions were noted during the first year of life. The lesions resolved with topical treatment and application of a mild keratolytic lotion.

Infantile acne also occurs in precocious puberty and adrenogenital syndrome. Exposure to halogenated compounds may lead to acne during the first year of life. In this case, the rash was progressive with the formation of pustules and granulomas. *Candida* dermatitis can resemble infantile acne.

9.55
Acne Vulgaris

Acne vulgaris in a 1-year-old boy. Of note was the papulopustular rash of the face which developed from closed (white) comedones. Acne vulgaris is an inflammatory process of sebaceous follicles. In this case, the probable cause was phenobarbital treatment. Acne may be brought on by a variety of medications, including adrenocorticotropic hormone (ACTH), corticosteroids, phenobarbitol, isoniazid, certain vitamin or mineral preparations, and iodine or bromide.

9.56
Photodermatitis

Summer prurigo in a 6-year-old boy after exposure to sunlight. The findings included pruritic papules on the face, which eventually became excoriated and crusting, leaving small superficial scars. The skin changes were restricted to the face, but they may also occur on clothed parts of the body. The lesions may persist for some time.

9.57
Xeroderma Pigmentosum

Xeroderma pigmentosum in a 7-year-old girl. Pigmented macules resembling freckles of various sizes were located on the face, the lips, and the conjunctiva. White atrophic spots were also noted. The child had extreme hypersensitivity to sunlight and regularly used sunscreen and other protective measures. Characteristic telangiectasia and small angiomas developed later in the course of the disease.

Xeroderma pigmentosa is a rare genetic disorder thought to be caused by hereditary endonuclease defect causing cellular DNA damaged by ultraviolet light to be left unrepaired. Skin malignancies (basal cell carcinoma, malignant melanoma) may appear in childhood.

Differential Diagnosis—Milder cases of xeroderma pigmentosum must be differentiated from simple freckles. Other entities to be considered are Peutz-Jeghers syndrome (page 228) and other photodermatoses.

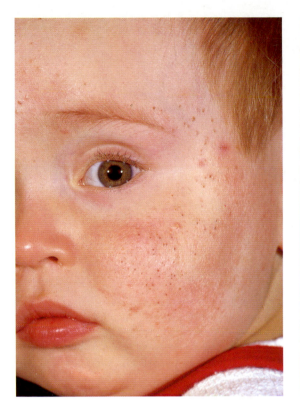 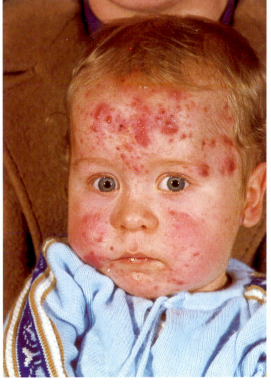

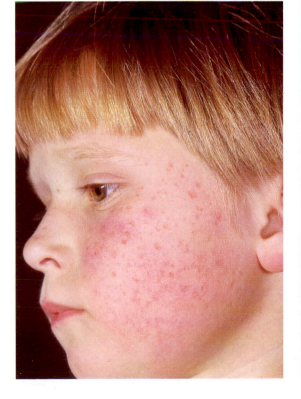 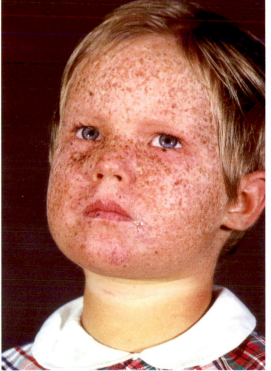

9.58

Flat Warts

Flat warts (verruca plana) on the dorsum of the hands of a 15-year-old girl. The numerous closely grouped round or oval light brown papules were 2–4 mm in size; the lesions healed after use of a tretinoin cream.

9.59

Insect Bites

Allergic skin reaction to insect bites in a 10-year-old boy. Numerous lentil-sized pruritic vesicles surrounded by a red halo were found on the forearm and elbow.

9.60

Steroid Acne

Steroid acne in a 15-year-old girl. Follicular papules and pustules were found symmetrically distributed in the axilla, on the neck, and on the back. The acne appeared 5 weeks after the start of oral corticosteroid therapy and resolved without scar formation.

9.61

Xanthoma Tuberosum

Xanthoma tuberosum in 2-year-old boy with Alagille syndrome. Numerous yellow nodules of varying size were found on the dorsum of the hand and on the dorsal surface of the fingers; the nodules were raised above the skin. Laboratory investigation demonstrated elevated direct bilirubin and cholesterol.

Histologically, xanthomas consist of accumulations of fibroblasts, reticulin fibers, and histiocytes. In addition to xanthoma tuberosum, there are eruptive xanthoma (extensive small yellow papules), tendinous xanthoma (found along extensor tendons), and xanthoma palpebrarum (xanthelasma).

9.58

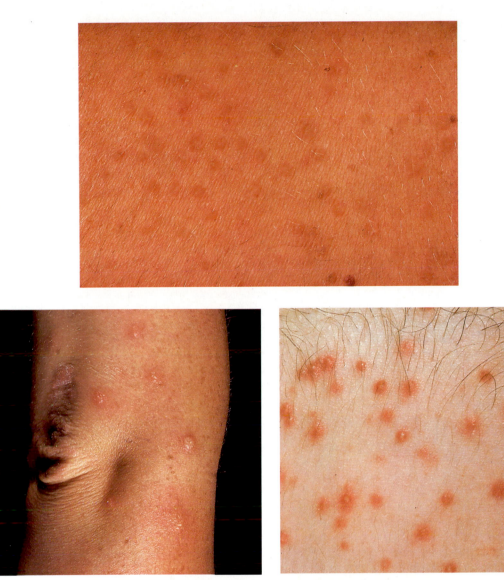

9.59   9.60

9.61

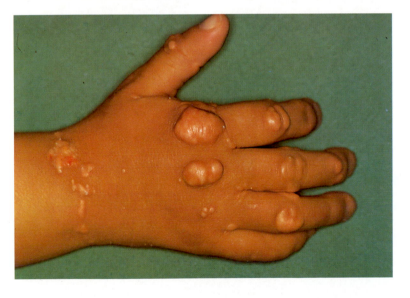

9.62 Calcinosis

Localized calcinosis (calcium deposition in connective tissue) in a 10-year-old-girl. Small, hard papules with irregular borders were found on the arms, the legs, and the torso. Deposition of calcium in the skin and subcutaneous tissue was confirmed by biopsy. Serum calcium and phosphorus levels were normal. The cause in this case was uncertain (idiopathic form).

Inflammatory processes as well as disorders of calcium and phosphorus metabolism may lead to calcinosis cutis. Calcinosis cutis may be the symptoms of the following diseases: hyperparathyroidism, renal disease, vitamin D intoxication (due to hypercalcemia), dermatomyositis (due to chronic inflammation), and scleroderma. Calcinosis cutis may also be caused by ruptured epidermal cysts (Malherbe's epithelioma) or local trauma (foreign bodies, hematoma, fat tissue necrosis). Hereditary diseases such as thyroid dysplasia ossificans and pseudohypoparathyroidism may also lead to localized dermal calcinosis. In calcinosis universalis, calcium deposition occurs symmetrically in the skin and musculature of the torso and extremities without previous trauma or metabolic illness. In later stages, erythema of the overlying skin and ulceration may occur.

9.63 Branchial Cleft Sinus

External branchial cleft sinus on the anterior aspect of the neck in a 14-year-old girl. Two cutaneous openings located at the anterior aspect of the sternocleidomastoid muscle were noted since birth. They appeared as slightly erythematous papules and produced no mucus.

Branchial cleft cysts or sinuses are the result of incomplete closure of the first and second branchial arches during embryonic development. The defects are usually unilateral. Mucous secretion sometimes occurs. The external branchial sinus can open into the pharynx and secrete saliva while the patient is eating. The external opening lies at the anterior edge of the sternocleidomastoid muscle (usually at the lower third). Unlike external sinuses, the internal branchial sinuses may have no connection to the skin. Complications related to the external branchial cleft sinus include secondary bacterial infection and cyst formation. Branchial cysts usually lie higher along the sternocleidomastoid muscle (upper third of the neck) and become manifest later in childhood. They may be confused with tuberculous lymphadenitis. Thyroglossal fistulas and cysts lie in the midline of the neck and may be attached to the base of the tongue. In addition to mucus, thyroglossal duct cysts may contain thyroid tissue.

9.64 Nevus Araneus

Nevus araneus (spider nevus) on the cheek of a 12-year-old boy. A radial mesh of dilated vessels is evident around a red point in the middle of the lesion (the central artery). The nevus becomes pale when pressure is applied to the central artery. These nevi are frequently solitary and vary in diameter from a few millimeters to several centimeters. They are commonly found on the face, the ear, the dorsum of the hand, and under the arms. These lesions are found in 15% of preschool age children and in up to 45% of healthy school-age children. Multiple spider nevi may be seen with pregnancy and in hepatic cirrhosis (in association with elevated plasma estrogen levels). Spiderlike telangiectasia are noted in Osler-Weber-Rendu disease (hereditary hemorrhagic telangiectasia). In Osler-Weber-Rendu disease telangiectasia usually develop during puberty and appear primarily on the face, the palms, the nail beds, the tongue, and the mucous membranes of the lips. These lesions may involve internal organs and may lead to severe hemorrhage and anemia.

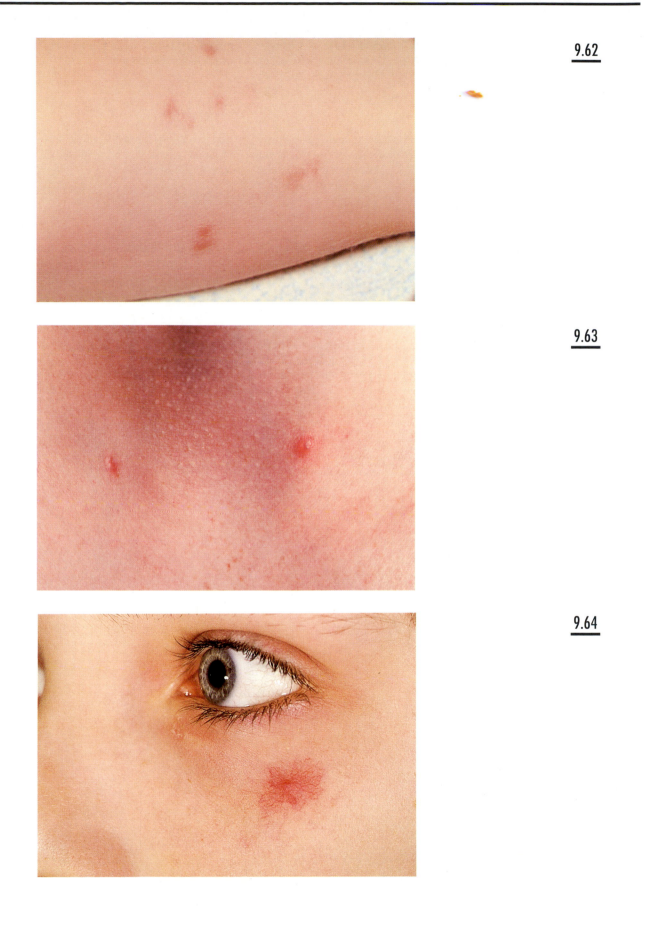

9.62

9.63

9.64

9.65

Nevus Spilus

Nevus spilus in a 15-year-old boy. The large, oval, hairless, light brown area of skin 6 × 12 cm in size was located on the left side of the abdomen. Numerous small dark-brown macules and slightly raised papules containing nevus cells were found within this area.

9.66

Nevus Sebaceus

Nevus sebaceus in a 6-month-old boy. An elongated, sharply demarcated, slightly raised orange area of skin, was located on the right cheek. The lesion caused no discomfort. Nevus sebaceus may increase in size during puberty and become verrucous due to hyperplasia of the sebaceous glands. In adulthood, secondary neoplasm (basal cell carcinoma) develop in 20% of the cases.

9.67

Verruca Vulgaris

Verruca vulgaris (simple wart) on the lower eyelid of a 12-year-old boy. The solitary, round, red-brown, hyperkeratotic papule had a diameter of 3.5 mm.

Differential Diagnosis—Molluscum contagiosum (rice-sized, pearly, umbilicated papules of soft consistency, which contain a doughy mass and usually occur as multiple lesions).

9.68

Dyshidrotic Eczema

Dyshidotic eczema in an 18-year-old young man. Intensely pruritic, deep vesicles were found on the fingers of both hands with thickening and scaling of the affected skin. The eczema began suddenly 3 weeks earlier. The cause was unknown. The ability to perspire was not affected. Dyshidrotic eczema is frequently found on the palms, soles, and interdigital area.

Differential Diagnosis—Contact dermatitis, fungal skin infections.

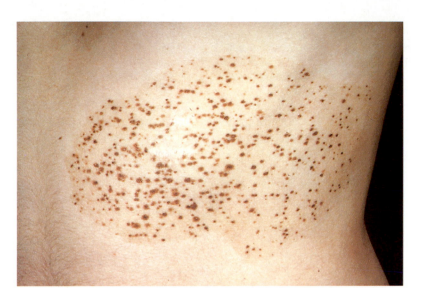

9.65

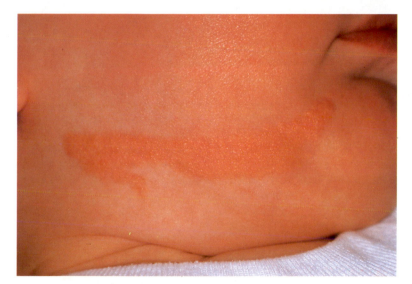

9.66

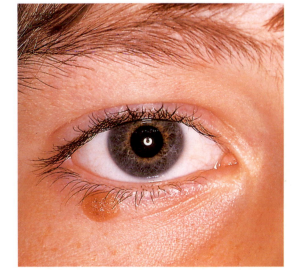
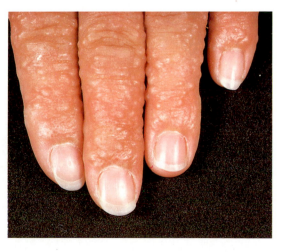

9.67 9.68

9.69

Nevus Flammeus

Nevus flammeus (port-wine nevus or flat hemangioma) on the right cheek and chin of a 1-year-old girl. The sharply demarcated, erythematous, macular lesion was irregular in shape. The lesion had been present since birth and demonstrated no tendency to regress.

Nevus flammeus occur frequently on the face, but may occur on other sites as well. If the neck is involved, it is known as Unna's nevus. Color may be varying shades of red. The lesion may involve the mucous membranes. Over time, nevus flammeus may become slightly raised or fade. Nevus flammeus may be associated with several syndromes including:

1. Sturge-Weber syndrome (page 296)
2. Klippel-Trenaunay-Weber syndrome (page 296)
3. Rubinstein syndrome, broad thumbs and toes, anti-mongoloid palpebral fissures, nevus on forehead (page 54)
4. Cobb syndrome (arteriovenous malformation of the spinal cord)
5. Beckwith-Wiedemann syndrome (nevus flammeus on the upper half of the face, page 334)
6. Patau syndrome (page 94).

In contrast to nevus flammeus, macular hemangioma (salmon patch) is usually present at birth and is localized to the base of the nose, the upper eyelids, or the upper lip. Salmon patches are poorly defined, bright red, and usually disappear during the first year of life.

9.70

Pigmented Nevus

Pigmented nevus (junctional nervus) in a 4-year-old boy. A superficial, discrete, brown, hyperpigmented lesion was noted on the left cheek. The lesion was not raised. In general pigmented nevi are benign; very seldom do malignant melanoma develop.

9.71

Nevus Sebaceous

Nevus sebaceous (Jadassohn) in a 2-year-old girl. The elongated, sharply demarcated, hairless, orange-yellow, elevated area of skin over the scalp was present since birth. Biopsy demonstrated hyperkeratosis, hyperplasia of the epidermis, deformed hair follicles and an abundance of sebaceous glands. Since malignant degeneration during adolescence may occur, the nevus was completely resected.

Nevus sebaceous may develop later in children and appear on the face, the ears, or the neck. Nevus sebaceous must be differentiated from epidermal nevus (nevus verrucosus), which appear in various forms. Nevus sebaceous must also be differentiated from ichthyosis hystrix. In ichthyosis hystrix, brown verrucose papules are arranged in a linear fashion. Histologic examination demonstrates epidermolytic hyperkeratosis, papillomatosis, and acanthosis.

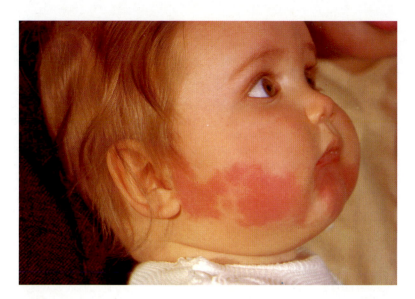

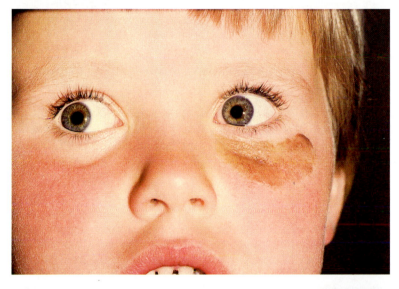

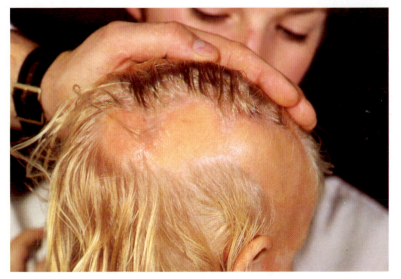

9.72

LEOPARD Syndrome

LEOPARD syndrome (multiple lentigines syndrome) in a 10-year-old boy. Physical findings included numerous dark-brown pigmented spots of varying size. The lentigines had been present since birth but had increased in number in the last few years. The mucous membranes were not affected. The boy had cardiac involvement, including pulmonic stenosis and the typical conduction disorders found on electrocardiogram (abnormal P waves, prolonged P-R interval, widened QRS complex). The child was of short stature due to severely delayed skeletal maturation. In this case, hearing was normal.

Typical findings in LEOPARD syndrome include diffuse multiple lentigenes, congenital heart disease, growth deficiency, as well as electrocardiographic conduction abnormalities. LEOPARD syndrome is an autosomal dominant disorder with strong penetrance and variable expressivity. LEOPARD stands for *L*entigenes, *E*KG disturbances, *O*cular hypertelorism, *P*ulmonary stenosis, *A*bnormalities of the genitalia, *R*etardation of growth, *D*efective hearing. Multiple lentigenes also occur in Peutz-Jeghers syndrome (with involvement of the mucous membranes) and in von Recklinghausen's disease (neurofibromatosis).

9.73

Congenital Giant Pigmented Nevus

Congenital giant pigmented nevus (giant hairy nevus) in a 1½-year-old girl. The extensive, sharply demarcated, hyperpigmented, hairy lesion was located on the back with many small pigmented lesions over other parts of the body. Histologically, the lesion was a compound nevus (both epidermal and intradermal).

Congenital giant pigmented nevi may be epidermal (junctional type) or intradermal. Malignant change (malignant melanoma) may occur in 10% of cases; therefore, giant pigmented nevi should be removed. Further complications include leptomeningeal melanocytosis that can lead to hydrocephalus, seizures, and developmental delay. In these cases, melanin-containing cells may be detected in the cerebrospinal fluid.

9.74

Intradermal Pigmented Nevus

Intradermal pigmented nevus in a 2-month-old infant. Several sharply demarcated, raised, dark-brown pigmented growths were noted at the base of the nose and below the left eye. The lesions were present at birth and had grown considerably since then. Histologic examination identified them as benign intradermal pigmented nevus.

9.75

Pigmented Nevus

Pigmented nevus (compound nevus) in a 3-day-old newborn. A palm-sized, slightly raised, dark-brown area of skin was noted on the anterior chest and abdomen. Histologically, the nevus was found to be a compound nevus (located in both the epidermis and the dermis). In contrast to a compound nevus, a junctional nevus lies on the epidermal surface only and is flat, smooth, and relatively small. Junctional nevi vary in color from light- to dark-brown and, over time, may become compound nevi. Pigmented nevi occur in 1 to 2% of all children. Junctional nevi are the most common. Intradermal nevi stand out more prominently from the body surface than compound nevi. Generally, these pigmented nevi get larger during adolescence but remain stable thereafter and may diminish in size after 60 years of age. Nevi may undergo malignant transformation. Lesions that demonstrate a rapid change in growth, or become otherwise symptomatic, should be removed because of the possibility of malignant degeneration.

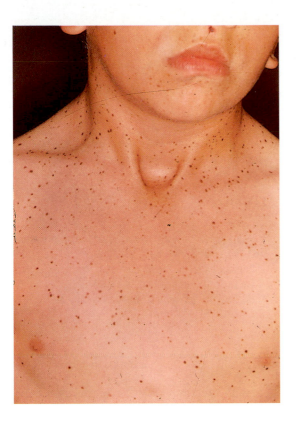

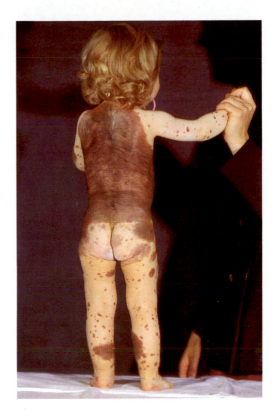

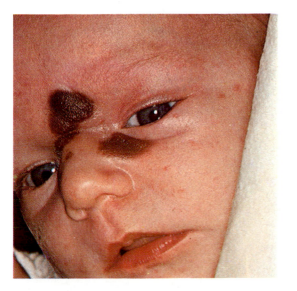

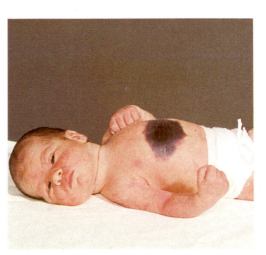

9.76

Nevus Sebaceous

Nevus sebaceous (Jadassohn) in a 10-month-old boy. Several, closely grouped, small, yellow nodules in front of the left ear were present since birth. After surgical removal, the diagnosis was confirmed histologically. Histologically, these lesions demonstrate hyperkeratosis, abnormal hair follicles, and an abundance of sebaceous glands.

Differential Diagnosis—For differential diagnosis see page 200.

9.77

Nevus Sebaceous

Nevus sebaceous (Jadassohn) in an 8-year-old boy. The lesion was an extensive, poorly defined, hardened, hairless area of the scalp above the parietal bone. The nevus was surgically removed (because of the risk of malignant degeneration) and the skin defect was covered by skin transplant.

9.78

Blue Nevus

Blue nevus in a 12-year-old girl. A pea-sized, dark blue, smooth nodule arose from the skin next to the right eye. The lesion developed during the first year of life and then ceased to grow. Despite the benign nature of the blue nevus, the lesion was surgically removed for cosmetic reasons. On histologic examination, deeply pigmented, spindle-shaped melanocytes were found in the dermis.

Blue nevi are usually solitary and found primarily on the face, neck, arms, upper leg, hands, and feet. They must be differentiated from cellular blue nevi, which are larger than 1 cm and found primarily on the thigh or sacral area. Since these lesions can become malignant, they must be surgically removed.

9.79

Congenital Pigmented Nevus

Congenital pigmented nevus in a 3-year-old boy. The lesion was a 3 × 7 cm hyperpigmented area of skin over the forehead. The lesion was notable for the abundant hair growth. After surgical removal, the skin was covered by a skin graft.

9.80

Halo Nevus

Halo nevus (leukoderma acquisitum centrifugum) in a 13-year-old girl. The lesion is unique in appearance; a central pigmented nevus is surrounded peripherally by a deeply pigmented area of skin (halo). The pigmented nevus was present since birth, whereas the deep pigmentation of the surrounding area first appeared at puberty. After 4 to 5 months, the pigmented nevus became pale, smaller, and disappeared. Repigmentation may occur.

Halo nevi may appear as solitary or multiple lesions. The depigmented halo is generally not greater than 5 mm in diameter. In the early stages, histologic examination may reveal a junctional or intradermal nevus; in later stages, a dense infiltrate of lymphocytes or histiocytes may be seen. Melanocytes are absent in the depigmented base. Therapy is usually not necessary, as halo nevi tend to resolve on their own. Malignant melanoma may look similar to halo nevi (including the depigmented base); in case of doubt, a complete removal and histologic examination should take place.

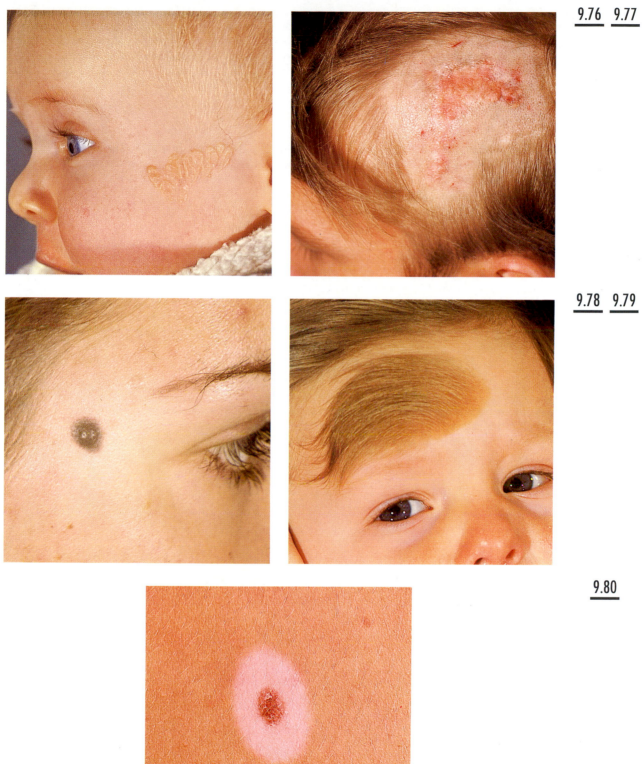

9.81

Schimmelpenning-Feuerstein-Mims Syndrome

Schimmelpenning-Feuerstein-Mims syndrome (linear sebaceous nevus syndrome) in a 14-year-old girl. Small, linearly arranged verrucous yellow-orange nodules were noted in the neck since the first year of life (linear nevus sebaceous). Multiple sebaceous nevi were also found on the scalp. In addition, the girl had numerous pigmented nevi on the arms and legs. The girl had a seizure disorder treated with anticonvulsants. Mental retardation was noted. Characteristic of Schimmelpenning-Feuerstein-Mims syndrome is the simultaneous occurrence of linear nevus sebaceous, multiple nevi of other types, seizure disorder, and mental retardation.

9.82

Malignant Melanoma

Nodular malignant melanoma in a 14-year-old girl. Findings included a 1.5-cm large, rapidly growing lesion that demonstrated central erosion.

Characteristic of malignant melanoma is the rapid growth, irregular or uneven pigmentation, and poorly defined border.

Differential Diagnosis—The differential diagnosis of melanoma includes granuloma telangiectaticum (pyogenic granuloma) and dysplastic nevi.

9.83

McCune-Albright Syndrome

McCune-Albright syndrome in a 13-year-old girl. Findings included patchy, poorly defined, round pigmented areas on the lower half of the body. These findings have been present since birth. Radiographs of the skeleton demonstrated typical features of fibrous dysplasia of the long bones and pelvis, as well as older spontaneous fractures in the neck of the left femur. Serum alkaline phosphatase was elevated. The girl had precocious menarche since the first year of life.

The findings in McCune-Albright syndrome include fibrous dysplasia of the bones with patchy pigmented cutaneous lesions and precocious puberty.

9.84

Sarcoidosis

Sarcoidosis of the skin in a 5-year-old boy. Findings included 1–2 mm large natural skin-colored nodules around the eyes. Pressure from a pleximeter revealed a brown-red infiltrate ("apple-jelly color"). Other organs were not affected.

Differential Diagnosis—The differential diagnosis includes molluscum contagiosum, milia, syringomyomas, and halinosis cutis et mucosae.

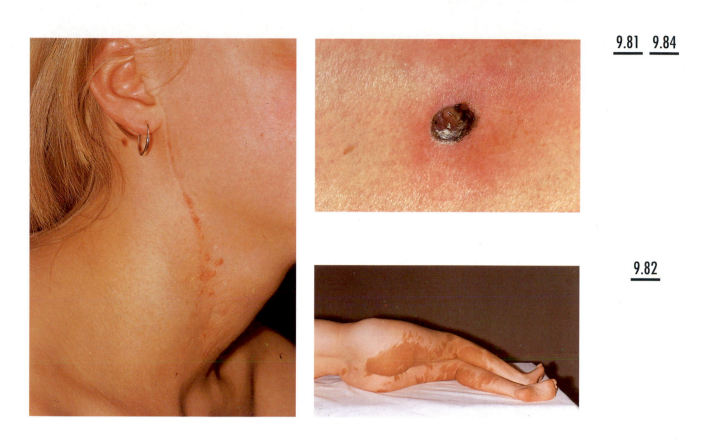

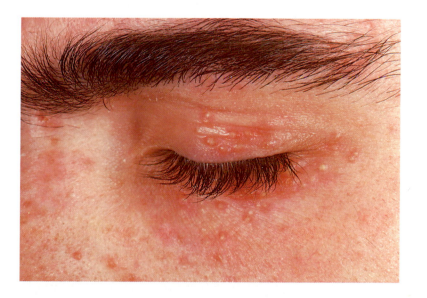

9.85

Shagreen Patches

Shagreen patches in a 14-year-old girl with tuberous sclerosis. Raised indurated areas of skin were noted on the lower back (the most frequent location). Shagreen patches are a typical finding in tuberous sclerosis. In addition, the girl had adenoma sebaceum of the face.

9.86

Pyogenic Granuloma

Pyogenic granuloma (granuloma telangiectaticum) in a 2-year-old boy. A pea-sized, red nodule which bled at times and was covered with a crusted surface was noted on the right cheek. The lesion had persisted for months without healing.

Pyogenic granuloma frequently occurs in children and is usually an isolated lesion found on the face, arms, or hands.

The lesion probably stems from an unobserved episode of trauma. Secondary infection leads to exuberant granulation tissue. Pyogenic granulomas grow rapidly at first, but then remain unchanged in size. It may be difficult to differentiate these lesions from small hemangiomas.

9.87

Pyogenic Granuloma

Pyogenic granuloma (granuloma telangiectaticum) on the underarm of a 10-year-old girl. The lesion was a bean-sized, broad-based, elevated red nodule with an irregular surface. The nodule was moist on its surface and its base had a narrow epithelial collar. The granuloma was excised because it was persistent and had a tendency to bleed. Microscopically, numerous granulocytes were found in the dense, capillary rich tissue. After surgical excision, histologic examination should always be performed to rule out neoplastic disorders (melanoma, Kaposi sarcoma, metastatic carcinoma).

9.88

Milia

Milia on the eyelid of a 16-year-old girl. Numerous firm, white papules, 1 mm in size were noted. Histologically, these are inclusion cysts of the pilosebaceous follicles which contain keratin. In newborn infants, they occur on the cheeks, forehead, nose, and nasolabial folds. They disappear within the first weeks of life without treatment. In older children and adults, they can persist for longer periods of time; lesions may be removed by making a small incision with a fine needle and expressing the keratin.

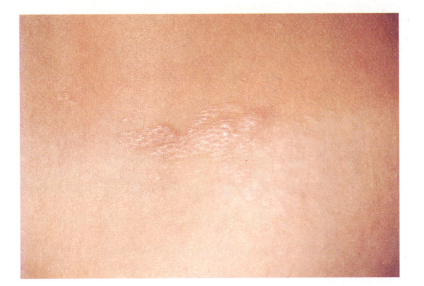

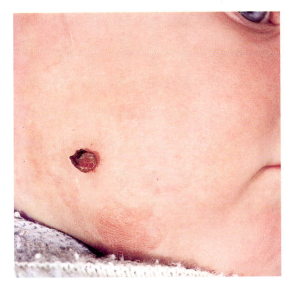
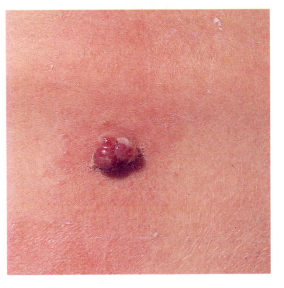

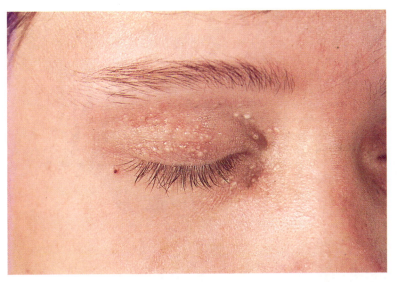

9.89

Histiocytoma

Histiocytoma (dermatofibroma) on the thigh of a 15-year-old girl. The lesion is a flat, round, hyperpigmented firm nodule, 1 cm in diameter, which contains histiocytes, fibroblasts, and capillaries. Histiocytoma is a benign tumor. In this case, the lesion was firm, but in other cases the lesions may be soft and pedunculated. They are usually solitary and primarily develop on the arms or legs, possibly as a result of trauma.

Differential Diagnosis—Differential diagnosis includes hemangiomas, epidermal cysts, juvenile xanthogranulomas, and neurofibromas.

9.90

Lymphocytoma

Lymphocytoma (lymphadenosis cutis benigna) of the underarm of a 4-year-old boy. The round, indurated, red-brown nodules, 2 cm in diameter, developed over the past several months. The etiology is uncertain. Many of these lesions regress spontaneously. Lymphocytomas may occur at any age, may be solitary or multiple, and occur primarily on the face, the earlobes, the scrotum, and the breast.

9.91

Spitz Nevus

Spitz nevus (spindle and epithelioid cell nevus, or juvenile melanoma) under the left eye of a 4-year-old boy. The pea-sized, red-brown, slightly raised nodule appeared suddenly under the child's left eye. Spitz nevi are usually solitary and are frequently located on the face, shoulders, and arms. Children ages 3 to 13 are most commonly affected. A Spitz nevus may grow rapidly and attain a diameter of 1.5 cm. The Spitz nevus is considered a variant of the compound nevus (page 202). After excision, there is no danger of spreading. The Spitz nevus must be differentiated from pyogenic granuloma (page 208), hemangioma, other pigmented nevi, malignant melanoma, and basal cell carcinoma.

9.92

Spitz Nevus

Spitz nevus (juvenile melanoma) in a 5-year-old girl.

9.93

Leiomyoma

Benign leiomyoma of the upper arm in a 7-year-old boy. Multiple firm, light-red nodules of varying size contain smooth muscle tissue. Characteristically, the child experienced paroxysmal bouts of pain. The pain, caused by muscle contractions, can be relieved through massage or cold compresses. Solitary lesions occur and may be treated with surgical excision.

9.94

Multiple Angioleiomyomas

Multiple angioleiomyomas in a 2-week-old girl. Of note were numerous bean-sized nodules under the skin on the back. These nodules were painless and easily mobile. Similar nodes were seen on the abdomen, the upper thigh, and the nape of the neck. The child died after 1 month due to hemorrhage. Before that, a skin biopsy led to the diagnosis of multiple benign angioleiomyomas. Autopsy demonstrated a 3-cm large angioleiomyoma in the area of the aorta with similar angioleiomyomas in the diaphragm, the myocardium, the pericardium, the pancreas, the small intestine, the thyroid gland, and the muscles of the lower arm. Histologic examination demonstrated no signs of malignancy. Angioleiomyomas are benign tumors that originate in the vasculature of the muscles. They usually appear as isolated lesions and are often localized to the legs.

Angioleiomyomas generally occur in the subcutaneous tissue and are partially surrounded by a capsule. These lesions may penetrate into the dermis.

Differential Diagnosis—The differential diagnosis of multiple angioleiomyomas includes cutaneous neurofibromas, dermatofibromas, piloleiomyomas, and leiomyosarcomas.

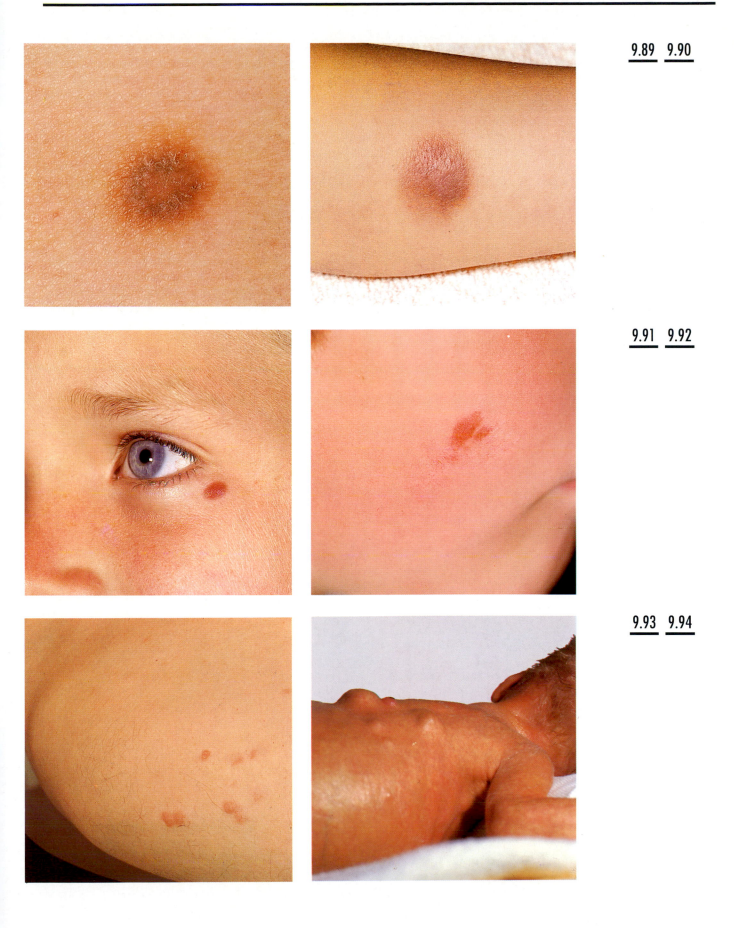

9.89   9.90

9.91   9.92

9.93   9.94

9.95

Ichthyosis Vulgaris

Ichthyosis vulgaris (X-linked ichthyosis) in an 8-year-old boy. Findings included large, brown, firmly attached scales on the neck, forehead, and other parts of the body including the flexor surfaces of the extremities but sparing the palms and soles. The condition first became manifest at 2 months of age. Response to therapy was poor.

Differential Diagnosis—X-linked ichthyosis must be differentiated from autosomal dominant hereditary ichthyosis vulgaris. In the autosomal dominant form, there is scaling over the back and extensor surfaces of the extremities. The flexor surfaces of the extremities and the face are apparently spared. The palms and soles are thickened and partially chapped. The initial manifestations of disease occur after the first year of life, and sometimes do not present until late childhood or adulthood. In contrast to hereditary X-linked ichthyosis, symptoms may improve with increasing age. In addition to hereditary autosomal ichthyosis vulgaris, there is also a rare acquired form of ichthyosis vulgaris. The acquired form can appear at any age and has been observed in patients with malignant disease (Hodgkin's disease). The skin changes do not differ from those seen in the hereditary form.

9.96

Lamellar Ichthyosis

Lamellar ichthyosis (congenital ichthyosiform erythroderma) in a 6-month-old girl. Diffuse erythema and scaling (without vesicle formation) over the torso, the flexor surface of the extremities, the palms and the soles, was noted since birth. Temporary improvement was achieved with symptomatic treatment.

Differential Diagnosis—The differential diagnosis of lamellar ichthyosis includes other forms of icthyosis and certain syndromes with ichthyosiform changes:
1. Sjögren-Larsson syndrome (ichthyosis, spastic diplegia, developmental delay)
2. Netherton syndrome (ichthyosis, abnormal breakage of hair, urticaria or angioneurotic edema)
3. Conradi-Hunermann syndrome (autosomal dominant syndrome with chondrodysplasia punctata "stippled" epiphyses, shortening of the long bones, joint contractures, ichthyosis)
4. Refsum syndrome (metabolic disturbance of phytic acid caused by α-decarboxylase deficiency leading to mild ichthyosis in the first or second decade of life, chronic polyneuritis, progressive paralysis, ataxia)

9.97   9.98

Lamellar Ichthyosis

Lamellar ichthyosis (congenital ichthyosiform erythroderma) in a 3-week-old boy. Skin changes included generalized erythema and scaling (including the flexor surfaces of palms and soles) with numerous dermal fissures. Bilateral eversion of the lid margin (ectropion) was noted.

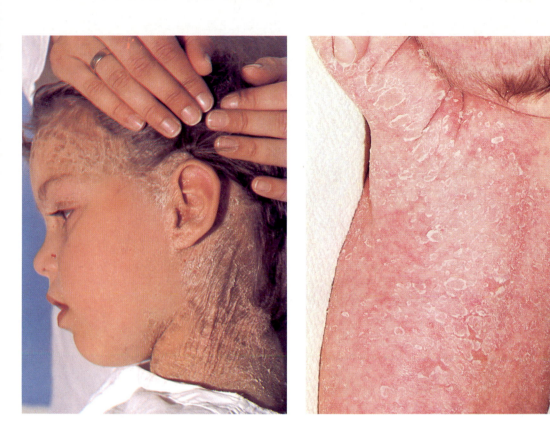

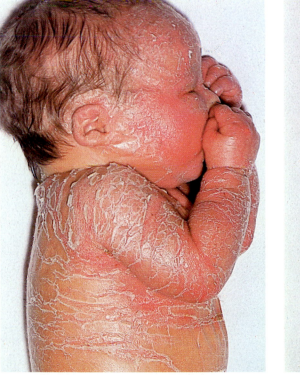
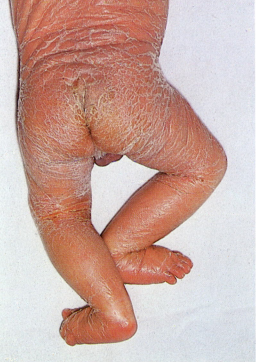

9.99
Congenital Ichthyosis

Congenital ichthyosis in a 1-day-old child ("harlequin fetus"), who died at 8 days of age. The skin over the entire body was thickened and fissured causing extreme disfigurement. The mouth was constantly held open and the lips everted. There was severe ectropion and chemosis. The hair was sparse and the nails were absent. Movement of the joints was severely limited. This severe form of ichthyosis (autosomal recessive inheritance) leads to death within a few days or weeks. This child died due to an aortic thrombus.

9.100
Congenital Ichthyosis

Congenital ichthyosis (ichthyosiform erythroderma) with unilateral cataract in a 4-week-old girl. The "white pupil" (due to cataract) of the left eye had been noted since birth. Ophthalmologic examination was performed to detect complications such as glaucoma and amblyopia ex anopsia.

Differential Diagnosis—The differential diagnosis of infantile cataracts includes:

1. Cataracts associated with hereditary dermatoses such as incontinentia pigmenti, Rothmund syndrome (atrophic telangiectatic dermatoses), and other ectodermal dysplasia syndromes
2. Cataracts associated with other malformations such as various trisomy and deletion syndromes, chondrodysplasia punctata, and Torsten-Sjögren syndrome
3. Inborn errors of metabolism including galactosemia, homocystinuria, Lowe syndrome
4. Intrauterine infection including rubella embryopathy or toxoplasmosis
5. Diseases of the eye that can secondarily lead to cataract (retinopathy of prematurity, uveitis, retinoblastoma)
6. Hereditary form (an isolated malformation).

9.101
Congenital Ichthyosis

Congenital ichthyosis (lamellar ichthyosis) in an 11-month-old girl. Since the age of 1 month, a generalized scaly erythroderma without vesicle formation was noted. The facial skin, like the skin over other parts of the body, demonstrated a diffuse erythema with patches of fine scaling. The flexor surfaces, the palms, and the soles were also affected. Because of the skin loss due to dermal scaling, the child had a constant loss of protein and was considerably underweight. Improvement followed symptomatic treatment with keratolytic lotions, bath oil, and emollients.

9.102
Ichthyosis Vulgaris

Ichthyosis vulgaris (autosomal dominant form) in an 8-year-old girl. Characteristic lamellar scaling of the extensor surfaces of the legs was noted. The flexor surfaces were not affected. The palms and soles were thickened and somewhat fissured. The father was likewise affected. The prognosis of ichthyosis vulgaris is relatively favorable with improvement in adulthood.

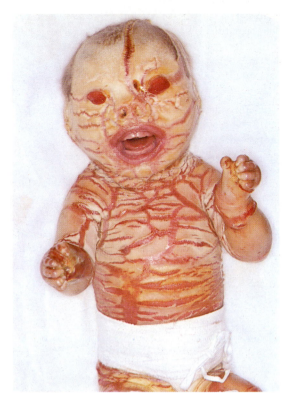

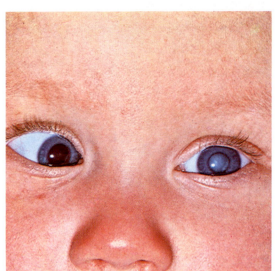

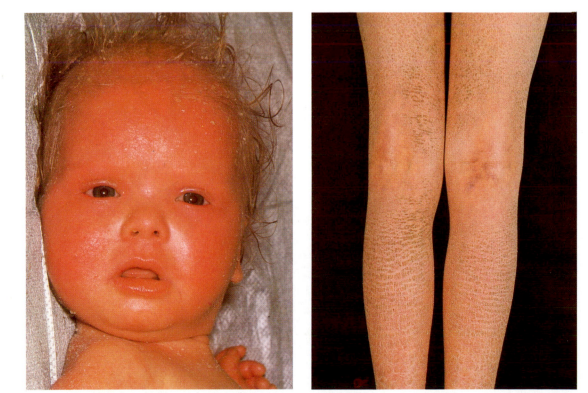

9.103

Pityriasis Rosea

Pityriasis rosea in a 14-year-old girl. Findings included a "herald patch," a solitary oval lesion on the back which was 3 cm and bright red. The lesion had a raised border and fine scales.

9.104

Pityriasis Rosea

Pityriasis rosea in a 14-year-old girl. Numerous dark-red, scaly papules of varying size were noted over the entire body, excluding the hands and feet. The lesions appeared in several stages, 5 to 10 days after the appearance of the herald patch. The lesions were smaller than the herald patch (< 1 cm), and were covered with fine, dry, silver scales. Spontaneous resolution occurred after 4 weeks.

9.105

Ichthyosis

X-linked recessive ichthyosis in a 16-year-old boy. Large brown scales were noted over the entire body, including the flexor surfaces of the extremities but sparing the palms and soles. The lesions were present since the first year of life. Corneal opacities were detected on slit lamp examination. X-linked recessive ichthyosis is caused by a deficiency of the enzyme steroid sulfatase. This patient had a poor response to symptomatic treatment.

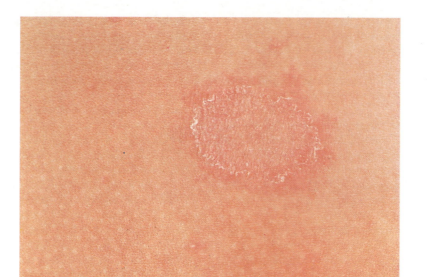

9.103

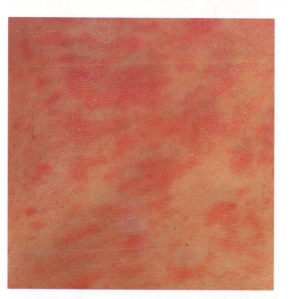

9.104

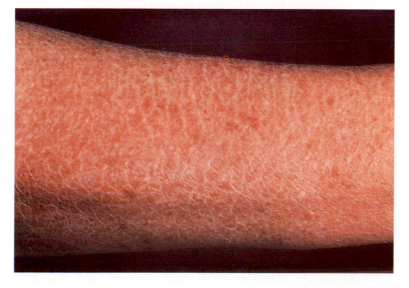

9.105

9.106–9.108

Psoriasis

Psoriasis in a 10-year-old boy. Shown is the generalized rash (Figure 9.106), an individual psoriatic lesion with slightly raised, red plaque covered with thick, shiny, silver scales (Figure 9.107), and discoloration of the nailplate with early onycholysis (Figure 9.108). In this case, the lesions were nonpruritic. Characteristic of psoriasis are the following findings:

1. Candle-spot phenomenon (the lesion becomes the color of candle wax with light scratching)
2. "Last membrane" phenomenon (the whole lesion can be lifted off with vigorous scratching)
3. Dew drop phenomenon or Auspitz sign (dot-shaped hemorrhages appear on the remaining skin surface which is now free from scales)
4. Koebner's phenomenon (loosening of the typical skin lesions by scratching with the fingernail)

In the case of this individual, psoriasis was noted in the fifth year of life. It was chronic and progressive in nature, with periods of spontaneous remission. Many family members were similarly affected.

Differential Diagnosis—The differential diagnosis of psoriasis varies depending on the morphology and location of the lesions as well as the patient's age. In cases where the diagnosis is uncertain, a skin biopsy should be performed. Typical findings of psoriasis include thickening of the stratum corneum with parakeratosis, hyperplasia of the epidermis with elongation of the rete ridges, microabscesses, vascularization of the dermis and infiltration of inflammatory cells. In cases in which psoriasis affects the scalp, fungal infection (tinea capitis) and seborrheic dermatitis must be ruled out. In cases of nail involvement, mycotic infection of the nails and lichen ruber planus must be considered. Chronic forms of psoriasis with extreme scaling must be differentiated from tinea corporis. Acute forms of psoriasis (with numerous disseminated small erythematous papules) must be distinguished from pityriasis rosea and secondary syphilis. Other forms of dermatitis associated with scaling must be considered. When psoriasis is localized to the anogenital area, *Candida* dermatitis (so-called diaper dermatitis), seborrheic dermatitis, and intertrigo must be considered. Guttate psoriasis, which occurs more frequently in children, can be confused with pityriasis rosea, secondary syphilis, and certain drug rashes.

9.109

Erythema Elevatum Diutinum

Erythema elevatum diutinum on the legs of a 10-year-old boy. Findings included red-blue, scaling, nodular lesions of varying sizes, some with central umbilication, ulceration, and crusting. The primary location is the extensor and flexor surfaces of the extremities and the hands. The course is prolonged and the cause is unknown.

Differential Diagnosis—Erythema elevatum diutinum may be differentiated from facial granuloma because of its location. Granuloma annulare, histiocytoma, and sarcoidosis can be differentiated by histologic examination. Lichen ruber planus (light red, shiny papules) and xanthoma (yellow-brown papules or nodules) are usually distinguished without difficulty.

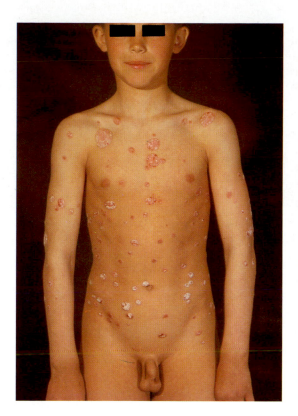

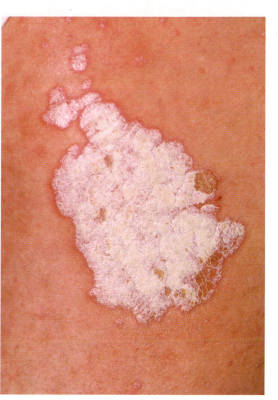

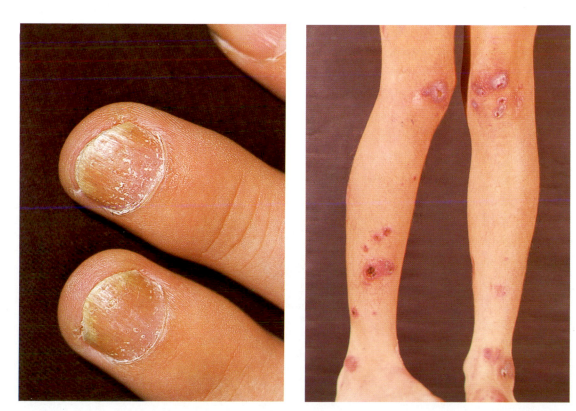

9.110 9.111
Lichenoid Pityriasis

Acute lichenoid pityriasis (Mucha-Habermann disease, varicelliform type) in a 6-year-old boy. Varicella-like lesions (small, red, slightly pruritic papules and vesicles, some with red-brown crusts) were noted over the entire body. The child was briefly febrile; otherwise his general health was unaffected. The lesions appeared on the anterior torso, upper arms, and thighs. They healed leaving pigmented, sunken scars. The mucous membranes were not involved. The illness may occur at any age. Acute lichenoid pityriasis is apparently a hypersensitivity reaction to an infectious agent.

Differential Diagnosis—Differential diagnosis includes viral rashes such as varicella, strophulus, and medication-induced rashes.

9.112 9.113
Lichenoid Pityriasis

Chronic lichenoid pityriasis (parapsoriasis guttata) in a 7-year-old boy. Generalized red, scaling, nonpruritic macules and papules of varying sizes were found over the entire body including the face. Characteristically, a red-brown papule is uncovered by scratching a scale. The course is prolonged, often lasting months or years. The cause of chronic lichenoid pityriasis is unclear. In the early stage, or if the lesions are not dense, the condition may be confused with viral exanthems or insect bites. Persistent cases must be differentiated from psoriasis guttate (light red lesions with silverly scales) and lichen ruber planus (sharply demarcated blue-red, flat papules with white opal striations, particularly on the flexor surfaces and often involving the mucous membranes).

9.114
Parapsoriasis

Plaque parapsoriasis in an 8-year-old girl. Numerous round, elongated, poorly defined pruritic, yellow-red, scaly patches of varying size were evident on the trunk and the extremities. Individual lesions were slightly raised. The course was chronic and responded poorly to treatment.

Differential Diagnosis—Plaque parapsoriasis must be differentiated from the early stages of mycosis fungoides or poikiloderma (atrophy of the skin) and nummular eczema.

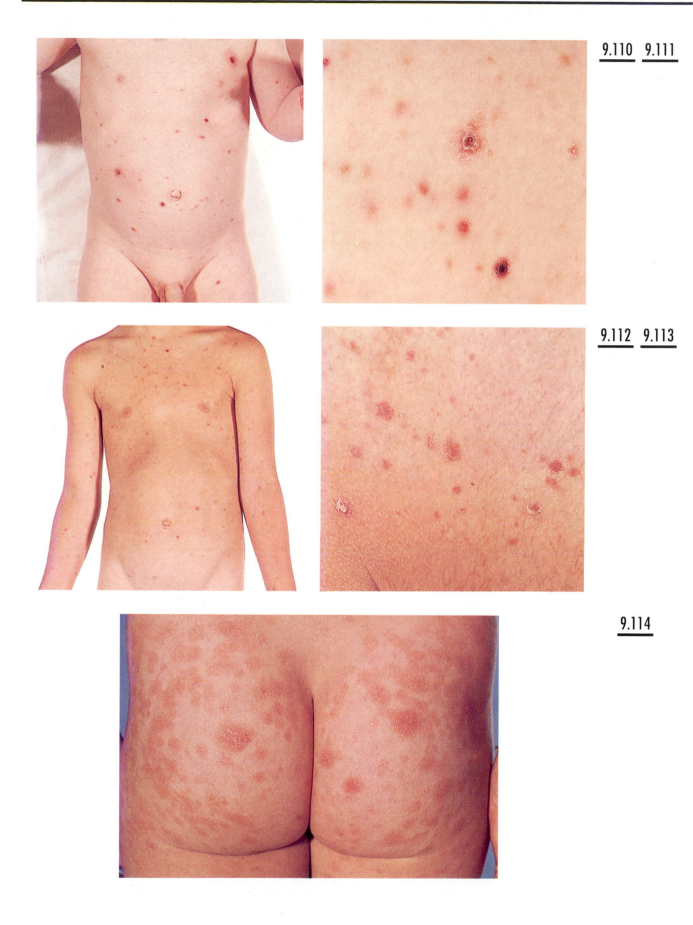

9.115–9.117

Papillon-LeFevre Syndrome

Papillon-Lefevre syndrome (keratoderma of palms and soles associated with periodontitis) in a 4-year-old boy. Of note is erythematous hyperkeratosis of the knees (Figure 9.116), the soles of the feet (Figure 9.117), and the palms. Anomalies of the nails and teeth as well as gingivitis and severe periodontitis occur (Figure 9.115). As a rule, this syndrome includes palmar and plantar hyperhydrosis, which can result in calcification.

This autosomal recessive hereditary syndrome must be distinguished from other syndromes that occur with keratoderma (excessive accumulation of stratum corneum):

1. Palmoplantar keratodermal simplex
2. Mal de Meleda (hyperkeratosis of the extensor surfaces of the extremities associated with developmental delay)
3. Keratoma hereditaria mutilans (associated with hyperkeratosis, autoamputation of the fingers, alopecia, deafness)
4. Hydrotic form of ectodermal dysplasia (page 274)

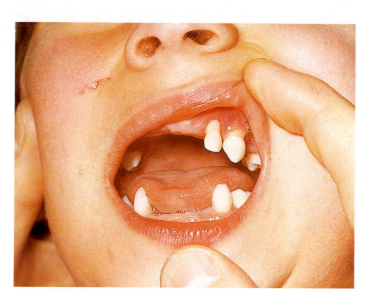

9.115

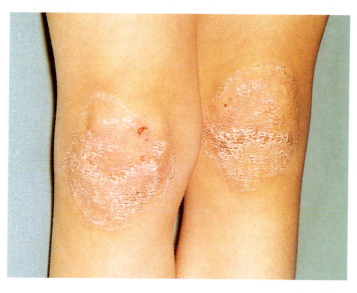

9.116

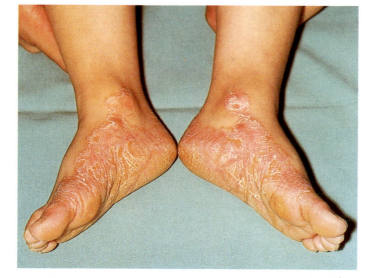

9.117

9.118 9.119

Urticaria Pigmentosa

Urticaria pigmentosa in a 1¼-year-old boy. Numerous brown, pigmented macules of varying size were noted over the skin and scalp. The lesions were pruritic and, in this case, were without vesicular changes. Rubbing the skin caused the formation of urticaria (Darier sign). The diagnosis can be confirmed through skin biopsy (revealing mast cell infiltration). Spontaneous remission usually occurs in adolescence.

9.120

Urticaria Pigmentosa

Urticaria pigmentosa in a 13-month-old girl. Red-brown macules and papules were noted over the entire body, especially the torso. When rubbed, these lesions became urticarial. When brought to the clinic at 12 years of age, only a few pigmented areas without urticaria remained.

Differential Diagnosis—Urticaria pigmentosa must be differentiated from papular urticaria (strophulus). In papular urticaria, the lesions on the extremities are more numerous than those on the torso and are rarely pigmented. Central facial lentigines (elevated dark-brown macules not to be confused with epithelides) are easily ruled out, as is healing lichen ruber planus. The nodular form of urticaria pigmentosa must be differentiated from xanthomas and juvenile xanthogranulomas.

9.121

Urticaria Pigmentosa

Urticaria Pigmentosa in a 4½-year-old boy. Numerous, poorly defined, irregular brown spots of varying size were noted. The child had no systemic complaints. As long as there are no signs of systemic mastocytosis (bone involvement, gastrointestinal involvement, or hepatosplenomegaly) the prognosis is good. Flushing and tachycardia occur more frequently in systemic mastocytosis (10% of cases) than in cases with isolated skin findings.

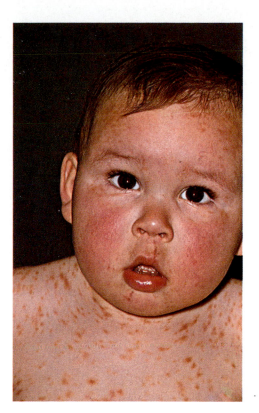

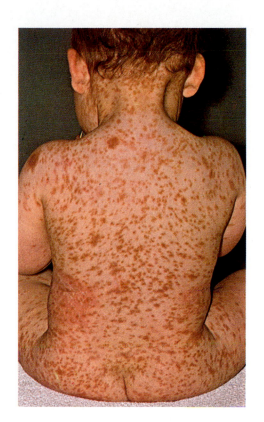

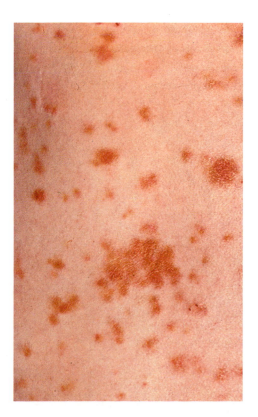

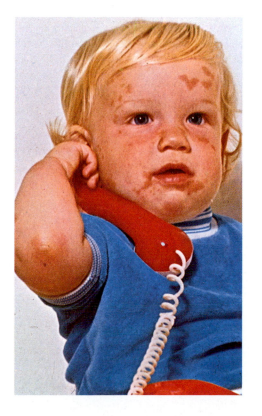

9.122

Urticaria Pigmentosa

Urticaria pigmentosa (bullous mastocytosis) in a 2-month-old girl. Partially crusted vesicles had been noted over the entire body since birth. Over time, these vesicles developed a brown hyperpigmentation. At first, the lesions were thought to be pyoderma, but skin biopsy led to the diagnosis of urticaria pigmentosa. Other areas of the body had macular or papular lesions that developed a dark-yellow or light-brown appearance. As a child, the father had also been diagnosed as having urticaria pigmentosa. The pattern of inheritance is unclear.

Vesicles, macules, papules, and nodular lesions may all be signs of mastocytosis in younger children. Lesions rarely appear after the age of 3 years.

Differential Diagnosis:—The differential diagnosis of urticaria pigmentosa includes juvenile pemphigoid, bullous impetigo, epidermolysis bullosa, incontinentia pigmenti, and bullous congenital ichthyosiform erythroderma.

9.123

Urticaria Pigmentosa

Urticaria pigmentosa in a 3-month-old boy. Several pruritic, maculopapular and vesicular lesions of varying size were noted on the extensor surface of the left thigh. There was no involvement of internal organs or systemic symptoms (diarrhea, tachycardia, flushing). Skin biopsy demonstrated infiltration of mast cells with intracellular metachromatic pigmentation.

Localized mastocytomas occur in about five percent of all cases of mastocytosis. The lesions may be solitary or in groups of vesicles. Lesions may be present at birth or may develop during the first few weeks of life. A generalized rash rarely follows.

9.124

Incontinentia Pigmenti Syndrome

Incontinentia pigmenti syndrome (Block-Sulzberger syndrome) in a 2-month-old girl. Linearly arranged vesicles and red nodules appeared on the flexor surface of both legs during the first month of life and remained for several months. The vesicles contained predominantly eosinophilic granulocytes. Between 6 and 12 months of age, red-brown, hyperpigmented lesions appear in a symmetrical distribution on the arms and legs. These lesions persisted. Fortunately, the child did not develop associated occular or central nervous system abnormalities which are seen in 30% of all patients. No treatment was necessary.

Differential Diagnosis—In the early vesicular stage, incontinentia pigmenti syndrome is difficult to differentiate from pemphigoid. Characteristic of incontinentia pigmentia is eosinophila and, on biopsy of the lesion, eosinophilic infiltrate. Other vesicular or bullous rashes must be ruled out, including epidermolysis bullosa and bullous impetigo. If only pigmentation is present, postinflammatory hypermelanosis (seen in papular urticaria, herpes zoster, lichen rubra planus, and medication induced rashes) as well as other hereditary pigmentation disorders must be differentiated.

9.122

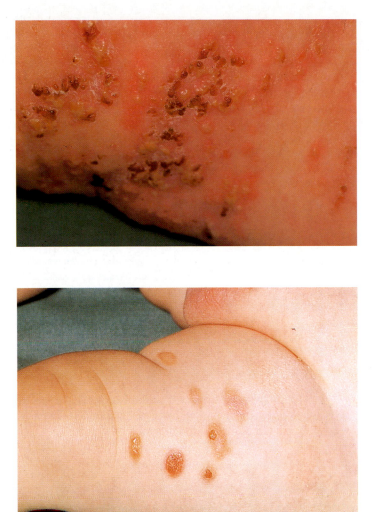

9.123

9.124

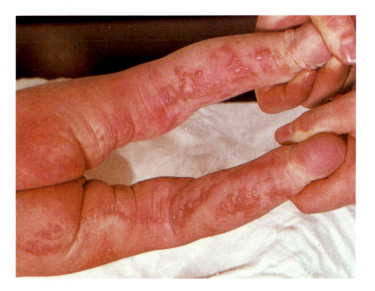

9.125a   9.125b

**Peutz-Jeghers
Syndrome**

Peutz-Jeghers syndrome in a 9-year-old boy. Numerous brown, melanin-containing macules of varying size were found in the areas surrounding the mouth and oral mucous membranes. The condition was present for years, but the diagnosis was made only after the child's father died of the same disease (due to intestinal problems). The boy suddenly developed an ileus due to an intussusception (the lead point being a large intestinal polyp). Further radiologic studies detected more polyps in the small intestine.

Differential Diagnosis—In cases of Addison's disease, the skin over various parts of the body, not only the mucous membranes, is hyperpigmented. Freckles, which may occur in fair-skinned people exposed to sunlight, are never located in the oral cavity. In the case of multiple lentigines syndrome, the mucosa is spared and polyposis of the gastrointestinal tract is absent. In Capute-Rimoin-Konigsmark syndrome (generalized lentigines with deafness) there are no pigmented lesions of the oral mucosa (an almost constant finding in Peutz-Jeghers syndrome). Cronkheit-Canada syndrome (polyposis associated with ectodermal defects including alopecia and nail atrophy) becomes manifest in the fifth or sixth decade of life, whereas the pigmented lesions of Peutz-Jeghers syndrome are either present at birth or develop in early childhood.

9.126a   9.126b

**Malignant
Melanoma**

Malignant melanoma in a 16-year-old boy. An irregular, round, poorly defined, ringlike, nonulcerative lesion (1.5 × 0.5 cm) was found on the back (Figure 9.126a). There was no metastasis to the lymph nodes (stage I). A wide excision of the lesion was performed. The clinical diagnosis was confirmed on histologic examination.

Malignant melanoma (nodular melanoma Figure 9.126b) in a 20-year-old man. A rapidly growing, tangerine-sized, round, red tumor with a brown border arose domelike above the skin. Thick plaques were visible at the peak of the dome. A similar pea-sized tumor was found beside the large tumor. This is a stage II malignant melanoma with regional lymph node metastasis. Many dysplastic nevi were also found on the back and rest of the body.

9.127

Turner Syndrome

Turner syndrome in a 12-year-old girl. Multiple pigmented nevi were noted on the legs. Other findings including pterygium colli, low hairline, shield-shaped thorax, and widely spaced nipples were noted at an earlier age, which led to the presumptive diagnosis of Turner syndrome. Karyotype demonstrated X-monosomy.

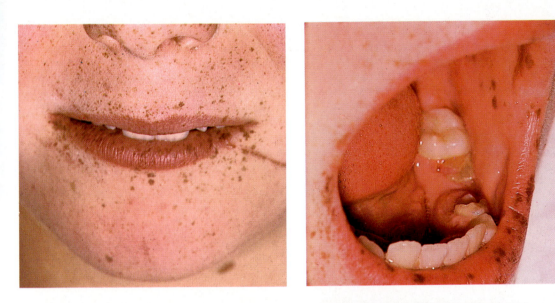

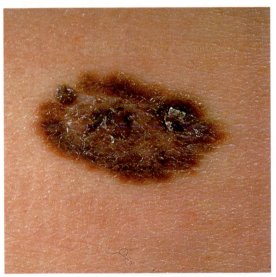
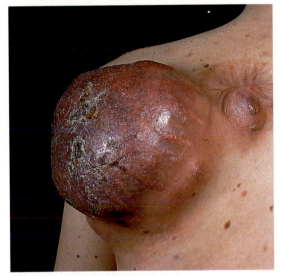

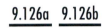

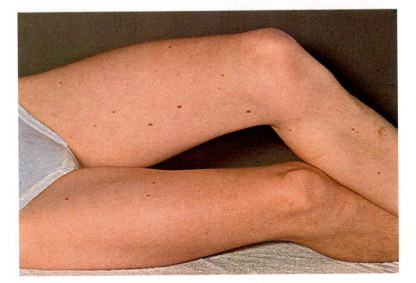

9.128–9.130

Ehlers-Danlos Syndrome

Ehlers-Danlos syndrome (cutis hyperelastica) in a 16-year-old boy. Findings included hyperelastic skin (Figure 9.128) and joints, which were hypermobile, leading to subluxation and gait problems (Figure 9.129). Flat scars with paper-thin scar tissue (Figure 9.130) were seen over the knees as were characteristic subcutaneous hematomas. The hematomas appeared after mild trauma and calcified on resolution.

Ehlers-Danlos syndrome is caused by a defect in collagen and has at least seven different forms that differ in regards to pattern of inheritance, degree of severity, and specific enzyme defect.

Differential Diagnosis—Milder forms of Ehlers-Danlos syndrome can be confused with inherited cutis laxa (diminished elastic tissue). In cases of cutis laxa, the skin hangs down in loose folds; upon being picked up, the skin does not return as quickly to its previous position as does the skin in individuals with Ehlers-Danlos syndrome. Hypermobile joints occur in Marfan syndrome (page 96) and with hydroxylysine-deficient collagen. Easily damaged skin with poor wound healing is characteristic of osteogenesis imperfecta.

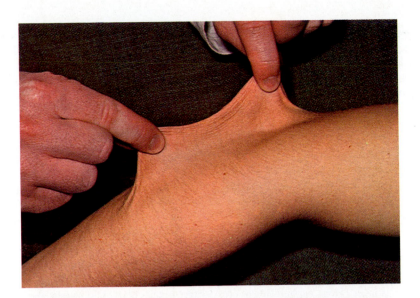

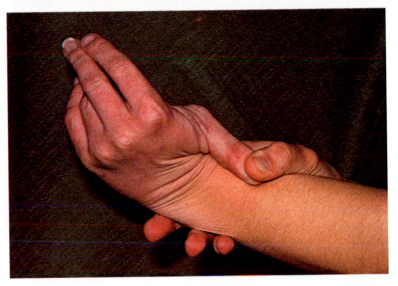

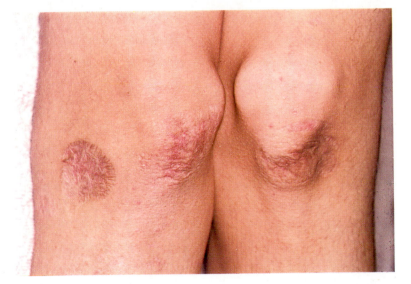

9.131
Epidermolysis Bullosa Simplex

Epidermolysis bullosa simplex in a 6-year-old girl. Ulcerated vesicles and bullae grouped closely together over the back were noted. The mucous membranes and the nails were not affected. The autosomal dominant form of epidermolysis bullosa becomes manifest shortly after birth. After only minimal trauma (rubbing of the skin), vesicles and bullae appear which are fluid-filled and break easily. Biopsy of the skin demonstrates disintegration of the cytoplasm of the cells in the basal layer of the epidermis.

9.132 9.133
Dystrophic Epidermolysis Bullosa

Dystrophic epidermolysis bullosa (recessive inherited form) in a 2-month-old boy. Findings included vesicle and bullous formation with extensive erosion after rupture of the vesicles. These areas gradually healed leaving behind atrophic scars, keloids, and contractures. The skin on the back and on the extremities was most affected. Nikolsky sign was positive (vesicle formation when the skin is rubbed). Dystrophy of the nails was noted leading to loss of some nails. Feeding was complicated by vesicles in the oral cavity. The child had a prolonged hospital course requiring hospitalization until 2 years of age. Frequent secondary bacterial infections required antibiotic treatment.

9.134 9.135
Dermatitis Herpetiformis

Dermatitis herpetiformis in an 11-year-old girl. Groups of vesicles and papules on erythematous base were symmetrically distributed on the extensor surfaces of the extremities, the buttocks, and the neck. The lesions were pruritic, partially excoriated and crusted over. Other affected areas include the knees, the elbows, the shoulders, and the scalp. Typical of dermatitis herpetiformis, the mucous membranes were not involved.

In small children with dermatitis herpetiformis, one finds larger vesicles often in the anogenital area. Excoriation can give rise to large, oozing areas. Dermatitis herpetiformis is chronic and progressive in nature and is frequently complicated by secondary bacterial infection. The etiology is probably autoimmune in nature.

Differential Diagnosis—Dermatitis herpetiformis must be differentiated from scabies, papular urticaria (strophulus), erythema multiforme (with vesicle formation), and atopic dermatitis.

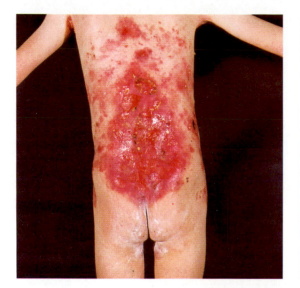

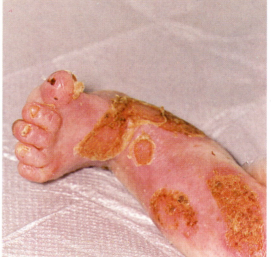

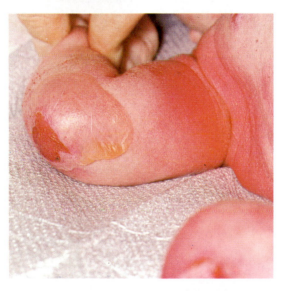

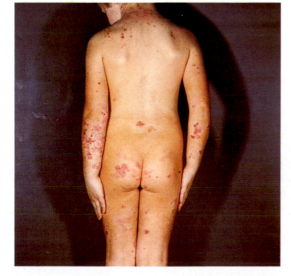

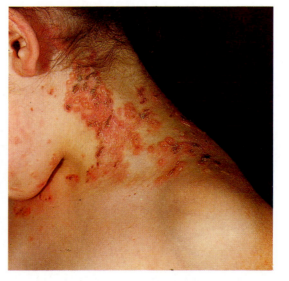

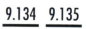

9.136

Ecthyma

Ecthyma in a 10-year-old boy. Crusted, pea-sized pustules on an indurated erythematous base were found on both knees. After loosening of the firmly attached crusts, a poorly defined, purulent ulcer was noted. Culture of these lesions isolated β-hemolytic group A streptococci. After persisting for several weeks, the lesions healed leaving a scarred area.

Ecthyma is frequently located on the legs. Autoinnoculation can cause new lesions to appear. Secondary infection with coagulase-positive staphylococci is possible. In cases of ecthyma gangrenosum, *Pseudomonas aeruginosa* can be detected in the ulcers (during *Pseudomonas* septicemia).

9.137

Bullous Impetigo

Bullous impetigo on the abdomen of a 4-year-old boy. The findings included large, broken, flaccid bullae associated with staphylococcal skin infection. The lesions healed without scarring. Bullous impetigo may also occur in the newborn.

9.138

Bullous Impetigo

Bullous impetigo on the knee of a 14-year-old girl. The large, ruptured bullae was previously filled with cloudy fluid and was now covered with a thin crust and had a narrow, erythematous border. This form of impetigo contagiosa is caused by *Staphylococcus aureus*.

Differential Diagnosis—In older children, the differential diagnosis of bullous impetigo includes erythema multiforme exuditivum, toxic epidermal necrolysis (Lyell syndrome), and other chronic bullous dermatoses. In the newborn, the differential diagnosis includes epidermolysis bullosa, urticaria pigmentosa (bullous mastocytosis), and dermatitis exfoliativa (Ritter's disease).

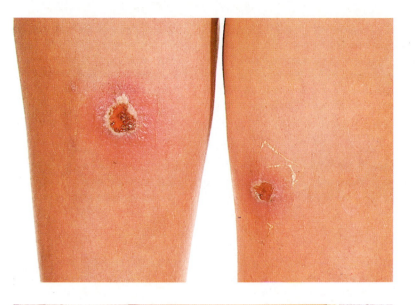

9.136

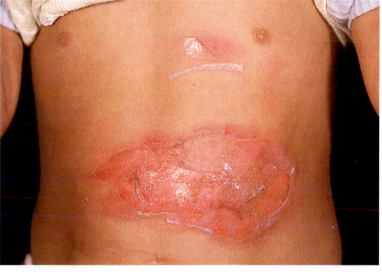

9.137

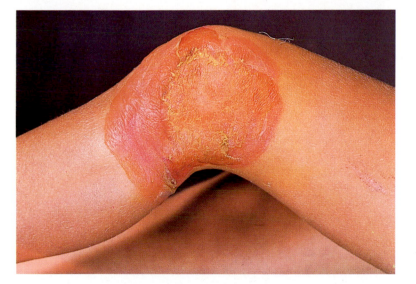

9.138

9.139

Herpes Zoster

Herpes zoster in a 17-year-old girl. Densely clustered, partially confluent, fluid-filled vesicles were evident on an erythematous base. The lesions varied in size and were distributed along a dermatome on half of the torso. The lesions did not cross the midline. After 2 to 3 days, the vesicles ruptured and crusted over. Unlike most adult cases of herpes zoster, the pain in this case was minimal. After treatment with acyclovir, the child gradually recovered. The girl had chickenpox (varicella) when she was 5 years old and now developed herpes zoster due to her compromised immune status (secondary to acute lymphoblastic leukemia).

9.140

Bullous Impetigo

Bullous impetigo in a 10-day-old boy. Several well-defined, flaccid pustules without surrounding erythema were noted on the extensor surface of the fingers. The pustules ruptured and contained *Staphylococcus aureus* (phage group 2). Because of the risk of staphylococcal scalded skin syndrome, systemic treatment with erythromycin was instituted.

9.141

Paronychia

Bacterial paronychia in a 13-year-old girl. A painful, erythematous swelling with a small collection of pus was noted at the base of the thumbnail. The infection was caused by *Staphylococcus aureus.*

In paronychia caused by *Pseudomonas aeruginosa,* a purulent green discharge is noted. Paronychia caused by *Candida* can become chronic and secondarily infected by bacteria. In a candidal infection, the nail is usually brittle and thickened with brown discoloration and fissures.

9.142

Ecthyma

Ecthyma (ecthyma gangrenosum) in an 18-year-old man with leukemia. After a bone marrow transplantation, the patient developed *Pseudomonas* sepsis. Ulcerated, indurated, erythematous skin lesions were noted over the entire body.

Normal children frequently get ecthyma simplex on the lower thighs after an insect bite or a skin abrasion. The initial lesion is a small vesicle or pustule which enlarges within several days, ruptures, and then is covered over with crust. After removal of the crust, a deep ulcer is visible, which heals slowly. Group A β-hemolytic *Streptococcus* is usually the causative agent.

9.139

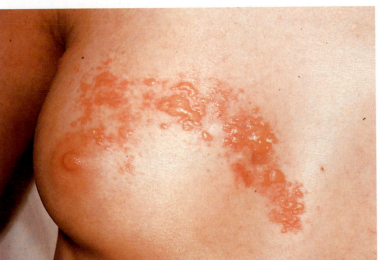

9.140 9.141

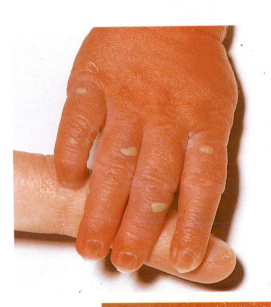

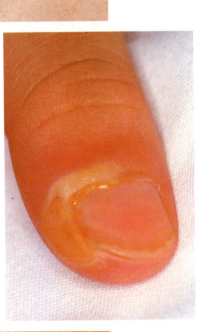

9.142

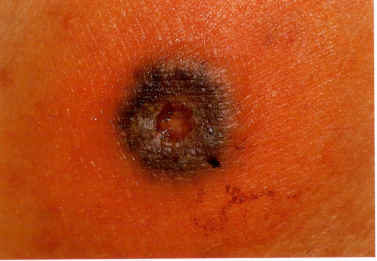

9.143

Erythema Chronicum Migrans

Erythema chronicum migrans (Lyme disease) in a 12-year-old boy. An expanding erythematous annular lesion was noted on the back. The rash appeared to emanate from a tick bite which had a 1 cm wide, indurated, dark red border.

Serum IgM antibodies against *Borrelia burgdorferi* were detected. The illness resolved after a 10-day course of treatment with doxycycline. No late complications were noted (arthritis, carditis, neurologic manifestations).

9.144

Lymphadenosis Benigna Cutis

Lymphadenosis benigna cutis in a 14-year-old girl. A solitary, firm, red, painless nodule, 1.5 cm in diameter, was noted on the right side of the nose after a tick bite. Serum antibodies against *Borrelia* were detected. The 4-week-old lesion resolved after a course of penicillin.

Clinically, lymphadenosis benigna cutis must be distinguished from pyogenic granuloma, malignant lymphoma, and angiolymphoid hyperplasia with eosinophilia. Histologically, lymphadenosis benigna cutis demonstrates a dense infiltrate of histiocytes and lymphocytes in a follicular arrangement.

9.145

Nummular Eczema

Nummular eczema in a 9-month-old boy. Numerous coin-shaped, erythematous, pruritic plaques, varying in size without well-defined borders were found on the upper thighs and on the extensor surfaces of the extremities. These lesions were chronic in nature and recurred despite local treatment.

Tinea corporis, in which the lesions have well-defined, raised borders, can be ruled out through microscopic examination and fungal culture.

9.143

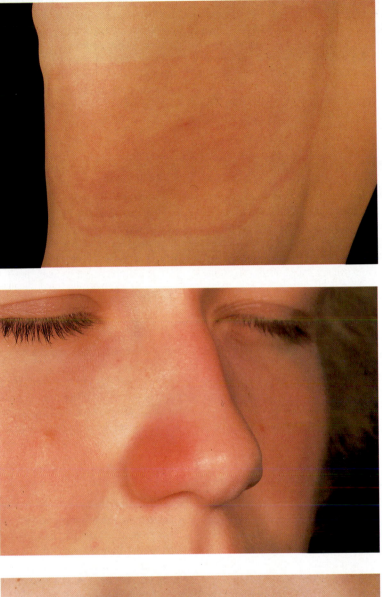

9.144

9.145

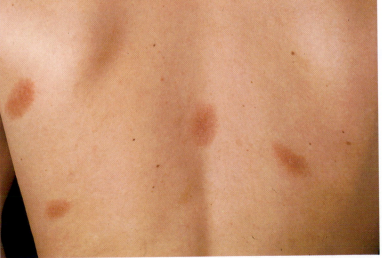

9.146
Impetigo Contagiosa

Impetigo contagiosa on the face of a 4-year-old boy. Numerous ruptured vesicles and pustules covered with a honey-yellow crust, are visible on the face, ears, and neck. Both group A β-hemolytic *Streptococcus* and *Staphylococcus aureus* were cultured. The condition began with the appearance of red macules that quickly changed into thin-walled vesicles and pustules.

Removal of the crusts revealed a red, oozing surface. The lesions responded quickly to antibiotic therapy. Hygienic measures must be emphasized in order to prevent spread of infection to other parts of the body (through autoinnoculation) or to other people.

Differential Diagnosis—The differential diagnosis of impetigo includes varicella, herpes zoster, and herpes simplex infections (which also may be secondarily impetiginized), as well as allergic, contact dermatitis.

9.147
Herpes Zoster

Herpes zoster in a 12-year-old boy. Findings included a crusting, vesicular rash unilaterally in the ophthalmic distribution of the trigeminal nerve (over the forehead, eye, and nose). The rash was associated with severe keratoconjunctivitis, pain, and high fever. Examination of the vesicle contents by electron microscopy revealed giant cells. Remission occurred with topical and systemic treatment with acyclovir. Infection involving the maxillary branch of the trigeminal nerve would affect the cheek and the ipsilateral palate; infection of the mandibular branch would affect the jaw and the ipsilateral aspect of the tongue.

Differential Diagnosis—The absence of neuralgia (especially in children) does not rule out herpes zoster. Immune suppressed patients can develop a generalized zoster infection that cannot be differentiated from varicella. In cases of herpes simplex infection, the skin lesions can mimic zoster so that differentiation is only possible serologically or through viral culture.

9.148
Eczema Herpeticum

Eczema herpeticum in a 15-month-old boy with a previous history of atopic dermatitis. Numerous vesicles which soon became pustular, ulcerated, and crusted, were found behind the ears, on the neck, and in other parts of the body. In addition, there was fever and regional lymphadenitis. Electron microscopy revealed intranuclear inclusion bodies (herpes simplex virus). Serum serology for herpes simplex virus was positive. Remission was achieved with systemic treatment with acyclovir.

The typical skin changes of eczema herpeticum not only occur in previously affected areas, but may spread widely. In cases of recurrent eczema herpeticum, systemic symptoms are lacking and local symptoms may be mild.

9.149
Filliform Warts

Filliform warts (verruca filiformes, a form of verruca vulgaris) on the lips of a 12-year-old girl. Several white, hard, protruding lesions of various size were noted on the lips. These lesions had a course irregular surface on a circumscribed base. Filliform warts occur primarily on the face (eyelids, lips) and on the neck. The causative agents are various human papilloma virus types in the papova group. The warts can be transmitted by direct contact and autoinnoculation.

Differential Diagnosis—Filliform warts must be differentiated from common warts (verruca vulgaris), juvenile flat warts (verruca plana), plantar and palmar warts, as well as warts of the mucous membranes (condylomata acuminata). Verrucous nevi can look like verruca filiformes or digitata, but are usually arranged in a linear fashion.

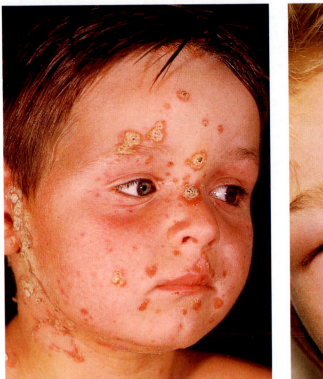
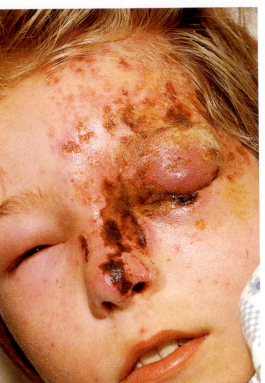

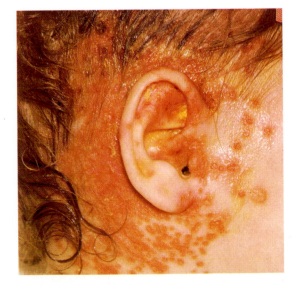
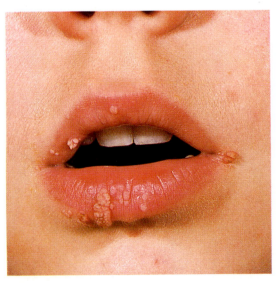

9.150

Cystic Acne

Cystic acne in a 14-year-old boy. A bright red, painful acne cyst 2 cm in diameter was noted on the right cheek. As a rule, cystic acne leaves behind a scar after healing.

9.151

Paronychia

Paronychia in a 12-year-old girl. The lateral aspect of the nail of the left index finger was inflamed, erythematous, swollen, and very painful. Due to worsening of the infection, the nail had to be removed. *Staphylococcus aureus* was cultured from the draining pus.

9.152

Pyogenic Granuloma

Pyogenic granuloma (granuloma telangiectaticum) in a 15-year-old boy. A bean-sized, broad based, dark red nodule was noted at the base of the nail. The lesion had a verrucous surface and bled when touched. Histologic examination ruled out an amelanotic malignant melanoma and confirmed the diagnosis of pyogenic granuloma.

Pyogenic granuloma is a benign vascular tumor originating from the dermis and containing abundant capillaries. It does not heal spontaneously and must be surgically removed. Pyogenic granuloma is most frequently found on the fingers, lips, mouth, trunk, and toes.

9.153

Herpetic Paronychia

Herpetic paronychia in a 4-year-old boy with acute, non-lymphocytic leukemia. Findings included swelling and erythema of the fingertips with vesicle formation on the left thumb and right second and third fingers. Herpes simplex virus was cultured from the contents of the vesicle. The boy, who still sucked his thumbs and fingers, had herpes labialis, which spread to the fingers.

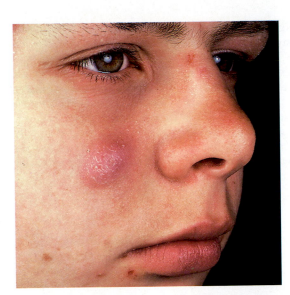

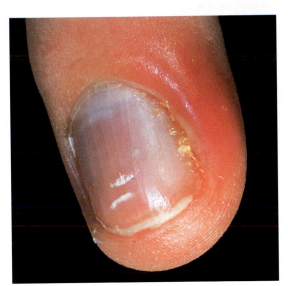
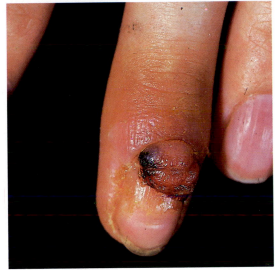

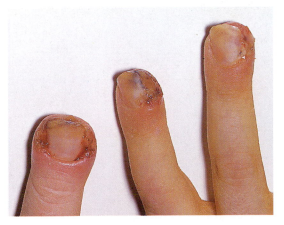

9.154

Aphthous Stomatitis

Aphthous stomatitis in a 15-year-old girl. On the inner aspect of the lower lip there was a solitary, bean-sized ruptured vesicle on a large erythematous base. The lesion was covered by a gray-white membrane. Removal of the membrane revealed an ulcer that was very painful and slow to heal.

The cause of aphthous stomatitis is uncertain and may be related to psychological stress, infection, or trauma. Aphthous stomatitis occurs more frequently in adults and may present as solitary or grouped lesions. As a rule they are localized to their anterior oral cavity and often recur.

Differential Diagnosis—In contrast to aphthous stomatitis, the ulcers of herpes simplex virus gingival stomatitis are numerous, associated with severe gingivitis, and cause regional lymphadenitis and high fever. Bednar's aphthae are usually localized to the lips and caused by trauma. In the case of solitary mucous membrane lesions, primary syphilis and tuberculous ulcerations must be ruled out. In Behcet syndrome, ulcers can be found on all mucous membranes (eyes, mouth, oropharynx, esophagus, stomach, intestines, genitals), and are often associated with erythema nodosum, arthritis, and central nervous system involvement.

9.155

Herpes Simplex

Herpes simplex viral infection of the perianal skin of a 12-year-old girl. Of note were several painful, ruptured vesicles covered by a gray-yellow membrane. The lesions were caused by autoinoculation (the original site of infection was the oral mucosa). The rash was accompanied by high fever and regional lymphadenopathy.

Differential Diagnosis—The differential diagnosis of herpetic lesions depends on the location of the lesions. In cases of vesicular or bullous lesions in the anogenital area, the following must be considered: juvenile pemphigoid, acrodermatitis enteropathica, impetigo, contact dermatitis, and diaper dermatitis.

9.156

Herpes Simplex

Recurrent herpes simplex viral infection of the skin of a 14-year-old girl. Grouped vesicles with local erythema were noted on the face. The girl was afebrile. The lesions resolved without scar formation after 1 week of local treatment with vidarabine.

Differential Diagnosis—Similar skin lesions may be seen with impetigo (with bacteria detected on culture) and herpes zoster.

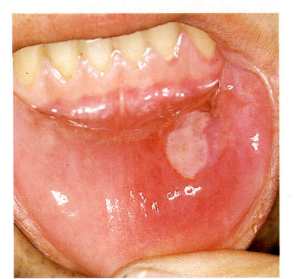

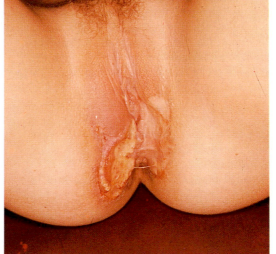

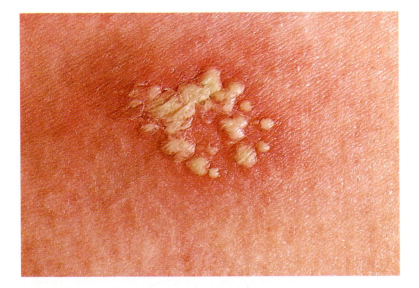

9.157

Aphthous Stomatitis

Aphthous stomatitis in a 4-year-old girl. Numerous ulcers (vesicles which were partially ulcerated and covered with a yellow pseudomembrane) were noted on the oral mucosa and the tongue. The gums were red and swollen. Fever and regional lymphadenopathy was noted. The ulcers were painful and caused the child to refuse food and drink. The lesions resolved after 8 to 10 days of symptomatic treatment.

Differential Diagnosis—Aphthous stomatitis must be differentiated from Coxsackie viral infection (hand-foot-and-mouth disease), Behcet syndrome (page 244), and Stevens-Johnson syndrome (page 172).

9.158

***Candida* Granuloma**

Candida granuloma of the lower lip of a 5-year-old boy (with congenital immunodeficiency). Findings included crusted plaques over the lips.

Differential Diagnosis—*Candida* granuloma must be differentiated from various forms of cheilitis. Cheilitis may be caused by exposure to chemicals (in lip ointments, lipsticks, toothpaste, and mouthwash) or may be due to allergy to foods such as oranges, artichokes, and mangoes.

9.159

Impetigo Contagiosa

Impetigo contagiosa around the mouth of a 2-year-old girl. The child had purulent vesicles around the mouth, which ruptured and became scabbed and crust covered. The lesions cultured *Staphylococcus aureus*. Due to the location of the lesions, eating was very painful and parenteral feeding was necessary for a short period of time.

9.160

Herpes Labialis

Herpes labialis (recurrent herpes simplex viral infection in a 7-year-old boy). A vesicle filled with watery fluid was found on the lower lip; in the left corner of the mouth, several closely grouped vesicles were noted. The lesions resolved 3 days later.

Differential Diagnosis—Cheilitis angularis (also known as perleche) may have numerous causes, including infection with *Staphylococcus aureus*, *Candida albicans*, or other skin diseases such as atopic dermatitis, and seborrheic dermatitis.

9.161 9.162

Coxsackie Viral Infection

Coxsackie viral infection (hand-foot-and-mouth disease) in a 5-year-old girl. Several vesicular and ulcerative lesions were noted in the oral cavity (Figure 9.161) and numerous 3- to 5-mm large pearl-gray vesicles on a narrow erythematous base were noted on both feet (Figure 9.162) and hands. Coxsackie virus A (type 16) was cultured from the vesicles. Fever and a generalized maculopapular rash were associated with these findings. After 1 week, the symptoms disappeared.

Typically, the oral lesions of Coxsackie hand-foot-and-mouth disease are larger than those seen in cases of herpangina. The lesions are scattered irregularly over the palate, the oral mucous membrane, and the tongue. The fever is mild and often lasts only a few days. As a rule, the vesicles on the hand and feet are oval and elongated. They occur primarily on the fingers and toes, the heels, and the palms and soles of the feet. The skin lesions disappear after 2 to 3 days. In young infants, a papular or vesicular generalized rash may occur.

Differential Diagnosis—Coxsackie infections must be differentiated from varicella, herpes simplex, papular urticaria, and scabies.

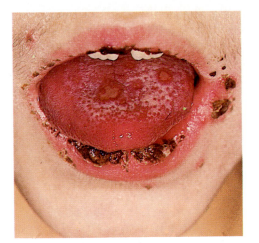

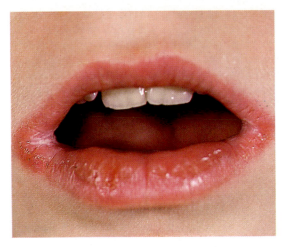

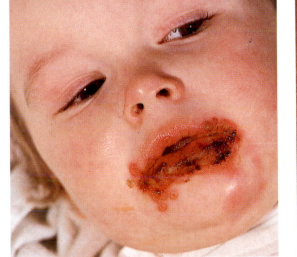

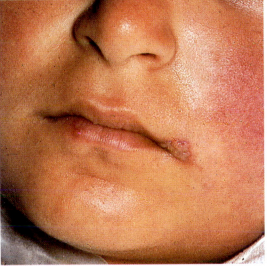

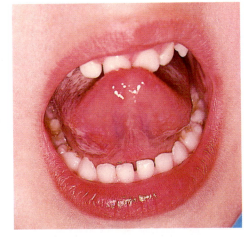

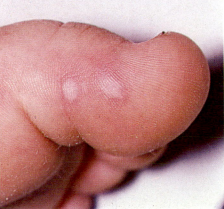

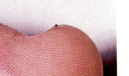

9.163

Molluscum Contagiosum

Molluscum contagiosum in a 14-year-old boy. Numerous 2- to 3-mm pearllike papules with central umbilication were noted on the arm and scattered on the face. Squeezing the molluscum lesion expressed a caseous substance that contained infected epidermal cells and eosinophilic inclusion bodies. Molluscum contagiosum frequently occurs on the face, eyelids, neck, axilla, and genital area. Molluscum contagiosum lesions are rarely solitary and may vary in size from a few millimeters to the size of a pea.

Differential Diagnosis—Microscopically, molluscum contagiosum can be differentiated from certain forms of warts which are similar macroscopically. It may be difficult to differentiate a solitary molluscum lesion from a granuloma telangiectaticum (page 208) or an epithelioma (seldom seen in children). In these cases, histologic examination is required.

9.164

Juvenile Xanthogranuloma

Juvenile xanthogranuloma in an 11-year-old girl. Numerous light-red, firm nodules of varying size were noted on the abdomen and genital area since birth. As is the case in juvenile xanthogranuloma, no hyperlipidemia was noted. Biopsy of the lesions demonstrated characteristic lipid-containing histiocytes and Touton giant cells (multinucleated, vacuolated giant cells with a ring of nuclei and a rim of foamy cytoplasm at the border). Areas frequently affected by juvenile xanthogranuloma are the scalp, the face, and the upper half of the torso. Solitary lesions are rare.

Differential Diagnosis—Juvenile xanthogranuloma must be differentiated from urticaria pigmentosa (papulonodular form), dermatofibroma (page 210), and xanthoma, associated with hyperlipidemia (page 360).

9.165 9.166

Gianotto-Crosti Syndrome

Gianotto-Crosti Syndrome (papular acrodermatitis) in an 18-month-old girl. The child had been ill with rhinitis and pharyngitis 2 weeks prior to the onset of the rash. Numerous red papules approximately 2 mm in diameter appeared on the cheeks and extremities but spared the torso. Areas of the rash were confluent. The eyes and mouth were not affected. Axillary and inguinal lymphadenopathy was noted; during the acute stage, hepatosplenomegaly was also noted. Serum transaminase, IgG, and IgM were elevated, and hepatitis B surface antigen was positive. The cutaneous symptoms resolved without treatment after 4 weeks.

Gianotti-Crosti syndrome is caused by hepatitis B virus.

The cutaneous findings in this case were characteristic regarding morphology, distribution, and duration. There may be no liver involvement. If hepatitis is noted, the infection is usually mild and the patient is anicteric (although progressive icteric forms have been noted). Recovery from hepatitis B infections (with regard to liver involvement) can take 6 months to 4 years.

Differential Diagnosis—Papular acrodermatitis may occur in other viral infections. It could be confused with lichen planus, erythema multiforme, Langhans' cell histiocytosis, and anaphylactoid Henoch-Schönlein purpura.

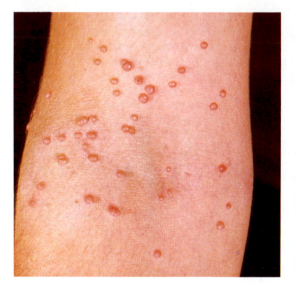
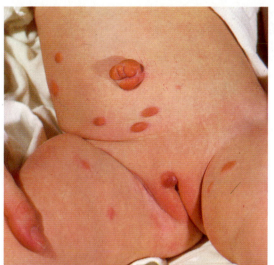

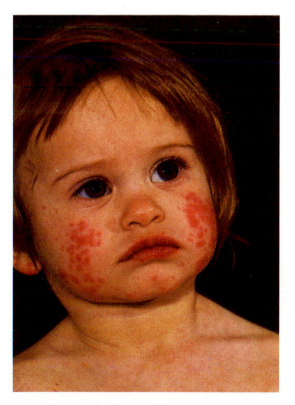
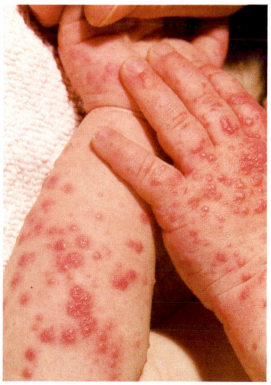

9.167 9.168
Candida Granuloma

Candida granuloma on the face and scalp of a 10-year-old boy. Extensive, crusted, erythematous lesions with partial scaling were noted on the face and scalp. Similar lesions were found on the underarms and lower thighs. The underlying cause of the infection was a severe, combined immune deficiency syndrome (Swiss type). Local treatment with nystatin was ineffective. Resolution followed systemic therapy with antifungal agents. *Candida* granuloma is an expression of chronic fungal infection associated with immune suppression. The face, scalp, as well as other parts of the body are frequently affected.

9.169
Chronic Candidiasis

Chronic candidiasis of the scalp and the ears in an 8-year-old boy with congenital immune deficiency syndrome. The scalp was thickened, erythematous, and scaly. *Candida* was identified as the causative agent through microscopic examination and fungal culture. It is important to differentiate this condition from infections caused by *Trichophyton* and *Microsporum*.

9.170
Tinea Corporis

Tinea corporis on the face of a 12-year-old boy. Numerous sharply outlined, partially confluent disc-shaped erythematous lesions with slight scaling were noted on the face. The border of the lesions was slightly raised, and the center was beginning to heal. *Trichophyton rubron* was detected microscopically and through culture (obtained from the edge of the lesion). The condition resolved after 3 weeks of topical tolnaftate treatment.

Differential Diagnosis—Differential diagnosis discussed on page 252.

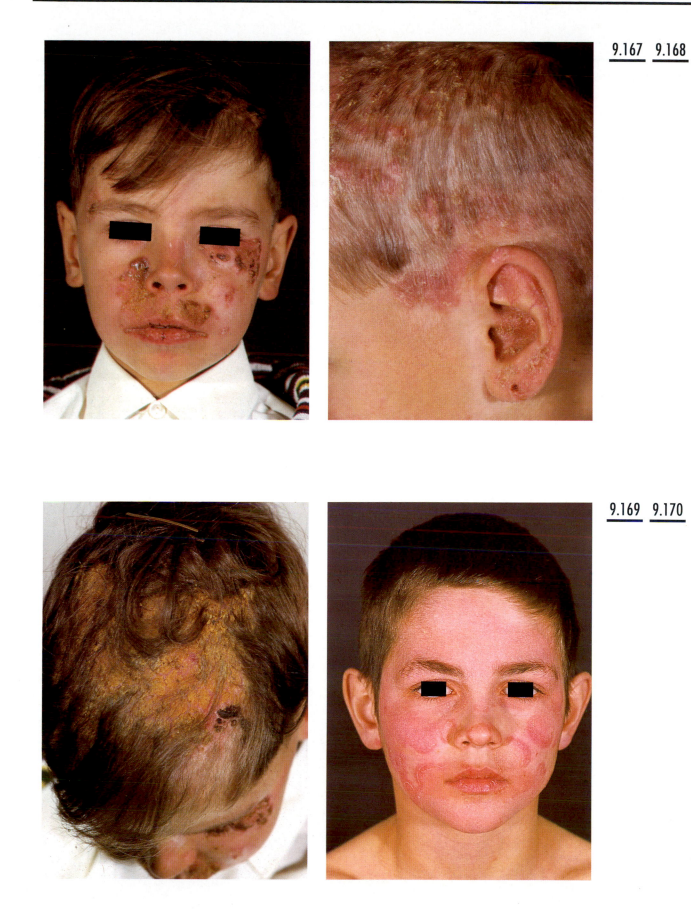

9.171

Tinea Corporis

Tinea corporis in an 8-year-old boy. Ring-shaped, slightly scaling erythematous lesions were found on the back. These lesions persisted for weeks and were caused by *Trichophyton mentagrophytes*. The specific agent causing tinea corporis cannot be identified from the skin changes alone. The most frequent agents associated with tinea corporis are *Trichophyton rubrum*, *Trichophyton mentagrophytes*, and *Microsporum canis*. In this child, the infection was apparently contracted through direct contact with his infected brother.

9.172

Tinea Corporis

Tinea corporis on the face of a 13-year-old girl. Dry, erythematous, scaly papules had spread centrifugally in the course of 4 weeks. The lesions healed without scar formation after topical treatment with miconazole nitrate.

9.173

Tinea Corporis

Tinea Corporis on the chin of a 3-year-old boy. The pruritic, scaling, erythematous rash was caused by *Microsporum canis* (detected by fungal culture). Tinea corporis must be distinguished from granuloma annulare (page 176), atopic dermatitis (particularly nummular eczema), psoriasis (page 218), seborrheic dermatitis, and pityriasis rosea. Initially, pityriasis rosea may look similar to tinea corporis, but pityriasis rosea has a different distribution and will heal without treatment in 6 to 9 weeks. When a fungal lesion is lichenified, it may be confused with lichen planus. Candidiasis and tinea versicolor (due to *Malassezia furfur*) must also be ruled out.

9.174

Tinea Corporis

Tinea corporis in a 9-year-old boy. Pruritic ring-shaped erythematous skin lesions on the neck and chest were caused by *Microsporum canis* (from contact with an infected dog). Characteristic of tinea corporis are the ring-shaped lesions with erythematous scaling borders. The lesions resolved after local treatment with clotrimazole.

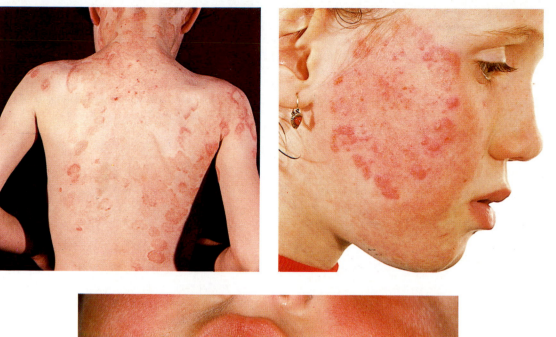

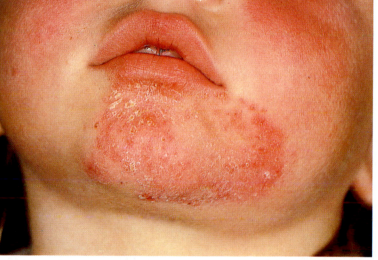

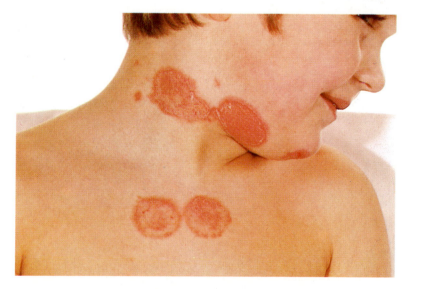

9.175

Tinea Capitis

Tinea capitis on the scalp of a 5-year-old boy. Confluent areas of alopecia with remains of broken, brittle hair were evident on the erythematous scaling scalp. The area was extremely pruritic. When examined with a Wood's lamp, the affected scalp appeared green. *Microsporum audouinii* was identified as the causative agent. Transmission of the fungus occurs by contact with infected hair or epithelial cells (for example, on a comb).

Differential Diagnosis—The differential diagnosis includes alopecia areata (page 276), trichotillomania (page 278), Menke syndrome (kinky hair disease) (associated with seborrheic dermatitis), psoriasis, and impetigo (with underlying crust formation). Pityriasis simplex capitis (scaling of otherwise normal skin) can occur together with alopecia areata. Pathologic scaling or hair loss exists in pityriasis amiantacea, which can appear secondarily on the scalp after bacterial dermatitis or lichen ruber planus.

9.176

Tinea Capitis

Tinea capitis on the scalp of a 10-year-old girl. Hair loss was noted in a 5 × 6 cm area which was inflamed and covered with silvery scales. The remaining hair in the center of the lesion appeared green in a Wood's lamp. The causative agent was *Microsporum canis*.

9.177

Tinea Capitis

Tinea capitis is a 7-year-old boy. Patchy alopecia was noted. The superficial infection on the scalp was caused by *Trichophyton tonsurans*. Typical of *T. tonsurans* infections, there were multiple centers that were angular rather than round. Microscopically, a chain of fungal spores inside the hair shaft could be identified (endothrix). The hair failed to fluoresce under a Wood's lamp (whereas in cases of favus caused by *Trichophyton schoenleinii*, a dark-green fluorescence is noted and with *Microsporum* infections, a light-green fluorescence is noted). The lesion resolved after eight weeks of therapy with systemic griseofulvin.

Differential Diagnosis—Discoid lupus, which can lead to localized hair loss, should be considered in the differential diagnosis.

9.178

Tinea Capitis

Tinea capitis with severe inflammatory response (kerion) in an 11-year-old boy. A palm-sized, swollen, erythematous area with pustules and honey-yellow crusting was noted on the scalp. The hair had fallen out from this area. Microscopically, fungal spores distributed around the hair shaft (ectothrix) were visible. Fungal culture demonstrated an infection with *Trichophyton verrucosum*.

9.179

Tinea Versicolor

Tinea versicolor in a 15-year-old girl. Irregular, small, red-brown macules covered with fine scales were noted. The lesions were partially confluent and nonpruritic. The thickened covering could be scraped off with a spatula ("wood-shaving phenomenon"). The lesions were located primarily on the neck, the chest, and the upper arms. The affected areas of skin did not tan when exposed to sunlight. Microscopically, small thick-walled spores and many short, thick hyphae were visible. Under a Wood's lamp, the affected hair had a golden yellow fluorescence.

Differential Diagnosis—Tinea versicolor must be differentiated from seborrheic dermatitis, parapsoriasis, ichthyosis vulgaris, and other fungal infections of the skin. Erythrasma (scaling erythematous macules in the groin and axilla which have a coral-red fluorescence under a Wood's lamp) occurs in adolescence and must be ruled out. Pityriasis rosea is similar in appearance, but differs from tinea versicolor in that it begins suddenly with a herald patch, is pruritic, and has a tendency toward lichenification.

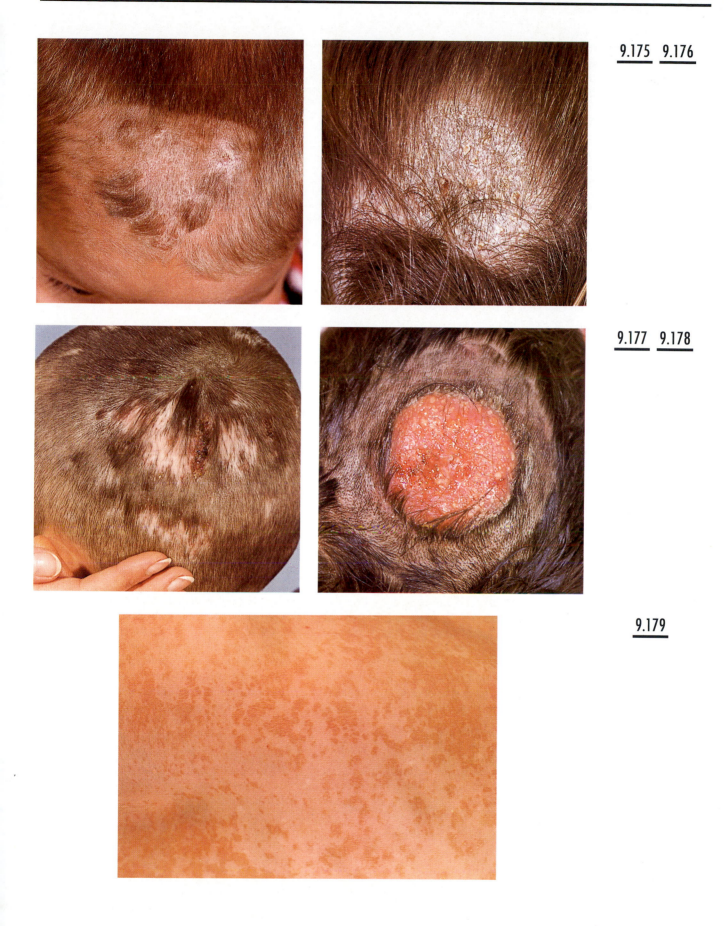

9.180

Scabies

Scabies in a 4-month-old child. An extensive, maculopapular, vesicular, and urticarial rash was noted on the trunk and extremities of this child. The lesions persisted for four weeks. Scabies is caused by an infestation with mites. Burrows, with a dark point at the entrance and a light point at the blind end, were noted. The child's mother had similar lesions. Confirmation of the diagnosis was made by detecting mites microscopically (after removing the mite from the burrow with a blunt needle and examining it under the microscope). Scabies frequently affects the flexor surfaces of the extremit-

ies, the interdigital spaces, the groin, and the axilla. In the infants and small children, the hands, the soles of the feet, the neck, and the face may also be affected. Scabies frequently leads to eczematization (with vesicle formation in infants and a papular rash in older children) and impetiginization (secondary bacterial infection causing pustules).

Differential Diagnosis—Skin lesions similar to scabies may be found in atopic dermatitis, pediculosis, and other forms of dermatitis.

9.181

Scabies

Scabies in a 4-year-old girl. Numerous intensely pruritic vesicles and papules were noted over the hand with interdigital eczematization. Treatment consisted of application of 1% γ-benzahydroxychloride and a complete change of undergarments and linen. A short course of corticosteroid cream was

necessary for the eczematized lesions. Despite killing the mites, pruritis can persist for some time. Concurrent treatment of infected family members is important in order to stop the spread of the infestation.

9.182

Scabies

Scabies in a 5-month-old infant. Many pruritic maculopapular lesions and some vesicular lesions were noted. Typical

burrows were seen on the dorsal side of the foot, on the sole, and over the flexor surface of the extremities.

9.183

Cutaneous Larva Migrans

Cutaneous larva migrans in a 16-year-old boy. Of note, was a 3–4 cm long, 2–3 mm wide, snakelike, erythematous band located on the dorsum of the foot. The lesion was intensely pruritic. Cutaneous larva migrans is caused by penetration of the hookworm larva into the deeper layers of the epidermis. The infection is usually the result of running barefoot

in sand contaminated by canine feces. Eczematization and impetiginization of the rash may occur. In this case, local treatment with thiabendazol was successful.

Differential Diagnosis—Differential diagnosis should include larva currens (caused by *Strongyloides stercoralis*) and myiasis (caused by the larvae of certain Diptera).

9.184

Tinea Pedis

Tinea pedis (athlete's foot) in a 15-year-old boy. Extensive fissures and maceration were found between the third and fourth toes of the right foot. The affected areas are intensely pruritic and odorous.

Tinea pedis is most frequently caused by *Trichophyton rubrum*, *Trichophyton mentagrophytes*, and *Epidermophyton floccosum*. These agents may be detected microscopically or in culture. Treatment consists of a fungicidal ointment.

Athlete's foot may be acquired at public swimming pools, showers, or by the use of footwear that does not permit free flow of air. Secondary bacterial infection is possible (erysipelas due to *Streptococcus*) as well as multiple fungal infections (*Trichophyton* or *Candida albicans*).

Differential Diagnosis—The differential diagnosis includes interdigital corns and calluses as well as erythrasma (without the fissures seen in interdigital mycosis).

9.185

Tinea Pedis

Tinea pedis in a 16-year-old girl. Maceration and extreme scaling was found in the interdigital areas. Fungi were detected microscopically.

Differential Diagnosis—Differential diagnosis includes contact dermatitis, atopic dermatitis, *Candida* dermatitis, dyshidrotic eczema.

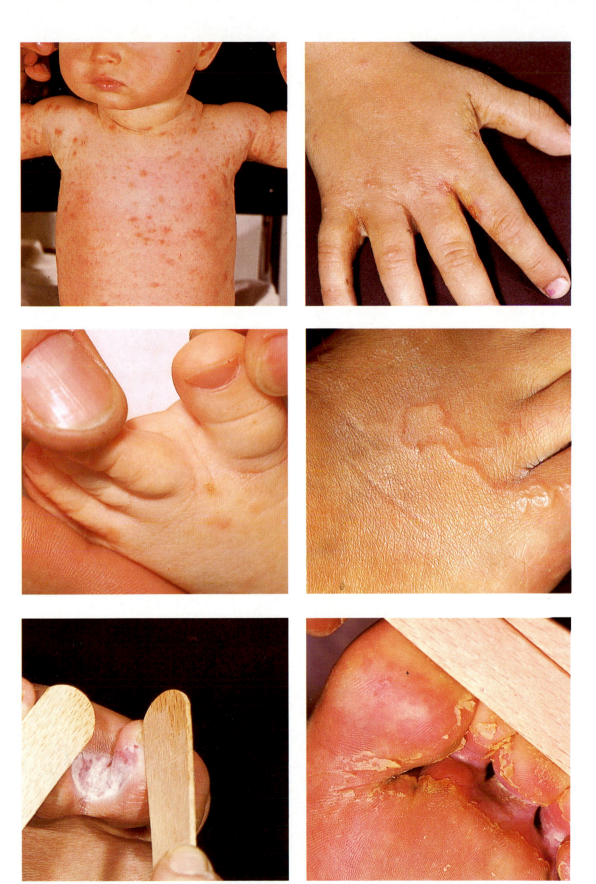

9.186

Pili Torti

Pili torti (twisted hair) in a 3-year-old girl. Short, extremely brittle hair had been present for 2 years. The hair was blonde and shiny. Microscopic examination demonstrated that the hair shaft was twisted along the long axis and indented and flattened at irregular intervals. No other family members were affected with pili torti. The mode of inheritance is variable (sporadic, autosomal dominant, or autosomal recessive).

Pili torti may be seen in Menke syndrome (kinky hair disease) (page 362). Menke syndrome is caused by excessive tissue binding of copper and is associated with retarded growth and development. In this case, the child's serum copper level was normal and the child's mental development was normal. Pili torti is also seen in Bjornstad syndrome (with congenital deafness) and Crandall syndrome (deafness and hypogonadism). Other causes of congenital hair anomalies include congenital trichorrhexis nodosa and monilethrix. Both of these conditions begin with brittle hair and may lead to partial alopecia. In cases of trichorrhexis nodosa, microscopic nodular swellings along the hair shaft are seen at irregular intervals. The hair can be easily broken at these nodules. In cases of monilethrix, the hair is dry, dull, and brittle. Microscopically, regular ball-shaped swelling are seen in the hair shaft between which the hair is thinned and friable. Trichorrhexis nodosa occurs as an acquired disorder that is caused by trauma (inappropriate combing). Monilethrix is an autosomal condition.

9.187

Pediculosis Pubis

Nits (eggs) of pediculosis pubis (crab lice) in the eyelashes of a 7-year-old boy. Numerous intensely pruritic macules, papules, and urticarial lesions were noted on the abdomen, upper thigh, and axilla. Both the eggs and crab lice were easily seen in the hairs with the aid of a magnifying glass. On the skin, the crab lice were visible as small brown dots resembling freckles. Paraffin oil was rubbed into the eyelids twice a day for a week, which caused the nits to fall out.

9.188

Pediculosis Capitis

Gray-white nits from pediculosis capitis in the hair of a 5-year-old girl. Impetiginized bites were seen on the temples, behind the ear, and on the neck. The lesions were intensely pruritic. The nits from the head lice were oval and covered, unlike the nits from crab lice. The nits of head lice cling to the hair firmly, unlike the scales of seborrheic dermatitis or the residue from hairspray. Differentiation of the nits from the hair findings in distal trichorrhexia nodosa is possible by means of microscopic examination. The nits were removed by careful combing of the hair with vinegar water. The child was treated with local application of a pyrethrin preparation as well as antibiotic therapy for secondary bacterial infection.

9.186

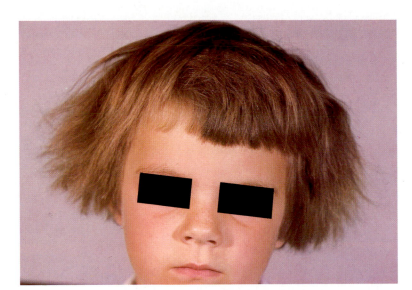

9.187

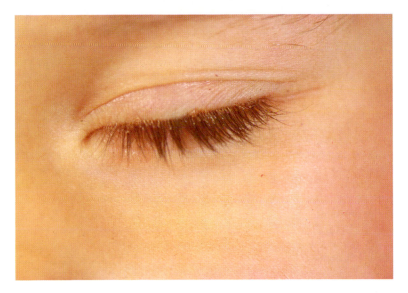

9.188

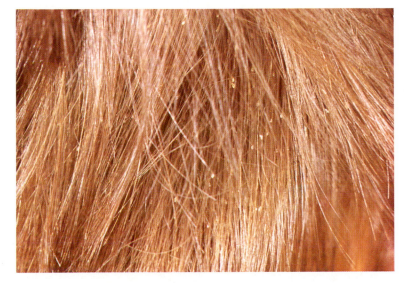

9.189

Geographic Tongue

Geographic tongue (lingula geographica) in a 10-year-old girl. Two large, irregularly shaped, well-defined red areas with slightly raised white borders were noted on the tongue. These lesions are formed by desquamation of the filiform papillae, causing the fungiform papillae to appear more prominent. Characteristically, the areas of desquamation mi-grated over the surface of the tongue during the course of several weeks. Histology demonstrates inflammatory changes, the cause of which is uncertain. The condition may last for several months or years. Fissures of the tongue are often noted. The sensation of burning may also occur.

9.190

Glossitis

Median rhomboid glossitis in an 18-year-old girl. A well-defined, pea-sized, smooth, red lesion was noted on the dorsum of the tongue, immediately anterior to the papillae vallatae. The lesion was associated with a burning sensation.

The affected part of the tongue is usually free of papillae and is rhombic or oval. The lesions are always found on the dorsal surface of the tongue and may have a verrucous surface. There may be transient inflammation and discomfort. Median rhomboid glossitis apparently stems from a developmental anomaly (persistence of the tuberculin impar). Other theories propose that median rhomboid glossitis (which usually does not appear until adulthood) is related to a hamartoma. Biopsy (performed in order to rule out carcinoma) can lead to significant bleeding.

9.191

Mucous Retention Cyst

Mucous retention cyst (mucocele) of the tongue in a 2-month-old boy. A taut elastic pea-sized growth that contained mucous was noted on the underside of the tongue. The lesion was removed surgically.

Mucous retention cysts frequently occur as a result of trauma. Traumatic disruption of the mucous gland duct leads to retention of secretions in the tissue. A border forms, consisting of granulation tissue or connective tissue, but seldom is truly epithelialized. The cysts often have a blue color and may be located on the lip, the floor of the mouth (ranula), the oral mucous membrane, or the tongue. They are sometimes mistaken for hemangiomas.

9.192

Lichen Planus

Lichen planus of the oral mucous membranes in a 17-year-old boy. Erythema of the oral mucous membrane (due to epithelial atrophy) with characteristic white papules forming a linear or reticulated network (Wickham's striae) were noted. Pruritic polygonal, flat, erythematous slightly shiny papules were also noted on the inner aspect of the upper thigh. Scratching in this area produced a linear array of papules (positive Koebner's phenomenon). The condition began suddenly and spread over the flexor surfaces of the hands and the underarm. The etiology is unclear. The diagnosis of lichen planus can be confirmed by skin biopsy. The disease can last for weeks or years and may recur. Topical corticosteroid preparations have proven successful. Antihistamines are often prescribed for relief of the pruritis.

Differential Diagnosis—Superficial *Candida* infections of the mouth must be considered. The changes in the oral mucous membranes can resemble those of systemic lupus erythematosus (which is chronic and progressive in nature). In adults, leukoplakia (white plaques which cannot be removed by rubbing) and syphilitic plaques (seen in secondary syphilis) should also be considered.

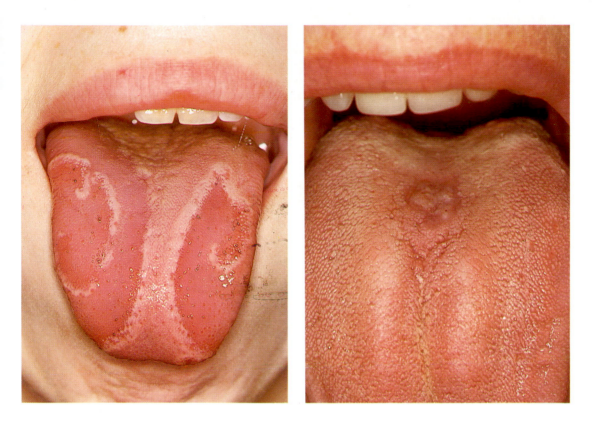

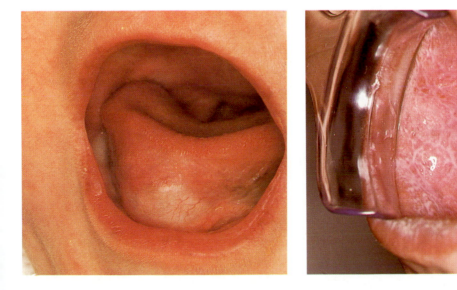

9.193

Subcutaneous Fat Necrosis

Subcutaneous fat necrosis in a 12-day-old newborn. The lesions were not detected until the ninth day of life. Extensive purple discoloration and swelling of the skin was noted over the back. The underlying tissue was diffusely hardened, but not painful.

Differential Diagnosis—Subcutaneous fat necrosis must be distinguished from sclerema neonatorum and "neonatal cold injury." With sclerema neonatorum, there is progressive hardening of the subcutaneous tissue associated with serious illness in the newborn. The involved areas are hard and nonpitting. The palms and soles of the feet are spared. In cases of neonatal cold injury, the face is reddened and there is pitting edema on the body. Neonatal cold injury occurs in the newborn after prolonged cold exposure.

9.194

Insulin Lipodystrophy

Localized insulin lipodystrophy in an 11-year-old with diabetes mellitus. Dimplelike depressions in the soft tissue of the upper thigh were caused by atrophy of subcutaneous adipose tissue due to frequent insulin injections.

9.195

Vitiligo

Extensive vitiligo (acquired pigment deficiency of the skin) on the back and on the extensor surface of the upper thigh in a 10-year-old boy. Numerous, irregularly shaped, white lesions with partially hyperpigmented borders were noted. The lesions had recently increased in size. The areas primarily affected include the face (especially the eyes and perioral areas), genitals, hands, feet, elbows, knees, and chest. When the scalp is involved, hair in the affected area may lose pigment. A familial incidence has been observed. The cause of vitiligo is unclear and may be related to trauma or to an autoimmune process. Vitiligo occurs more frequently in patients with hyperthyroidism, adrenal insufficiency, and diabetes mellitus. The course is variable. Spontaneous remission is possible.

Differential Diagnosis—The differential diagnosis includes the following:

1. Nevus anaemicus (congenital deficiency of terminal blood vessels in circumscribed area)
2. Nevus achromicus (poorly defined, bright yellow skin lesions due to deficient melanin formation)
3. Multiple depigmented skin lesions associated with tuberous sclerosis (page 306)
4. Partial albinism (congenital, autosomal dominant condition with white forelock and depigmented skin on forehead)
5. Waardenburg syndrome (cutaneous hypopigmentation, page 278)
6. Hypomelanosis of Ito (incontinentia pigmenti achromicans: bizarre, depigmented skin pattern, present since birth, associated with ocular abnormalities and central nervous system disorders)
7. Acquired skin disorders associated with hypopigmented macules such as pityriasis alba, tinea versicolor (page 254), scleroderma (page 166), and lichen sclerosis (page 116).

9.196

Keloid

Keloid developed after second-degree burns on the hands of an 11-year-old boy. The lesion was a 4×6 cm, firm, red scar with stretched shiny skin, causing restriction of finger movement.

Keloids may develop during wound healing. Frequently, keloids are located on the sternum, the neck, the face, or the ear (after ear piercing). Treatment consists of repeated injections of corticosteroids as well as surgical excision and skin transplantation. In contrast to keloids, hypertrophic scars remain restricted to the wound area.

9.197

Perniosis

Perniosis (skin changes caused by the inability to adjust to temperature fluctuations) in a 15-year-old girl. Two silver dollar-sized, blue-red, doughy pruritic swellings (erythrocyanosis crurum puellarum) were noted on the outer aspect of the lower right leg. Perniosis is a vascular response to cold injury. The onset is sudden with gradual remission over the course of 2 weeks. In children, the prognosis is generally good.

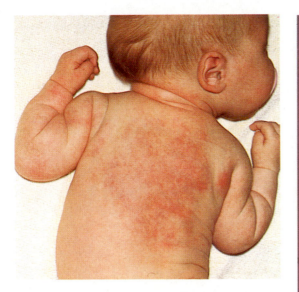

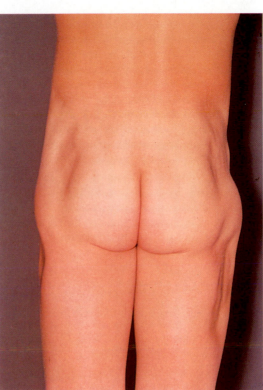

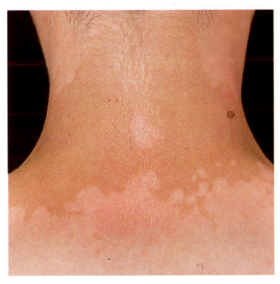

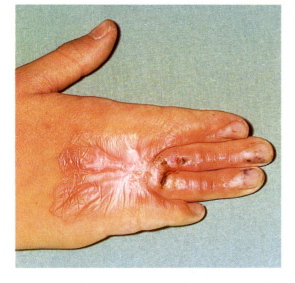

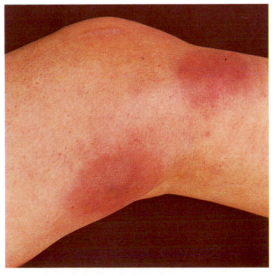

9.198
Acanthosis Nigricans

Benign acanthosis nigricans in a 10-year-old girl. The affected skin had a velvety texture with hyperpigmentation and was found on the shoulders, the nape of the neck, the axilla, the groin, and the inner aspect of the thighs and knees. Mucous membranes were not affected.

Benign acanthosis nigricans is a congenital anomaly inherited as an autosomal dominant trait. At first, the skin is dry, rough, and deeply pigmented; later, the skin is thickened and covered by small papillomatous elevations and develops a gray-brown or black discoloration. Benign acanthosis nigricans must be differentiated from malignant acanthosis nigricans (which occurs in conjunction with adenocarcinoma) and from pseudoacanthosis nigricans (which occurs in obese individuals). In cases of Addison's disease, hyperpigmentation of the skin is not associated with changes in skin texture. Erythrasma, which is found on flexor surfaces and is symmetric in distribution, is easily recognized by typical red fluorescence under a Wood's lamp.

9.199   9.200
Pseudoxanthoma Elasticum

Pseudoxanthoma elasticum in a 12-year-old girl. Numerous flat, yellow papules, 1–3 mm in size, were linearly arranged in the folds of the neck. The lesions increased in number and gave the skin a velvety texture. Lesions were also found in the axilla, groin, and the flexor aspects of the elbows and knees. In this case, the mucous membranes of the oral cavity, rectum, and vagina were not involved. Pseudoxanthoma elasticum may be associated with visual disturbances, or other ophthalmologic problems as well as circulatory problems including hypertension.

The underlying defect in this hereditary disease is unknown. Four different forms of the disorder have been described. Degenerative changes and calcium deposition occur in the elastic fibers of the skin and blood vessels. No specific therapy for the disorder is known. The diagnosis is confirmed through biopsy.

9.201
Pseudoxanthoma Elasticum

Pseudoxanthoma elasticum in an 18-year-old man. Fundu-scopic examination of the eye revealed characteristic yellow, vessellike branching streaks (angioid streaks) caused by the degeneration of Bruch's membrane. Vascular involvement was noted in other organs including the brain, the heart, and the extremities. Typical skin changes were present (numerous yellow papules). This is an example of the autosomal dominant inherited type I form of the disease, which has an unfavorable prognosis.

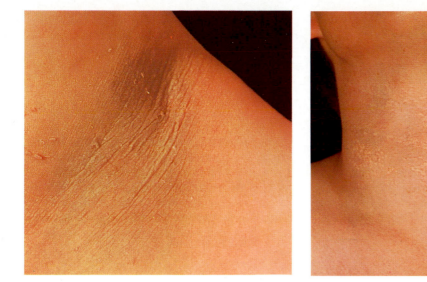

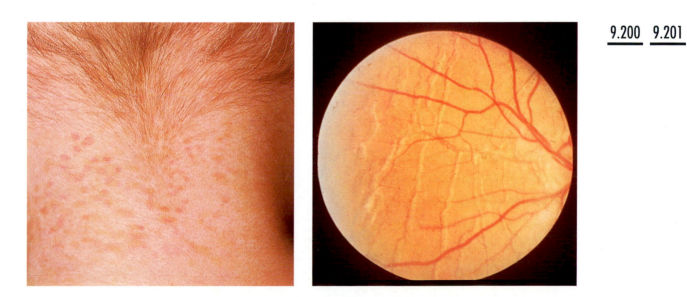

9.202

Erythema Elevatum Diutinum

Erythema elevatum diutinum in a 13-year-old boy. Numerous red, partly rounded, nodular lesions with central indentation were noted on the forearms, hands, and legs. The skin findings were chronic and progressive in nature, and are probably related to an allergic condition.

Differential Diagnosis—Differential diagnosis includes granuloma annulare, hypertrophic lichen planus, and sarcoidosis.

9.203

Erythema Annulare Centrifugum

Erythema annulare centrifugum in a 14-year-old girl. Numerous partly ring-shaped, erythematous, and edematous lesions of varying size were noted. The centers of these lesions tended to fade, and the lesions spread centrifugally. The lesions were located on the covered parts of the body where one is prone to perspiration. Erythema annulare centrifugum

(or marginatum) develops rapidly and can last for weeks or months. The cause is usually unclear. It occurs in approximately 10 percent of rheumatic fever cases. Because the border of the erythematous lesions can be slightly scaly, erythema annulare centrifugum must be differentiated from a fungal skin infection (either microscopically or by culture).

9.204

Erythema Annulare Centrifugum

Erythema annulare centrifugum in a 10-year-old boy. Several small, erythematous, slightly scaly lesions were noted on the

left shoulder; later, the lesions became ring- and garland-shaped.

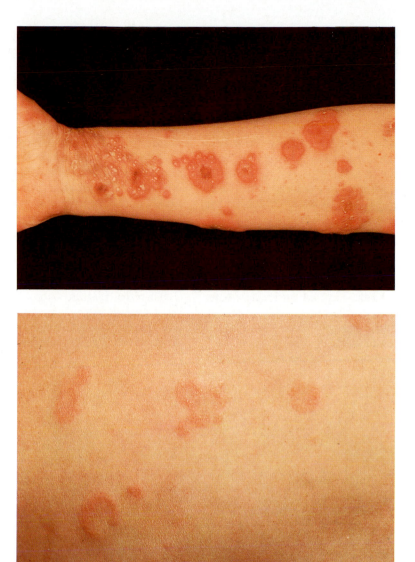

9.202

9.203

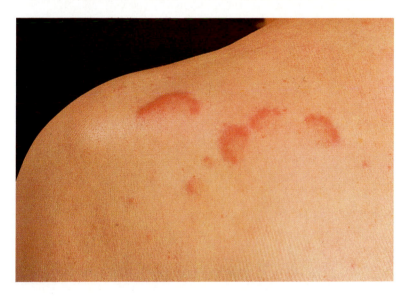

9.204

9.205

Cirrhosis of the Liver

Cirrhosis of the liver due to glycogen storage disease type IV in a 1-year-old girl. Palmar erythema was present on both hands as a result of vasodilation and increased circulation. The diagnosis of glycogen storage disease type IV was confirmed histologically and through enzyme studies. Cirrhosis of the liver with portal hypertension was confirmed at autopsy.

9.206 9.207

Lesch-Nyhan Syndrome

Lesch-Nyhan syndrome in a 4-year-old boy. The findings included chronic damage to the lower lip caused by biting (Figure 9.206), mutilation of the fingers, and marked shortening of the right index finger due to scar contracture (Figure 9.207). These injuries were all due to self-inflicted bite wounds. The child was severely mentally retarded, had cerebral palsy, short stature, and self destructive behavior. The diagnosis was confirmed by the detection of hyperuricemia in the absence of hypoxanthine guanine phosphoribosyltransferase activity in the erythrocytes.

9.208

Juvenile Xanthogranuloma

Juvenile xanthogranuloma in a 4-month-old boy. Multiple, poorly defined, yellow-brown, flat nodules suddenly appeared in the area of the head and trunk and persisted for over one month. Histologic examination revealed lipid containing histiocytes and Touton giant cells. Spontaneous regression of the lesions occurred later in the course of illness.

Juvenile xanthogranulomas are harmless but should not be overlooked, since there is an apparent association with neurofibromatosis.

Differential Diagnosis—The differential diagnosis includes papulonodular urticaria pigmentosa, dermatofibromas, leukemic infiltrates, histiocytosis X, and xanthomas associated with hyperlipoproteinemia.

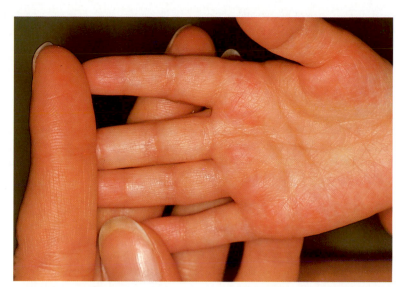

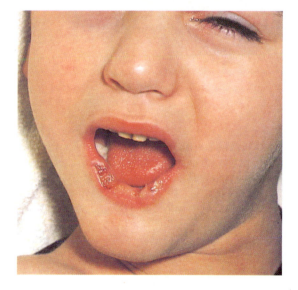

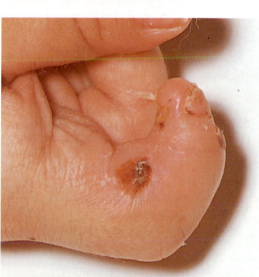

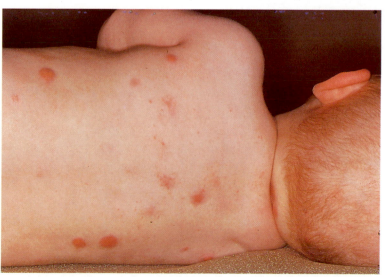

9.209

Atrophoderma Vermiculatum

Atrophoderma vermiculatum (keratosis pilaris with resulting atrophy) in a 2-year-old infant. Linear erythematous lesions with hyperkeratosis were noted on the right cheek. Atrophic skin remained after the hyperkeratotic areas were removed.

9.210

Keloid

Keloid on the neck of a 5-year-old boy. The elongated, erythematous, elevated, sharply demarcated lesion limited movement of the neck. The lesion formed due to excessive reaction of the connective tissue to minimal trauma in a particularly predisposed individual. Keloids occur frequently in the area of the sternum or the ear.

9.211

Anhidrotic Ectodermal Dysplasia

Anhidrotic ectodermal dysplasia (Christ-Siemens-Touraine syndrome) in a 9-year-old boy. The findings included hypoplasia of the eyelashes and eyebrows, fragile wrinkled skin over the eyelids, hypodontia, and swelling of the lips. The hair was sparse and the skin was dry. There was a striking discrepancy between the light hair on the head and the dark pigmentation of the iris. The child also had hyperhydrosis (caused by hypoplasia of the sweat glands) with intolerance to heat and hypoplasia of the sebaceous glands. The boy's physical and mental development were normal.

Differential Diagnosis—Differential diagnosis includes many of the other ectodermal dysplasia syndromes.

9.212

Cheilitis

Cheilitis granulomatosa (Miescher's cheilitis) in a 15-year-old boy. Swelling of the upper lip without involvement of the cheeks, chin, eyelids, or forehead was noted. Initially, the swelling would appear and resolve spontaneously. Later, the lips remained swollen. In other cases, the lower lip and one or both cheeks may be swollen. The swelling, accompanied by fever, is at first mild and brief. Later, the swelling is constant. After several years, spontaneous remission may occur. Cheilitis granulomatosa may be seen in several syndromes. In Melkersson-Rosenthal syndrome, cheilitis granulomatosa occurs in conjunction with facial paralysis and fissuring of the tongue. The findings in Melkersson-Rosenthal syndrome are due to a chronic granulomatous inflammation of uncertain etiology. This syndrome may be related to Boeck's sarcoidosis. Isolated cheilitis granulomatosa is perhaps a manifestation of Melkersson-Rosenthal syndrome. Cheilitis may also be mistaken for angioneurotic edema.

Differential Diagnosis—Constant or recurrent swelling of the lips occurs in Ascher syndrome (with abnormal lip formation, swelling of the eyelid, and thyroid enlargement). In cases of cheilitis glandularis, the lower lip is swollen and has numerous pinhead-sized openings from which saliva can be expressed.

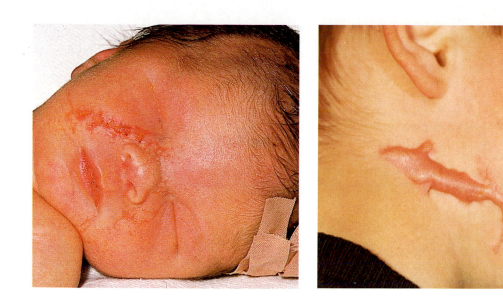

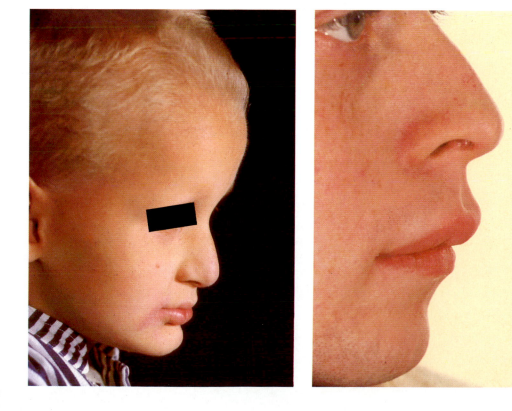

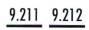

9.213

Panniculitis

Panniculitis in a 9-month-old girl who was treated with corticosteroids for infantile spasms. A poorly defined, 2×3 cm erythematous hardening of the skin was noted over both cheeks. Close inspection revealed several subcutaneous nodules with erythema of the overlying skin. The lesions were noted 2 weeks after the end of corticosteroid treatment. The lesions are typical of post-corticosteroid panniculitis. This inflammatory reaction resolved spontaneously after 3 weeks without scar formation.

In post-corticosteroid panniculitis, multiple nodules may appear on the face, arms, or torso. During the first year of life, panniculitis can be caused by exposure to cold (primarily on the face). A few hours or days after exposure to the cold, erythematous, indurated plaques may appear. Panniculitis is also seen in Weber-Christian syndrome, in which the lesions are 1–6 cm in size, erythematous, painful nodules located on various parts of the body. The nodules are frequently accompanied by fever and arthralgia. The lesions disappear slowly over the course of several weeks, leaving behind dimples in the skin (atrophy of adipose tissue).

Differential Diagnosis—Differential diagnosis of panniculitis includes diseases that cause granuloma formation in the subcutaneous tissue as well as certain vasculitides (such as erythema nodosum, page 160).

9.214

Erythema Infectiosum

Erythema infectiosum in an 18-month-old girl. Findings included a butterfly shaped erythematous rash on the face (erysipelas-like reddening with a raised border) accompanied by a garland-shaped maculopapular rash over other parts of the body, particularly the arms. The rash was not associated with fever.

9.215

Adenoma Sebaceum

Adenoma sebaceum associated with tuberous sclerosis in a 12-year-old boy. A seizure disorder had been diagnosed since the age of 1 year. The skin changes on the faces, which first appeared in adolescence, consisted of small telangiectatic papules, 1–3 mm in diameter and spread from the nasolabial fold to the cheeks and chin. In other cases, the papules may be larger and yellow in color. Other cutaneous manifestations of tuberous sclerosis included multiple depigmented nevi and a subungual fibroma on the right great toe. These findings were associated with mental retardation. Other organs including the brain, the eye, and the kidneys were affected by the disease.

Differential Diagnosis—Adenoma sebaceum may be difficult to differentiate from acne vulgaris. Acne vulgaris does not usually occur until adolescence and forms comedones and pustules. In cases of benign trichoepithelioma (epithelioma adenoides cysticum), numerous round, natural skin-colored papules appear on the cheeks at puberty. The lesions may become larger and take on a yellow or red appearance.

9.216

Systemic Lupus Erythematosus

Systemic lupus erythematosus in a 15-year-old girl. An extensive, well-defined, scaling, butterfly-shaped rash was noted on both cheeks; irregularly outlined erythematous areas were also noted on the bridge of the nose and at the hairline. Associated symptoms included persistent fever, arthralgia and arthritis, hepatosplenomegaly and generalized lymphadenopathy. Laboratory investigations revealed antinuclear antibodies and anti-DNA antibodies; serum complement was low. Immunohistologic examination of the skin revealed immunoglobulin and complement deposition at the dermo-epidermal junction.

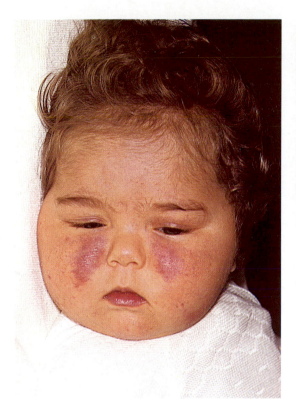

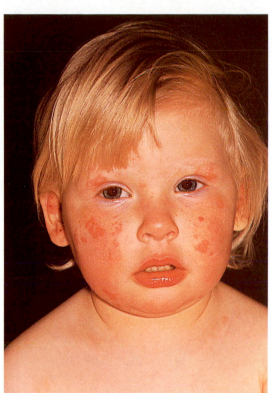

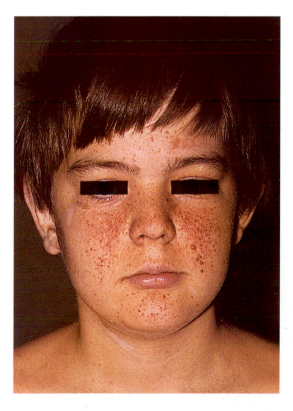

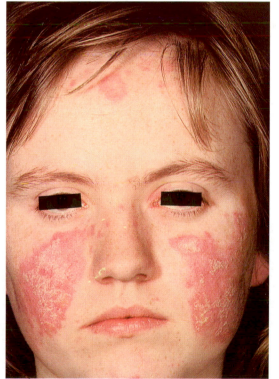

9.217

Accessory Skin Tag

Accessory skin tag in a 7-year-old boy. The skin tag was pea-sized, smooth, and firm. The skin tag was broad-based and contained cartilage.

9.218

Microtia

Microtia (rudimentary ear pinna) and atresia of the external auditory canal in a 2-month-old girl. The child also had nevus flammeus (port-wine nevus) on the forehead above the bridge of the nose. No abnormalities of the inner ear were noted, nor were there any other associated deformities. The cause of the ear deformity was unknown.

9.219

Congenital Microcephaly

Congenital microcephaly and protruding ears in an 18-month-old girl. Microcephaly (OFC: 28 cm at birth) and poorly formed, low-set ears were noted. Mental development was severely delayed. No other deformities were noted and there were no signs of intrauterine infection or chromosomal anomaly. At 3 years of age, surgery was performed to correct the ear deformity.

Microcephaly may be secondary to intrauterine infections or specific chromosomal anomalies (Down syndrome, trisomy 13 or 18). Hereditary microcephaly (recessive inheritance) may present with findings similar to this case.

9.220

Ectodermal Dysplasia

Ectodermal dysplasia (hypohidrotic form) in a 10-month-old boy. The child was brought to the clinic because of unexplained fever and failure to thrive. The sparse hair over the head and body, the absence of eyelashes, the thin, dry skin, decreased tearing and decreased perspiration (detected through pilocarpine electrophoresis) were characteristic of hypohidrotic ectodermal dysplasia. Radiologic examination revealed abnormal dentition. Other findings included thick, swollen lips, hyperpigmentation of the periorbital skin, and low-set ears. The child developed chronic atopic rhinitis and intermittent hoarseness (due to hypoplasia of the mucous glands in the respiratory tract). At several times during hospitalization, febrile episodes without signs of infection occurred. These febrile episodes were the result of hyperthermia from hypohydrosis. The child failed to grow normally, in part due to intolerance to milk. Other family members had ectodermal dysplasia. This family is an example of classic ectodermal dysplasia syndrome (Christ-Siemens-Touraine syndrome). Other forms of ectodermal dysplasia include ectodactyly-ectodermal dysplasia clefting syndrome (EEC syndrome) and Goltz Gorlin syndrome.

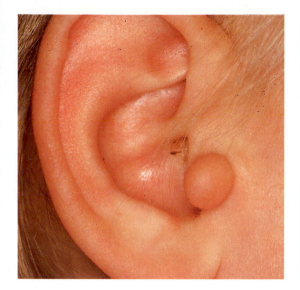

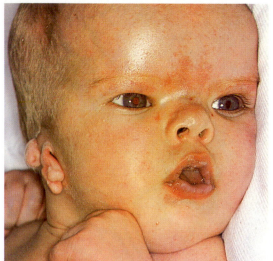

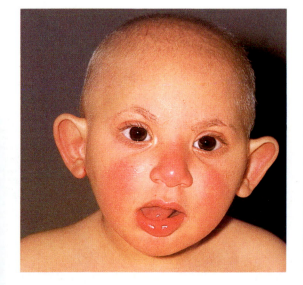

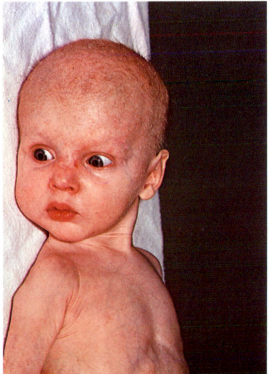

9.221

Alopecia Areata

Alopecia areata (localized hair loss) in a 6-year-old girl. The hair follicles of the affected area were still intact. Without any specific treatment, the hair grew back after 2 to 3 months. At first, the new hair was lighter than the rest of the scalp hair; later, the hair color was similar.

The prognosis of alopecia areata differs depending on the cause. A small number of cases will be alopecia totalis (loss of all scalp hair). In cases where there is scar tissue or the follicles are destroyed by infection, physical damage, or malignancy, hair loss is irreversible.

Differential Diagnosis—In cases of alopecia areata, the following processes must be ruled out: trichotillomania (behavioral abnormality leading to hair-pulling, page 278), traction alopecia (trauma caused by pigtails, ponytails, hairbands, or other hair treatments), tinea capitus (page 254), severe atopic or seborrheic dermatitis and other scalp infections.

9.222

Alopecia Areata

Alopecia areata (idiopathic form) in a 6-year-old boy. Hair loss was noted at the edge of the scalp (ophiasis) on otherwise unaffected skin. These findings occurred suddenly and the cause was unclear. Despite local corticosteroid therapy, there was no improvement. In general, the prognosis is unfavorable. Often this type of alopecia areata may progress to alopecia totalis.

9.223

Alopecia Totalis

Alopecia totalis in a 2-year-old boy. Hair loss over the entire head (including eyebrows and some eyelashes) occurred within a short period of time. The following were excluded as causes of the diffuse hair loss: toxins (such as thallium), medications (chemotherapeutic agents), metabolic and endocrine disorders, severe systemic infection, central nervous system disease (encephalitis, cranial trauma), and tumors.

In cases of alopecia universalis, hair is lacking not only on the head but also on the rest of the body. Treatment of total or universal alopecia is almost always unsuccessful if no specific cause has been identified. However, if a primary disease process can be identified and treated, the alopecia can be corrected if the hair follicles are not permanently damaged.

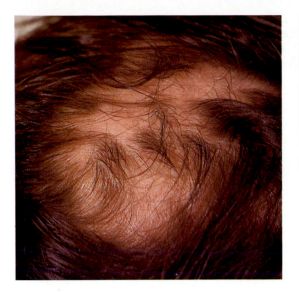 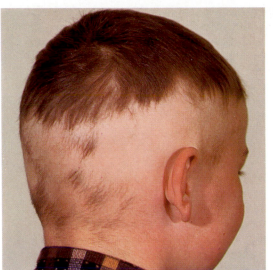

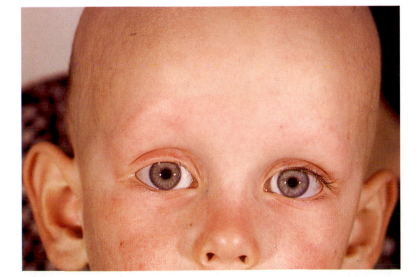

9.224 9.225

Trichotillomania

Trichotillomania in a 14-year-old girl. Diffuse alopecia of the head resulted from foreful compulsive tearing out of hair. Some eyelashes were also missing. In some cases, a skin biopsy is necessary to confirm the diagnosis. The findings on biopsy demonstrate normal hair follicles, juxtaposed with damaged follicles, parafollicular hemorrhage, partial follicular atrophy, and catagen transformation of the hair.

Differential Diagnosis—Differential diagnosis of trichotillomania includes tinea capitis and alopecia areata. If this behavior is not modified, hair follicles can be irreversibly damaged resulting in persistent alopecia.

9.226

Partial Albinism

Partial albinism (poliosis circumscripta) in a 6-year-old girl. A white forelock, resulting from the absence of melanocytes, had been present since birth. Unlike most cases, there was no hypopigmented area of scalp at the site of the forelock. In partial albinism, depigmented areas of skin can occur on the torso and the extremities (with the exception of the back, hands, and feet). The term "partial" refers to the distribution of the skin changes.

Differential Diagnosis—Poliosis, frequently in the area of the eyebrows and eyelashes, occurs in 80% of cases with Vogt-Koyanagi syndrome (uveitis, hearing impairment, and vitiligo). In resolving alopecia areata, the hairs that grow back are often depigmented. Poliosis is also present in cases of tuberous sclerosis. Vitiligo, an acquired pigment disorder of the skin, is often first seen in areas exposed to sunlight. The irregularly defined white macules seen in vitiligo often have hyperpigmented borders. On the affected areas of the scalp, the hairs are usually normally pigmented; only after prolonged periods do they begin to lose their pigmentation. For further comments and differential diagnosis of vitiligo, see pages 262 and 306.

9.227

Partial Albinism

Partial albinism (poliosis circumscripta) in a mother and child. The only anomaly was the white forelock. The associated findings of Waardenburg's syndrome (acrocephaly, facial dysmorphism, occular anomalies, abnormal dentition, deafness) were not noted. Isolated poliosis circumscripta, like Waardenburg's syndrome, is inherited as an autosomal dominant trait.

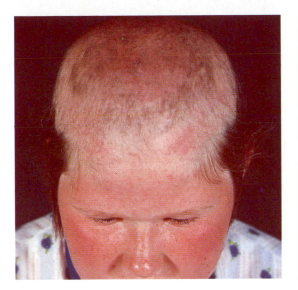

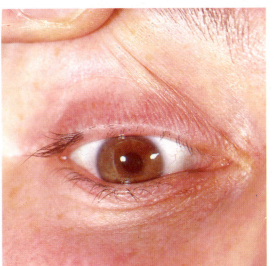

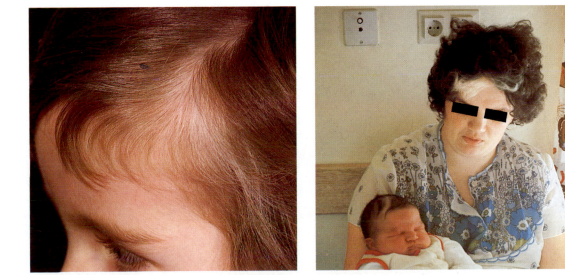

9.228

Verruca Vulgaris

Verruca vulgaris next to the fingernails of a 12-year-old boy. The findings included numerous, painful, periungual, gray-yellow papules with hyperkeratosis and rough surfaces which had already undermined the nailbeds. Nail growth was disturbed in this area. Treatment consisted of topical application of liquid nitrogen.

These viral lesions are frequently located on the fingers, dorsum of the hands, knees, elbows, and face. Both verruca vulgaris (common warts) and verruca plana (juvenile flat warts) may be found in these locations. Juvenile flat warts are small (less than 3 mm), slightly raised and red-brown. Flat warts are recognized by their linear arrangement along excoriations. They can be spread to the scalp by combing.

Differential Diagnosis—Warts involving the area near the fingernails must be distinguished from periungual fibromas, which may be seen in tuberous sclerosis.

9.229

Damaged Nails

Nail changes in a 5-year-old nail biter. Damage can be seen both to the nail and to the skin surrounding the area. As a complication of this traumatic injury, paronychia and warts may occur.

Habitual nail-biting is related to aggressive behavior. It occurs widely among older children and can persist as a habit into adulthood. Nail-biting is thought to be repression of aggressive impulses, which may unconsciously manifest in this fashion. Nail damage can also occur by constant rubbing of the fingernails or by frequent application of certain nail cosmetics.

9.230

Paronychia

Herpetic paronychia in a 4-year-old boy with acute non-lymphocytic leukemia. The findings included edematous swelling and erythema of the fingertips with vesicle formation on the left thumb and right second and third fingers. Herpes simplex virus was cultured from the vesicular contents. The boy, who still sucked his thumb and fingers, had herpes labialis, which led to infection of the fingers.

9.228

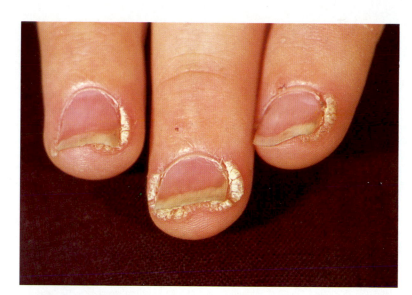

9.229

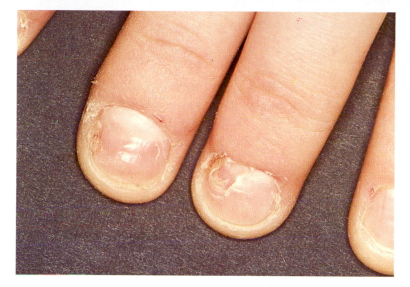

9.230

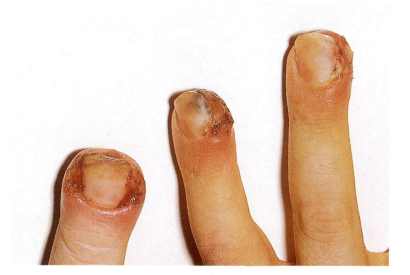

10.1 Leukemia

10.1.1 Acute Nonlymphocytic Leukemia

Acute nonlymphocytic leukemia (ANLL) in a 6-year-old boy. Of note was proptosis of the left eye due to infiltration and proliferation of myeloblasts within the orbit. Three weeks before these symptoms, the child had fever, sore throat, and extensive cervical lymphadenopathy. When the symptoms failed to respond to antibiotic therapy and proptosis developed, the child was admitted to the hospital. Peripheral blood smear and bone marrow aspirate demonstrated acute nonlymphoblastic leukemia, myeloblastic type (positive peroxidase and sudan B black stain). The child responded poorly to chemotherapy. Remission could not be achieved and the child died of sepsis 2 months later.

Differential Diagnosis—For the discussion of differential diagnosis of exophthalmos, see pages 282 and 316.

10.1.2 Acute Nonlymphocytic Leukemia

Acute nonlymphocytic leukemia (ANLL) in a 13-year-old boy. Swelling and ulceration of the gums occurred because of leukemic infiltration. Simultaneous enlargement of the right submandibular gland was also noted. Gingival and glandular swelling regressed after an intensive two week course of chemotherapy (induction phase).

Differential Diagnosis—For differential diagnosis of gingival swelling, see pages 106 and 148.

10.1.3 Acute Lymphocytic Leukemia

Acute lymphocytic leukemia (ALL) in a 10-year-old girl. Petechial hemorrhages were found on the soft and hard palate due to thrombocytopenia. In addition to petechiae, ecchymotic skin lesions were noted. In this case, the skin and mucous membrane hemorrhages were the initial symptoms that led to the diagnosis of ALL.

10.1.4 Acute Lymphocytic Leukemia

Acute lymphocytic leukemia (ALL) in a 10-year-old boy. A large, skin hemorrhage (suffusion) was noted over the lower thigh. Over the remainder of the body one could see ecchymoses (small circumscribed patchy skin hemorrhages) and petechiae. Therapy led to complete remission. After 5½ years, this boy is still in remission.

10.1.5 Mees' Lines

Mees' lines on the fingernail of a 7½-year-old boy. He had been treated with chemotherapeutic agents (including vincristine, daunorubicin, and cyclophosphamide) for several weeks due to acute lymphocytic leukemia. The transverse white bands on the fingernails and toenails are commonly seen nail changes due to chemotherapy.

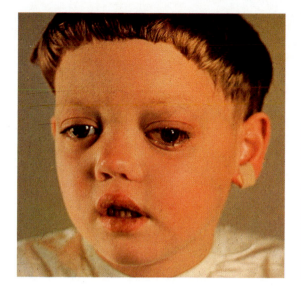

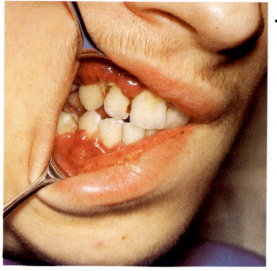

10.1.1   10.1.2

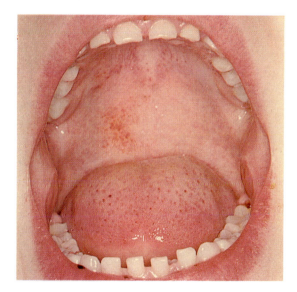

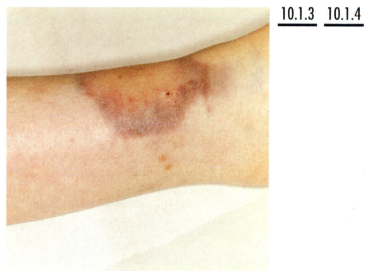

10.1.3   10.1.4

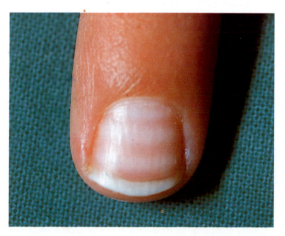

10.1.5

10.1.6
Acute Nonlymphocytic Leukemia

Acute nonlymphocytic leukemia in a 5-year-old girl. The initial symptoms of disease were skin hemorrhages. Chemotherapy led to partial remission. After 5 months, the child developed marked abdominal distention due to ascites (with hepatosplenomegaly and profound anemia). Hypoproteinemia was also noted. Despite multiple blood transfusions, the child died due to persistent internal bleeding.

10.1.7
Acute Lymphocytic Leukemia

Acute lymphocytic leukemia in a 7-year-old boy with chronic candidiasis. Several firm, white, poorly defined plaques which could be removed with great difficulty, were found on the tongue. Candida albicans was detected microscopically and by fungal culture. Lesions such as these are seen in immune suppressed individuals. Typical findings seen in cases of thrush differ in that the lesions are softer and scraping usually results in punctate hemorrhages on an erythematous base.

10.1.8
Acute Lymphocytic Leukemia

Acute lymphocytic leukemia in a 10-year-old boy with *Candida* dermatitis of the face. Round, scaly, pruritic, erythematous lesions (approximately 2 cm in diameter) were noted over the face. The child had similar skin lesions over the scalp and body. In addition, an extensive lesions that was resistant to therapy was located in the mouth. *Candida albicans* could be detected microscopically and by culture. Lesions such as these are seen in immune suppressed individuals with chronic mucocutaneous candidiasis.

10.1.9
Acute Lymphocytic Leukemia

Acute lymphocytic leukemia (ALL) in a 7-year-old girl with herpes zoster. Groups of vesicles of various size were found on the right hand. These vesicles were either filled with serous fluid or ulcerated and covered with a hemorrhagic crust. The illness began with a febrile episode during induction chemotherapy for acute lymphocytic leukemia (ALL). Within a few days, red papules developed on the hand. These papules changed to vesicles and persisted for 2 weeks. No other skin lesions were noted and secondary bacterial infection did not occur. The girl previously had chickenpox (varicella) at 3 years of age.

Herpes zoster is caused by the varicella/zoster virus in patients who have previously had chickenpox. The virus may persist in neural tissue and reactivate when the patient is immunocompromised. Herpes zoster occurs in 2–3% of patients with malignant disease undergoing chemotherapy and is of particular concern due to the risk of generalization. Recurrent episodes may occur.

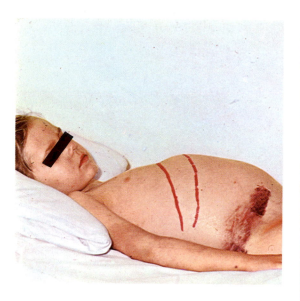

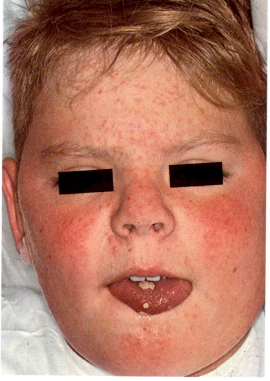

10.1.6   10.1.7

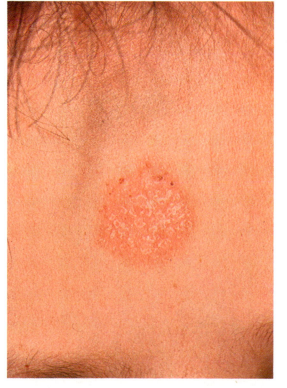

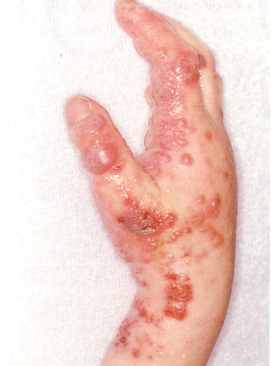

10.1.8   10.1.9

10.2 Bleeding Disorders

10.2.1

Hemophilia A

Hemophilia A (factor VIII deficiency or classic hemophilia) in an 11-year-old boy. Findings included an egg-sized hematoma in the subcutaneous tissue over the right hip due to minor trauma. Smaller, patchy skin hemorrhages were noted on the arms and legs.

10.2.2

Hemophilia A

Hemophilia A in a 9-year-old boy. The child had severe hemophilia A with a factor VIII level less than 1%. Ecchymosis around both eyes and bruising over the forehead was noted. Frequent hemarthrosis (particularly of the knees) occurred. In children with hemophilia, hemorrhage can occur in the eye, conjunctiva, iris, retina, and vitreous body. To control the bleeding manifestations of hemophilia A, factor VIII concentrate was given at home.

10.2.3

Hemophilia A

Hemophilia A with hemorrhage in the left knee joint (hemarthrosis) in a 14-year-old boy. The findings included warm, fluctuant swelling of the left knee, which caused restriction in movement. The child was febrile to 39° C. After administration of factor VIII and immobilizing the joint, the effusion regressed and physical therapy could begin. After this episode of hemarthrosis, regular replacement therapy was introduced in order to prevent further hemorrhage into the joint space.

Differential Diagnosis—For a discussion of the differential diagnosis of knee joint swelling, see page 158.

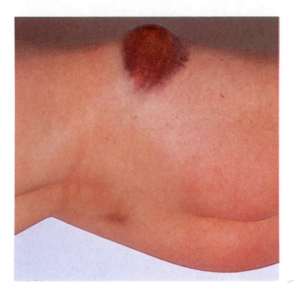

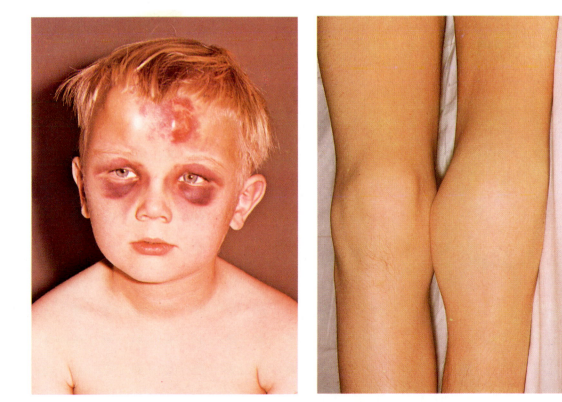

10.2.4 Waterhouse-Friderichsen Syndrome

Waterhouse-Friderichsen Syndrome in a 16-year-old girl with meningococcal sepsis. Ecchymotic, purpuric and petechial lesions were noted over the body especially on the legs. Severe circulatory collapse was also noted (cold extremities, hypotension, thready pulse, disorientation). Diplococci were visible in granulocytes in the blood smear. Laboratory investigations demonstrated disseminated intravascular coagulation (thrombocytopenia, decreased fibrinogen, increased fibrin split products, and decreased factors V and VIII). In septic patients, superficial skin hemorrhages can also be caused by hypoprothrombinemia (due to liver damage). Petechial and ecchymotic lesions may be seen in septic patients without consumption coagulopathy due to direct interaction of the pathogen and platelets. If only petechial lesions are seen in a septic patient, a vasculitic process should be considered.

10.2.5 Idiopathic Thrombocytopenic Purpura

Idiopathic thrombocytopenic purpura in a 3-year-old girl. Petechial skin hemorrhages were noted over the entire body, especially on the arms and legs. At 10 days before the appearance of the petechial rash, the child had an acute upper respiratory infection and had been treated with a sulfonamide medication. Laboratory investigation revealed thrombocytopenia (platelet count: 1,000/μl), prolonged bleeding time, and abnormal clot retraction. Bone marrow aspirate revealed an increased megakaryocyte count. The condition responded to 6 weeks of prednisone therapy.

Differential Diagnosis—Thrombocytopenic skin hemorrhages may be associated with:

1. Decreased number of megakaryocytes in the bone marrow (in cases of bone marrow aplasia or bone marrow infiltration)
2. Normal number of megakaryocytes in the bone marrow (in cases of Wiskott-Aldrich syndrome)
3. Normal or increased numbers of megakaryocytes in the bone marrow (in autoimmune disease or in consumption coagulopathy)

Petechial and ecchymotic skin hemorrhages may also occur in disorders of platelet function such as thrombasthenia.

10.2.6 10.2.7 Henoch-Schoenlein Purpura

Henoch-Schoenlein purpura in a 7-year-old boy. Findings included closely grouped petechial lesions on the extensor surface of the upper thigh and buttocks; similar but less numerous lesions were noted on the extensor surfaces of the arms and on the face. Other manifestations of this allergic vasculitis included edema, arthralgia, hemorrhagic lesions in the intestinal mucosa, and nephritis. Laboratory investigation demonstrated normal coagulation studies and platelet count.

Differential Diagnosis—Purpuric lesions similar to those seen in Henoch-Schoenlein purpura may be caused by severe septicemia (in combination with thrombocytopenia and consumptive coagulopathy), polyarteritis nodosa, idiopathic thrombocytopenic purpura, and thrombasthenia.

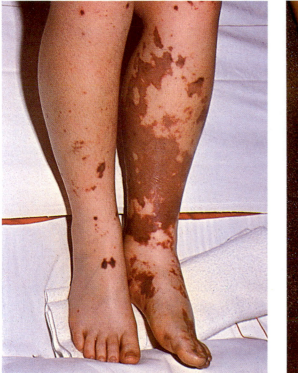

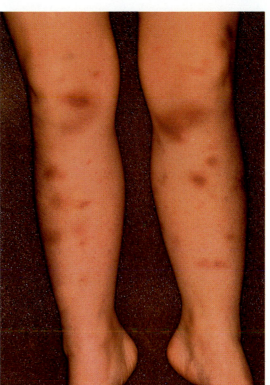

10.2.4   10.2.5

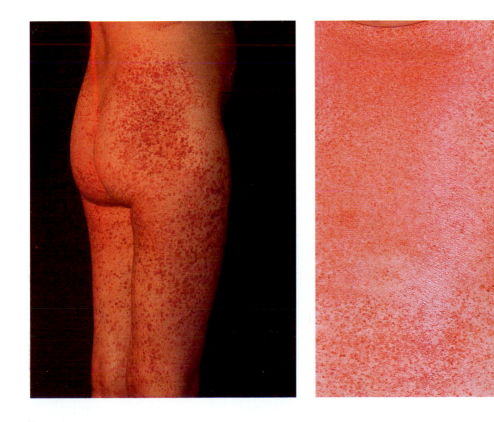

10.2.6   10.2.7

10.2.8
Henoch-Schoenlein Purpura

Henoch-Schoenlein purpura in a 9-year-old boy. At 10 days before the onset of the rash, the child had a streptococcal infection with high fever. During the days that followed, joint swelling, edema, and petechial skin hemorrhages began to appear. Edematous swelling of the eyelids was noted. On the fourth day of illness, the patient had colicky abdominal pain and bloody stools. Rapid improvement followed treatment with prednisone, but the illness recurred when treatment was discontinued. Remission was achieved after 4 weeks of illness.

Differential Diagnosis—Differential diagnosis includes other processes, which may present with petechial or purpuric lesions. These include thrombocytopenia, disseminated intravascular coagulation, and various vasculitic processes. Vasculitis may be due to either viral or bacterial infection such as in the hemorrhagic exanthem of measles, scarlet fever, and chickenpox. In cases of polyarteritis nodosa (an inflammatory condition of the medium and small arteries), skin changes similar to anaphylactoid purpura are present but are usually more severe in nature. Polyarteritis nodosa includes neurologic symptoms (paresthesia, pain, muscle weakness) and cardiac symptoms (myocardial infarction, cardiac failure) not seen in anaphylactoid purpura. When the central nervous system is involved, seizures and encephalitis may result. Hepatosplenomegaly is frequently seen. The disease is usually fatal.

10.2.9
Polyarteritis Nodosa

Polyarteritis nodosa in a 14-year-old boy. Petechial skin hemorrhages were found on the arms and legs and isolated hemorrhages were noted on the face and trunk. The onset of disease was sudden with high fever and muscle pain. Neurologic symptoms (paresthesias) and hematuria were noted later in the course. As the disease progressed, involvement with coronary arteries was noted. Coronary arteritis leads to tachycardia, myocardial infarction, and cardiac failure. Tissue obtained from renal biopsy supported the diagnosis of polyarteritis nodosa.

10.2.10   10.2.11
Henoch-Schoenlein Purpura

Henoch-Schoenlein purpura in an 11-month-old boy. Of note were urticarial lesions on the face, which developed central purpuric areas. Lesions were also found elsewhere on the body, especially on the extensor surface of the extremities. The skin lesions responded to 5 days of prednisone therapy (Figure 10.2.11) but recurred after treatment was stopped. Prior to the appearance of the skin lesions, the child was noted to have bronchitis. The platelet count and other coagulation studies were normal.

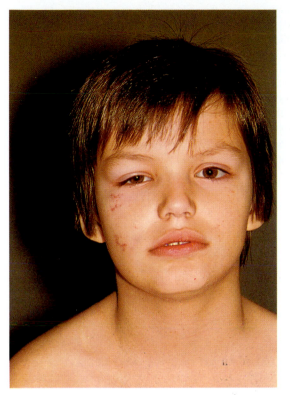

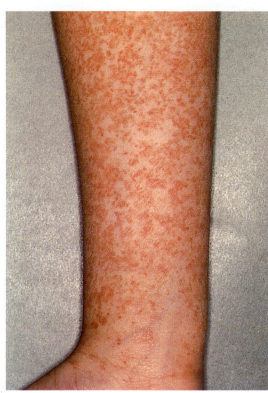

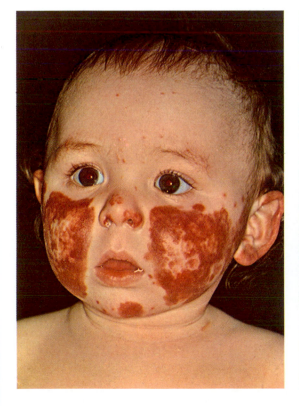

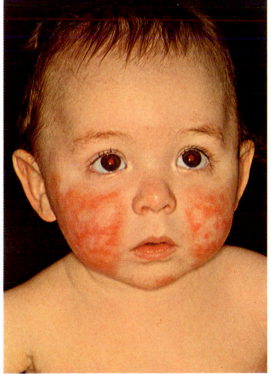

10.2.12
Polyarteritis Nodosa

Gangrene of both feet secondary to polyarteritis nodosa in a 3-year-old girl. The illness began with high fever and blue-purple discoloration of the hands and feet. The extremities were cool and peripheral pulses were diminished. Due to coronary artery involvement, the child developed hypertension and severe cardiac failure (tachycardia, hepatomegaly). Laboratory investigation revealed leukocytosis, elevated ESR and sterile blood cultures. During the first week of hospitalization, the foot began to blacken; starting first with the toes and then spreading over the entire foot (dry gangrene). With appropriate treatment, the cardiac failure improved and the circulatory problems in the hands regressed.

Despite therapy, the child had both feet amputated. After exclusion of other causes (embolic phenomenon, mercury poisoning, other autoimmune processes), prednisone therapy was begun for suspected polyarteritis nodosa. Treatment was continued intermittently for years because circulatory problems in the legs recurred shortly after therapy was discontinued.

Differential Diagnosis—Gangrene can occur in conjunction with bacterial sepsis, disseminated intravascular coagulation, arterial emboli, systemic lupus erythematosus, scleroderma, and acrodynia (mercury poisoning).

10.2.13
Purpura Fulminans

Purpura fulminans in a 12-year-old girl. At 2 weeks after a viral illness (herpes stomatitis), numerous ecchymotic and purpuric lesions were noted on both legs and buttocks. As the condition progressed, fever, swelling, and discoloration of the entire right leg (as well as vesicle formation on the

foot) were noted. Laboratory evaluation revealed thrombocytopenia and decreased factor V level. Eventually, dry gangrene of the right foot occurred leading to amputation of the lower leg.

10.2.14
Gas Gangrene

Gas gangrene in a 14-year-old girl. The findings included dry mummification (blackening) of the right foot and distal third of the tibia. Gas gangrene is caused by an anaerobic infection of the soft tissue. In this case, the child was infected

with *Clostridium perfringens* (originating from necrotizing enteritis). Clostridia was identified on blood culture. Septicemia was treated with intensive antibiotic therapy. The leg had to be amputated at the thigh.

10.2.15
Urticaria Pigmentosa

Urticaria pigmentosa (mastocytosis) in a 2-year-old girl. Numerous, poorly defined, confluent brown nodules and vesicles were noted on both lower legs. The lesions appeared suddenly after the administration of aspirin during the course of a febrile illness. The lesions were intensely pruritic. If the lesions were rubbed, wheals would form (positive Darier

sign). The diagnosis of urticaria pigmentosa had been made earlier based on clinical presentation and skin biopsy. The surface of the skin lesions on the legs had the typical "orange peel" texture.

Differential Diagnosis—For differential diagnosis of urticaria pigmentosa, see page 226.

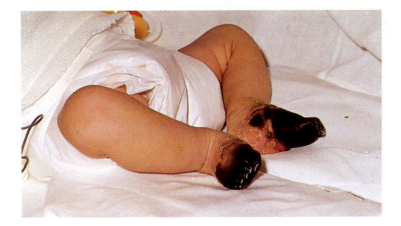

10.2.12

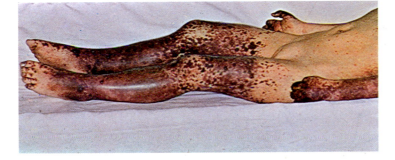

10.2.13

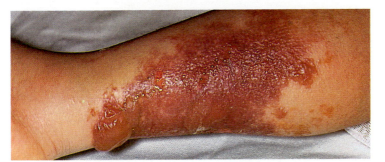

10.2.14

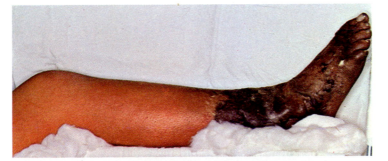

10.2.15

11.1
Nevus Flammeus

Nevus flammeus in a 2-month-old boy. An extensive, patchy, sharply demarcated red skin lesion was noted at the hairline. The findings had been present since birth. A nevus flammeus located on the neck is commonly known as "Unna's nevus."

Nevus flammeus occurs on the neck of 40% to 70% of all newborns and is a harmless anomaly, which often persists throughout life. Nevus flammeus found on the eyelids or base of the nose usually disappear in early childhood. The port-wine nevus (flat hemangioma), like the nevus on the neck, usually persists. Port-wine nevi are usually asymmetric, found on the face or upper half of the torso, and do not extend over the midline. Port-wine nevi may be associated with Sturge-Weber syndrome or Klippel-Trenaunay-Weber syndrome.

11.2
Nevus Flammeus

Unilateral nevus flammeus (port-wine nevus or flat hemangioma) on the upper lip of a 5-week-old boy. There was no indication of angiomatous change of the leptomeninges that may be seen in Sturge-Weber syndrome.

11.3
Cavernous Hemangioma

A large cavernous hemangioma (strawberry nevus) in a 3-month-old boy. The nevus had grown considerably since birth, extending into the scalp and closing the right eye. Cavernous hemangiomas may go through a period of growth followed by a stationary phase and later involution. In this case, both resection and radiotherapy were deemed impossible, so no specific therapy was instituted. The decision was made to wait for spontaneous regression, which usually begins in the first year of life. In other cases, prednisone may be used to hasten involution.

11.4
Kasabach-Merritt Syndrome

Kasabach-Merritt syndrome in a 3-year-old boy. A giant cavernous hemangioma of the left thigh extended to the scrotum and lower abdomen. The laboratory investigation revealed severe thrombocytopenia, fragmented erythrocytes, and consumption of coagulation factors. These findings were due to platelet entrapment in the cavernous hemangioma. Skin hemorrhage or bleeding into internal organs did not occur. Consumption of platelets and coagulation factors spontaneously improved when the blood vessels leading into the hemangioma became thrombosed.

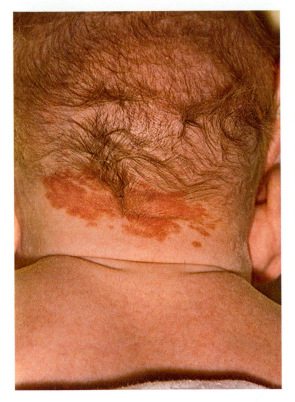
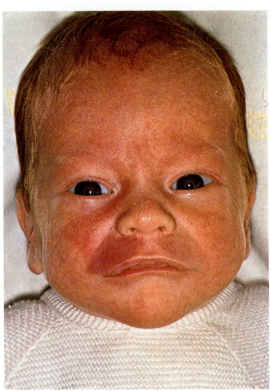
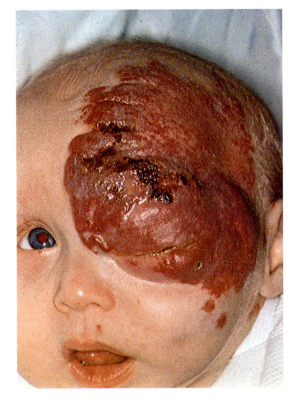
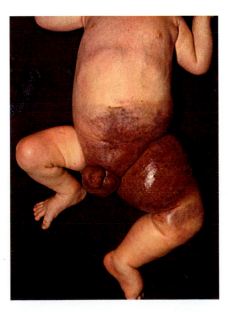

11.5
Sturge-Weber Syndrome

Sturge-Weber syndrome (encephalotrigeminal angiomatosis) in a 4-year-old boy. Unilateral nevus flammeus involving the area of distribution of the maxillary branch of the trigeminal nerve was noted. At 3 months of age, the boy underwent surgery for glaucoma due to choroid angioma. Thus far, there have been no signs of central nervous system involvement (seizures, hemiparesis, intracranial calcification, mental retardation).

Differential Diagnosis—The various oligosymptomatic forms occur such as Milles syndrome (facial nevus and choroid angioma). In Fegeler syndrome (posttraumatic nevus flammeus) unilateral nevus flammeus occur in a trigeminal distribution associated with swelling of the forehead and cheek, hyperesthesia of the affected area of the face, and ipsilateral paresis of the extremities following trauma. In Bonnet-Dechaume-Blanc syndrome (neuroretinoangiomatosis) unilateral angiomas of the retina and unilateral cerebral arteriovenous malformations may occur. In Van Bogaert-Divry syndrome (corticomeningeal diffuse angiomatosis), pigmentation disorders, net-like telangiectasias, retinal angiomas, and severe central nervous system defects occur. Maffucci syndrome is characterized by multiple capillary or cavernous angiomas of the skin and internal organs, associated with multiple endochondromas and asymmetric dyschondroplasia of the bones of the extremities.

11.6
Sturge-Weber Syndrome

Sturge-Weber syndrome in a 14-year-old boy. Nevus flammeus was found on the left side of the face (stopping at the midline), the back, and the left buttock. Choroid angiomas were also noted but did not lead to glaucoma. The child had serious central nervous system involvement leading to severe mental retardation and intracranial vascular calcification (in the leptomeninges of the parietooccipital area ipsilateral to the nevus flammeus). No hemiparesis was noted. Seizures, which had been noted since the age of 3 months, were controlled with anticonvulsant medication. The facial nevus faded as the child grew older.

11.7
Klippel-Trenaunay-Weber Syndrome

Klippel-Trenaunay-Weber syndrome in a 10-year-old boy. The findings included macrosomia of the entire left arm, enlargement of the third, fourth, and fifth fingers, and ipsilateral nevus flammeus on the volar side of the hand, upper arm, and shoulder. The surface temperature of the left arm was elevated. A vascular bruit could be appreciated over the involved area. No other deformities were noted. Due to multiple arteriovenous fistulas, high output cardiac failure occurred (requiring treatment with cardiac glycosides).

Differential Diagnosis—For discussion of the differential diagnosis of macrosomia, see page 74.

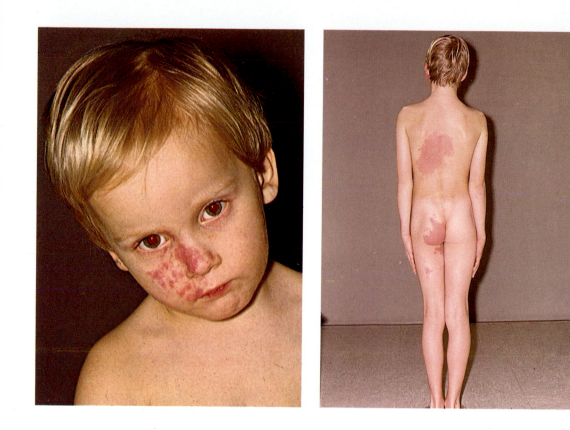

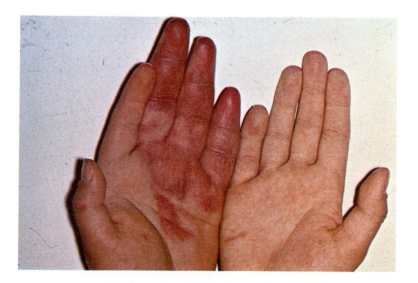

11.8

Lymphangioma

Lymphangioma in a 6-day-old newborn. The findings included swelling of the cheek without pain or erythema. The swelling was soft, diffuse, and easily compressible. The diagnosis of localized lymphangioma was made at the time of surgery.

Localized lymphangiomas occur most frequently in the axilla, neck, upper arm, and perineum. Lymphangiomas may occur on the tongue resulting in macroglossia, or on the lips, resulting in macrocheilia. They can grow into the mediastinum and compress the trachea. Cystic lymphangiomas (cystic hygroma) can become so large as to present difficulties at birth. Cystic hygroma should be surgically resected as soon as possible since spontaneous regression cannot be expected. Recurrence after complete removal is rare. Lymphangiomas may be difficult to differentiate from deeply located hemangiomas.

11.9

Dermoid Cyst

Congenital dermoid cyst in a 6-week-old infant. Findings included a cherry-sized, smooth, spherical, pedunculated tumor growing from the right nostril. The cyst originated from the nasal septum. After surgical removal, histological examination confirmed the diagnosis of congenital dermoid cyst (page 318).

Dermoid cysts lie in or near the midline and may be located in the area of the nose. Dermoid cysts involving the nose may recur.

11.10

Cavernous Hemangioma

Superficial cavernous hemangioma (strawberry nevus) in a 1-year-old child. Of note was an extensive, sharply demarcated, cystic, compressible blue-red mass on the nose. The surface of the lesion was uneven. The growth had been present since birth but had recently begun to increase in size. The mass did not obstruct nasal breathing. No therapeutic intervention was attempted since spontaneous regression frequently occurs. Prednisone therapy can prevent further growth or cause involution of the mass.

11.11

Cavernous Hemangioma

Deep cavernous hemangioma in a 4-month-old girl. The findings included extensive swelling in the area of the hard and soft palate extending into the right orbit. After 1 year, gradual regression of the hemangioma occurred without therapy.

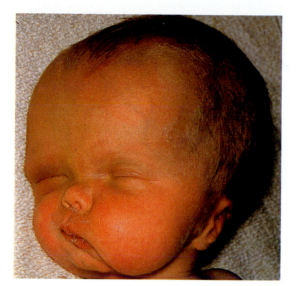 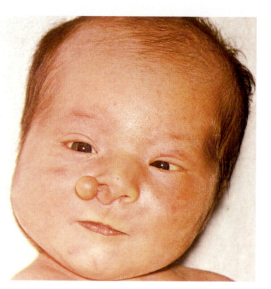

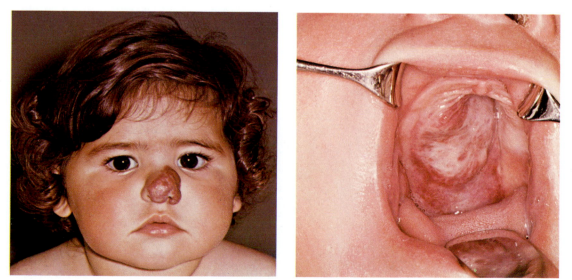

11.12

Lipoma

Giant lipoma on the back of a 4-year-old boy. Findings included a soft, superficial swelling in the subcutaneous tissue above both shoulder blades and on the right side of the chest extending down to the pelvic rim. At first, these findings were thought to be due to a lymphangioma. An extensive subcutaneous lipoma was demonstrated at the time of surgery. The lesion was removed with no recurrence.

11.13

Lymphangioma

Lymphangioma on the right shoulder of a 2-year-old boy. This soft, fist-sized swelling was not clearly differentiated from the surrounding tissue. The mass had been present since birth and was noted to be growing during the previous year. The mass caused no restriction of movement. The treatment of choice is surgical excision, which can be technically difficult due to infiltration of the lymphangioma.

Simple localized lymphangioma can be differentiated from more deeply embedded cavernous lymphangioma (page 298). Special forms of lymphangioma include cystic hygroma (page 302), and lymphangiohemangioma (which has vascular and lymphatic tissue). Cavernous lymphangioma and cystic hygroma are the most frequent. When localized to the mouth, pharynx, or mediastinum, lymphangioma can cause airway obstruction.

11.14

Myositis Ossificans Progressiva

Myositis ossificans progressiva in a 6-year-old boy. Numerous, subcutaneous, bone-hard swellings were noted in the paravertebral and right scalpular area. Involvement of the back and axilla led to restriction of movement of the right shoulder. Characteristic calcification was detected radiographically in the area of the axilla, neck, and lumbar spinal column. The condition began during the previous year with localized painful swelling of the soft tissue of the back. After a short time, these swellings turned to extensive, hard indurations. As the disease progressed, ankylosis of numerous joints occurred due to calcification of tendons and muscle (including torticollis due to calcification of the sternocleidomastoid muscle).

11.15

Myositis Ossificans Progressiva

Myositis ossificans progressiva in a 6-year-old boy (shown in Figure 11.14). Myositis ossificans progressiva (progressive ossification of muscles) is frequently associated with other congenital abnormalities. Associated findings include lateral deviation of the big toe with prominence of the first metatarsal phalangeal joint (hallux valgus). Deformities of the big toe or thumb (brachydactyly) are frequent osseous malformations in myositis ossificans progressiva. Other congenital anomalies include hypogonadism, deafness, and hypodontia. The child was followed for 7 years. During this time, there was progressive dysplasia of the connective tissue leading to progressive ossification and restriction in movement of both the arms and the back.

Differential Diagnosis—Differential diagnosis of myositis ossificans progressiva includes:
1. Myositis ossificans circumscripta (seen in areas of trauma)
2. Calcinosis circumscripta or universalis (page 196)
3. Lipoid calcinosis (cholesterol accumulation, calcium deposition, and granuloma formation in muscles)
4. Progressive scleroderma (localized or widespread calcification of soft tissue)
5. Dermatomyositis or chronic polymyositis (Wagner-Unverricht syndrome)

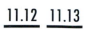

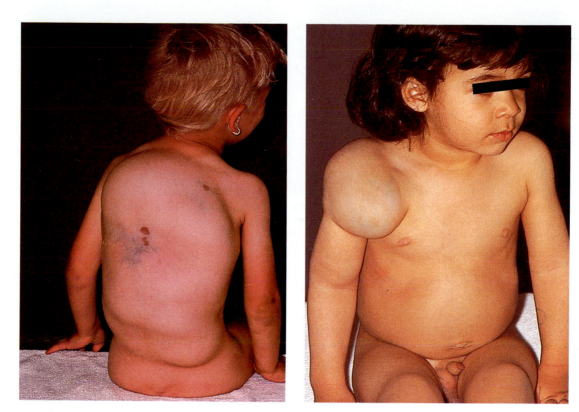

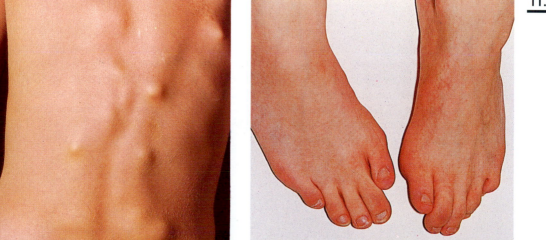

11.16
Cystic Hygroma

Cystic hygroma in a 2-month-old boy. A well-defined, firm, nonpainful, apple-sized swelling was present since birth. At first, the mass did not appear to enlarge. At the time of surgical resection, a multicystic mass with thin, transparent walls containing an amber yellow fluid was found. Complete removal was successful with no recurrence.

Cystic hygroma can also be located in the axilla, the popliteal space, the groin, and the retroperitoneum.

Differential Diagnosis—Cystic hygromas must be differentiated from cavernous and simple lymphangioma (page 298). When located in the neck, cystic hygroma must be differentiated from thyroglossal duct cyst, brachial cysts (page 196), dermoid cysts, lipomas, malignant lymphoma, and tuberculous lymphadenitis.

11.17
Non-Hodgkin's Lymphoma

Non-Hodgkin's lymphoma in a 9-year-old girl. The child presents with persistent cervical lymphadenopathy. The nodes were painless and the child was afebrile. No hepatosplenomegaly was noted and examination of the peripheral blood smear was normal. Lymph node biopsy demonstrated non-Hodgkin's lymphoma. Bone marrow involvement was noted.

After 2 weeks of chemotherapy, the enlarged lymph nodes were no longer palpable.

11.18
HIV Infection

HIV infection in an 11-year-old boy with severe hemophilia A (factor VIII deficiency). Findings included bilateral egg-sized cervical lymphadenopathy. Since 1 year of age, the child required frequent infusions of factor VIII concentrate. Serologic testing demonstrated HIV infection.

11.19
Thyroglossal Duct Cyst

Thyroglossal duct cyst in a 6-year-old boy. The plum-sized, soft swelling in the midline of the neck between the hyoid bone and the thyroid cartilage had been present for some time, but had recently grown in size and was beginning to cause difficulty in swallowing. A fistulous opening (remnant of the persistent thyroglossal duct) was not detected. The cyst was removed surgically.

Enlargement of the middle lobe of the thyroid, thyroid tumor, and dermoid cyst must be considered in the differential diagnosis.

11.20
Perimandibular Abscess

Perimandibular abscess in a 12-year-old boy. The findings included diffuse, fluctuant, erythematous, painful swelling in the submandibular region. The swelling had appeared suddenly and was treated by incision and drainage. Culture was positive for both aerobic and anaerobic organisms. The abscess was caused by an inflamed tooth, which was removed.

11.21
Chronic Cervical Lymphadenitis

Chronic cervical lymphadenitis, caused by atypical myobacteria (scrofula) in a 4-year-old girl. The findings included an egg-sized swelling of the lymph nodes, erythema of the overlying skin in the submental area, and cherry sized, nonpainful, movable, preauricular lymph nodes. The involved lymph nodes later became fluctuant and formed fistulous tracts. Complete excision led to healing. Histologic examination of the excised nodes demonstrated granuloma formation and caseous necrosis. Culture demonstrated myobacteria resistant to several antituberculous drugs (INH, rifampin, PAS, streptomycin). Although this was an infection with atypical mycobacteria, skin testing with old tuberculin proved positive (cross-reaction).

11.16   11.17

11.18   11.19

11.20   11.21

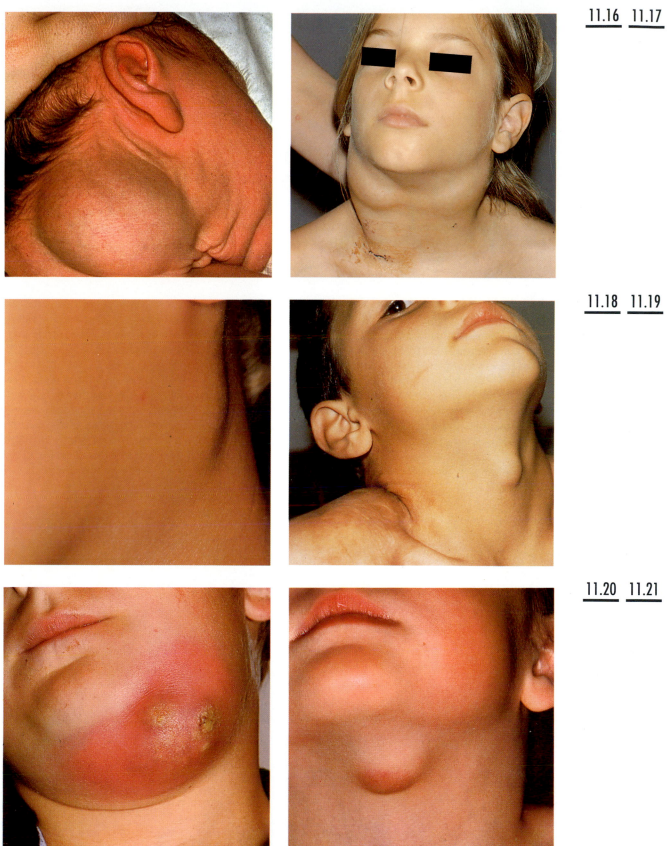

11.22

Cavernous Hemangioma

Deep cavernous hemangioma of the skin in a 4-day-old newborn. The findings included a tangerine-sized, soft, movable, nonpulsatile mass on the right half of the forehead. Radiographic examination of the skin demonstrated that there was no bony defect (ruling out encephalocele, cranial meningocele). Histologic examination of the mass demonstrated

that this was a large cavernous hemangioma and not a malignant lesion.

Differential Diagnosis—Differential diagnosis includes encephalocele and meningocele as well as other vascular tumors such as angiosarcoma and hemangioendothelioma.

11.23

Teratoma

Benign teratoma on the neck of a 3-month-old boy. The mass was a fist-sized, sharply demarcated, firm swelling on the anterior aspect of the neck which had been present since birth. The diagnosis of benign teratoma was made after surgical resection. During pregnancy, maternal serum alpha fetoprotein was not elevated (elevated AFP is seen in ⅔ of all malignant teratomas). Radiographic examination detected calcium shadows corresponding to rudimentary teeth.

Teratomas usually occur in the midline. During the first year of life, teratomas are frequently located in the sacrococcygeum. In early childhood, teratomas may be seen in the testicles; by school age they are frequently found in the ovaries. In addition, teratomas may also occur in the anterior mediastinum, retroperitoneum, cranium, and neck. Other locations are rare.

11.24a 11.24b

Sacrococcygeal Teratoma

Sacrococcygeal teratoma before resection (on the fourth day of life) and after resection (on the 20th day of life). The tumor was originally presumed to be benign. Surgical removal of the teratoma was accomplished without having to remove the coccyx. At 1 month of age, urinary retention was noted. Radiographic examination revealed a tumor in the pelvis which compressed both ureters. A second operation was performed to remove a presacral malignant teratoma, apparently related to remaining tissue of the original tumor. After removal of the tumor, the child was treated with both radiation and chemotherapy. The child has been free of any recurrence.

Sacrococcygeal teratoma may be either benign or malignant. The incidence of malignancy is dependent upon the patient's age. Before the fourth month of life, the malignancy rate is 6%; between the fourth month and the fifth year, the malignancy rate is 50%. Sacrococcygeal teratoma must be differentiated from other tumors of the sacrococcygeal area such as lipoma, neuroblastoma, other neurogenic tumors, cystic lymphangioma, and hemangioma. Meningocele or meningomylocele may frequently occur in the sacrococcygeal area, but can frequently be distinguished on physical examination.

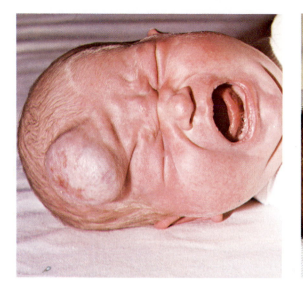
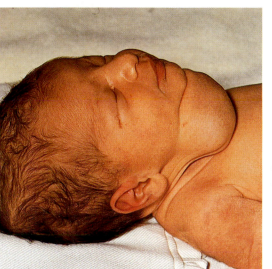

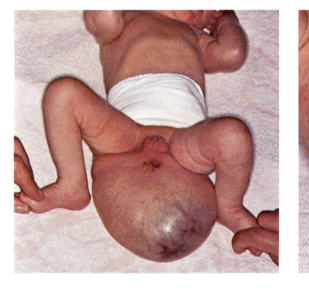
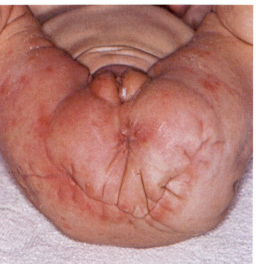

11.25

Tuberous Sclerosis

Tuberous sclerosis in a 3½-year-old girl. Multiple depigmented macules were noted on the upper arm. In addition, adenoma sebaceum was noted on the face and shagreen patches were noted on the leg. Computed tomography revealed tumorlike nodes in the cerebral cortex along the left lateral ventricle. The course was further complicated by seizures which began at 5 months of age.

There are many cutaneous changes associated with tuberous sclerosis. Depigmented macules (elongated white spots 1–3 cm in length) are easily recognized with a Wood's lamp and are principally located on the torso and limbs. Depigmented macules are frequently seen in tuberous sclerosis. Cafe-au-lait spots may also occur; however, they are not as numerous as those seen in neurofibromatosis. The most frequent skin finding in tuberous sclerosis is adenoma sebaceum (small red-brown nodules on the face) and shagreen patches (raised indurated skin lesions).

11.26

Vitiligo

Vitiligo in a 3-week-old infant. Findings included numerous, irregular, sharply demarcated depigmented macules over the back. The skin lesions were incidental findings during an admission to the hospital for bronchopneumonia.

Vitiligo is an acquired defect in pigmentation. The cause is unknown. Hereditary factors or an autoimmune response may play a role. The affected skin is lacking in pigment and melanocytes. Therapy is usually unsatisfactory.

Differential Diagnosis—Differential diagnosis discussed on page 262.

11.27

Tuberous Sclerosis

Tuberous sclerosis in a 14½-year-old boy. The findings include a periungual fibroma with resulting nail dysplasia. Periungual fibromas may not develop until puberty. They are smooth, firm, flesh-colored, 5–10 mm large lesions. In addition to periungual fibromas, other findings of tuberous sclerosis were present (depigmented macules, seizure disorder, mental retardation).

11.28

Tuberous Sclerosis

Tuberous sclerosis in a 10-year-old girl. Shagreen patches were noted over the lower back. These lesions were poorly defined, yellow, indurated areas of skin with a texture resembling orange peel. The findings of shagreen patches allowed for early diagnosis of tuberous sclerosis.

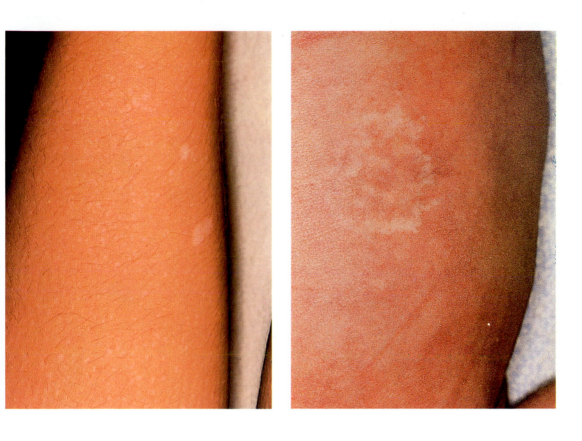

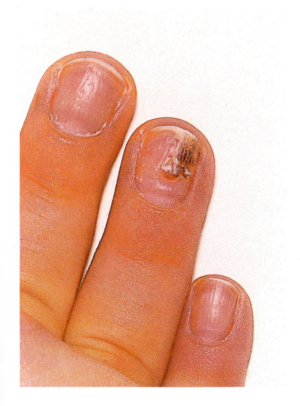

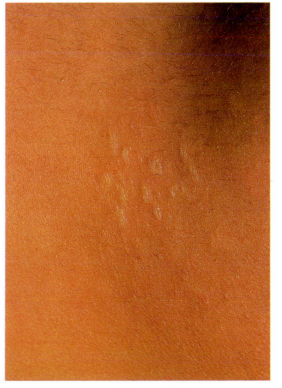

11.29–11.32
Acute Graft Versus Host Disease

Acute graft versus host disease (GVHD) in a 13-year-old boy, 2 months after an allogenic bone marrow transplantation for aplastic anemia. Initially, a generalized, erythematous maculopapular rash with fine desquamation was noted (Figure 11.29 and 11.30). Later, rough lamellar desquamation (Figure 11.31) and detachment of the nails (Figure 11.32) was seen. There was no blister formation. The liver was also affected by acute GVHD; presenting with nausea, vomiting, right upper quadrant pain, and abnormal liver function tests. After 4 weeks of treatment, the child was discharged from the hospital.

The cutaneous manifestations of acute GVHD must be distinguished from drug eruptions and viral exanthem. Pain caused by pressure on the palms and soles, periungual edema and edema of the ears are all cutaneous manifestations of acute GVHD. Diagnosis of acute GVHD can be confirmed by skin biopsy. At an advanced stage of GVHD, bullous changes appear especially at pressure points. Cutaneous manifestations of chronic GVHD can begin forty days after bone marrow transplantation. The findings in chronic GVHD may include violet papules resembling lichen planus or morphea-like lesions which can become confluent and restrict movement of the joints.

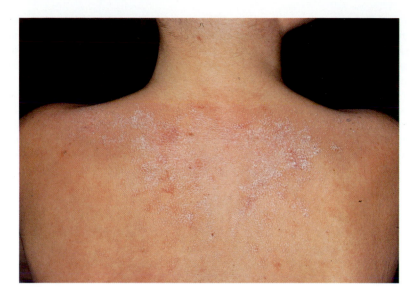

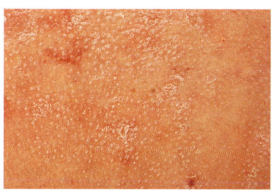 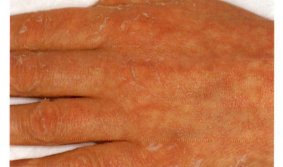

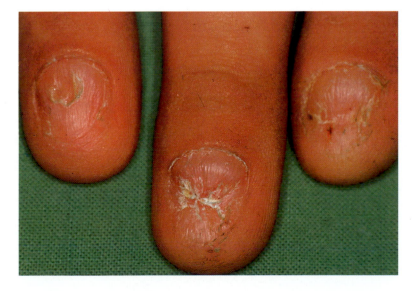

11.33 11.34
Neurofibromatosis

Neurofibromatosis (von Recklinghausen's disease) in a 13-year-old girl. Findings included numerous cafe-au-lait spots of various size on the torso and cutaneous neurofibromas on the legs. These findings appeared at approximately eleven months of age. Subcutaneous fibromas were palpable along the larger peripheral nerves. In addition, there was enlargement of the right leg due to extensive growth of the neurofibromas (plexiform neuroma).

Cafe-au-lait spots are seen in 90% of patients with neurofibromatosis. These skin lesions are caused by hyperpigmentation of the basal epidermal cells. They develop within the first year of life. Since cafe-au-lait spots may occur in healthy children, they are considered diagnostically important only when more than six spots, greater than 1.5 cm in diameter are noted. Cafe-au-lait spots may also be seen in cases of tuberous sclerosis (page 306).

Cutaneous neurofibromas are soft, red nodules which can attain considerable size. These nodes are sessile at first, but later the nodes become pedunculated. They are often present in great numbers. The oral mucous membranes are affected in 5 to 10% of the cases. The lesions may also involve the palate, the tongue, and the lips.

11.35
Neurofibromatosis

Neurofibromatosis (von Recklinghausen's disease) in a 4-year-old boy. A cherry-sized, subcutaneous fibroma was found on the right thigh. In addition, there were numerous cafe-au-lait spots and multiple subcutaneous nodules (arranged like a string of pearls on the neck). The disease is inherited in an autosomal dominant fashion. In this family, both the mother and sister had neurofibromatosis.

11.36
Neurofibromatosis

Neurofibromatosis (von Recklinghausen's disease) in a 15-year-old girl. Findings included a giant, infiltrative, brown pigmented tumor (plexiform neuroma) on the chest and left upper arm. In addition, many cutaneous neurofibromas were noted on the torso and several cafe-au-lait spots were seen on the extremities. Histologic examination of the neuroma revealed abundant, loose connective tissue with Schwann cells and mast cells confirming the clinical diagnosis.

Sarcomatous degeneration of neurofibromas may occur as the disease progresses in approximately 5% of patients. In addition, pheochromocytomas and optic gliomas may be observed.

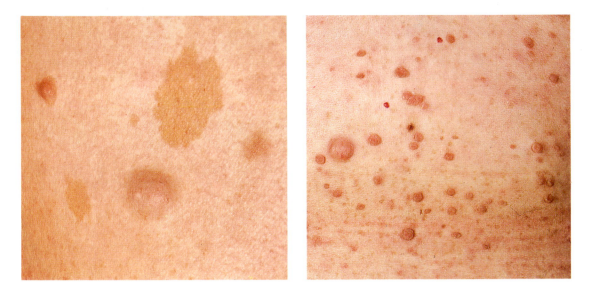

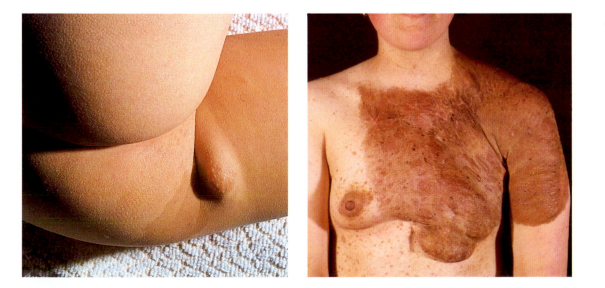

11.37

Mucocele

Mucocele (mucous cyst) on the maxillary gingiva of a 4-week-old girl. Of note was a solitary, cherry-sized protuberance of the mucous membrane which was filled with clear fluid. These cysts are believed to occur after traumatic rupture of a salivary duct. Treatment consists of surgical excision. Retention cysts of the salivary glands are called mucoceles; retention cysts of the sublingual glands are called ranula (because of the similarity to the inflated bladder of a frog's throat).

Differential Diagnosis—Differential diagnosis of cysts located on the gums include dentigerous cysts, dysontogenic cysts, epulis (see below), and "chocolate cysts" (juvenile bone cysts).

11.38

Ranula

Ranula in a 2-week-old girl. Two bean-sized, well-defined, taut blue mucous retention cysts were noted on the floor of the mouth under the tongue. These were connected with the ducts of the submaxillary salivary glands. Therapy consisted of surgical removal. Ranula can displace the tongue, rupture easily, and lead to secondary bacterial infection.

Differential Diagnosis—Differential diagnosis includes epidermoid cysts in the floor of the mouth.

11.39

Epulis

Epulis in a 4-day-old girl. Findings included a plum-sized, pedunculated tumor of firm consistency originating from the gingiva. Recurrence after resection is possible. The cause of congenital epulis is unclear and probably not consistent.

11.40

Epulis

Epulis in a 2-day-old newborn. Findings included an apple-sized, firm tumor with a nodular surface. The mass was connected to the lower ridge of teeth by a pencil-thin pedicle and protruded from the mouth. Surgical removal was accomplished on the same day. The diagnosis of epulis was confirmed by histologic examination. There was no recurrence after surgical resection.

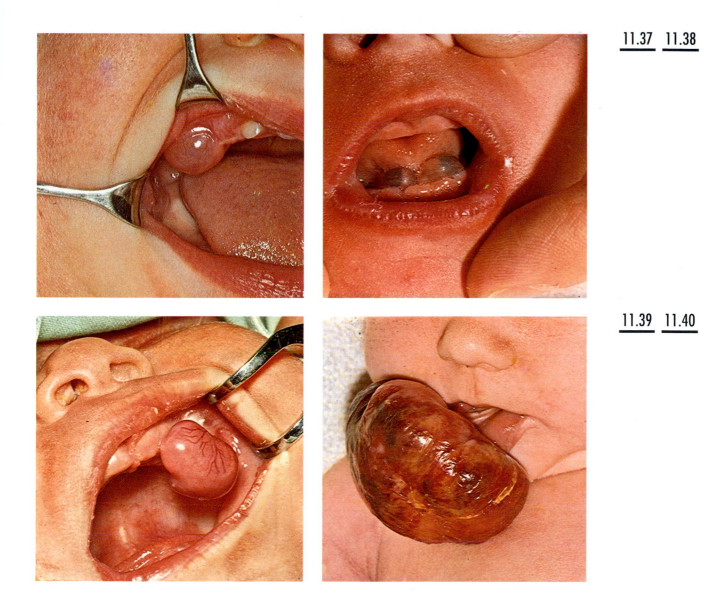

11.41

Neurofibrosarcoma

Neurofibrosarcoma in a 15-year-old girl who had symptoms of neurofibromatosis (von Recklinghausen's disease). The tumor had infiltrated the underlying tissue, causing the right side of the neck to become diffusely swollen. Surgical operation achieved only partial resection. Histologic examination of the tissue demonstrated that this was a neurofibrosarcoma.

The possibility of sarcomatous degeneration must always be considered in neurofibromatosis, particularly if there is rapid enlargement of the node, pain, or ulceration.

11.42

Mucoepidermoid Carcinoma

Mucoepidermoid carcinoma of the parotid gland in a 16-year-old boy. A firm, nontender mass, which was difficult to distinguish from the surrounding area, was noted in the area of the left parotid gland. Regional lymph nodes were not swollen. The tumor was completely removed. Relapse or metastasis did not occur. Histologically, mucoepidermoid tumors can be separated into well differentiated and undifferentiated forms. Mucoepidermoid tumors can be locally invasive, but only rarely metastasize.

Differential Diagnosis—Unilateral, persistent swelling in the parotid area can be caused by other parotid tumors, particularly mixed parotid tumor (pleomorphic adenomas), as well as hemangiomas and lymphangiomas. Parotid swelling can also be caused by obstruction of the duct by salivary calculus. In these cases, a calcium shadow can be detected radiographically. Recurrent parotitis can be unilateral or bilateral, and is not associated with pain. The cause of this condition is unknown; recurrent parotitis resolved after several episodes without specific treatment.

11.43

Horner Syndrome

Horner syndrome in a 3-month-old girl. Ptosis, miosis, and enophthalmos were present since birth. There was no heterochromia of the iris on the affected side. A tumor on the left side of the neck was noted at the age of 2½ months. Elevated levels of homovanillic acid (HVA) and vanillylmandelic acid (VMA) were noted. The tumor was removed and chemotherapy was initiated. Histologic examination confirmed the diagnosis of neuroblastoma originating in the sympathetic trunk in the cervical region with metastasis to the lymph nodes. The girl recovered fully.

11.44

Parotitis

Parotitis (mumps) in a 15-year-old girl. The findings included painful, nonerythematous swelling of the parotid glands. The patient complained of pain when chewing and dryness of the mouth. Serum and urine amylase levels were elevated (without any evidence of pancreatitis). The complement fixation reaction from mumps was positive in the second week of illness.

Differential Diagnosis—Differential diagnosis for parotid swelling includes:

1. Cervical lymphadenitis with preauricular involvement (differentiated by physical examination).
2. Suppurative parotitis (painful, erythematous swelling of the parotid gland. Pressure on the parotid gland causes pus to be expressed through the duct).
3. Recurrent parotitis (mildly painful swelling which resolves spontaneously. The etiology is unknown, possibly due to allergy).
4. Salivary calculus (intermittent swelling of the glands due to obstruction. Calcium shadows can be detected radiographically).
5. Parotid tumors (unilateral chronic swelling caused by hemangiomas, lymphomas, mixed parotid tumors).
6. Mikulicz's disease (seen in leukemia, tuberculosis).

11.45

Mastoiditis

Mastoiditis in a 6-year-old boy. The right ear was displaced anteriorly and downward. The area behind the ear was painful and swollen. The child originally had acute otitis media, which went untreated, leading to perforation of the tympanic membrane and mastoiditis. Cultures obtained from the periosteal abscess contained pneumococci. The child improved after systemic antibiotic therapy.

Differential Diagnosis—Inflammation and swelling in the postauricular area can stem from lymphadenopathy secondary to superficial skin infection in otitis externa.

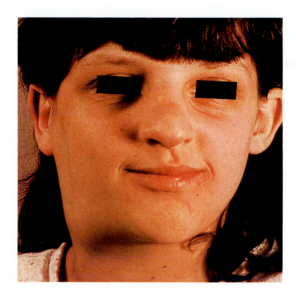 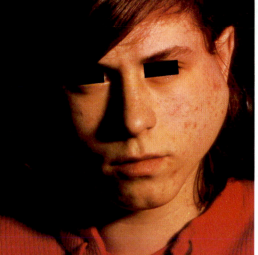

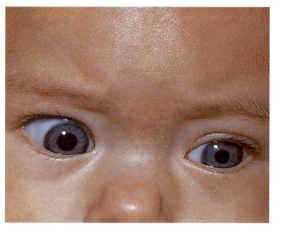

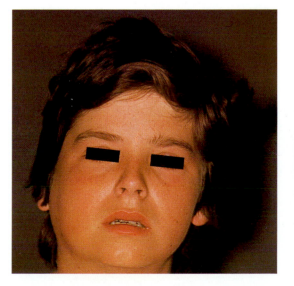 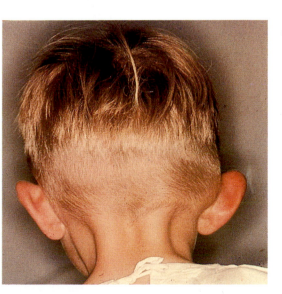

11.46

Retinoblastoma

Retinoblastoma in a two year old boy. The figure demonstrates the child after enucleation of the left eye. The first symptom of retinoblastoma was an acute increase in intraocular pressure in the left eye. Extensive infiltration of the tumor was noted in the soft tissue of the orbit, the cheek, the parotid gland, as well as the liver, lymph nodes, and vertebrae. The right eye was not affected. Despite surgical intervention, radiation, and chemotherapy, the child died 5 weeks later.

Although retinoblastoma can present at birth, retinoblastoma usually presents within the first or second years of life. This tumor of the posterior retina may involve one or both eyes. If the disease is bilateral, it is thought to follow an autosomal dominant pattern of inheritance. In cases of inherited retinoblastoma, other malignancies may also develop (osteogenic sarcoma).

Differential Diagnosis—The differential diagnosis of childhood orbital tumors includes leukemic infiltrates, teratoma, rhabdomyosarcoma, tumors of the optic nerve, malignant lymphoma, angioma, hemangioma, other vascular anomalies (arteriovenous malformation), neurofibromatosis, tuberous sclerosis, histiocytosis X, orbital cysts, meningocele, and encephalocele. For discussion of pseudoglioma, see page 318.

11.47

Neuroblastoma

Neuroblastoma in a 1-year-old child. Proptosis and ecchymosis of the orbit were due to retrobulbar metastases which involved the orbit, the sphenoid bone, and the maxillary sinus. Horner syndrome (page 314) and opsiclonus were not present. The liver and numerous lymph nodes in the neck and groin were enlarged due to metastasis of the tumor. Radiographic studies demonstrated extensive metastasis to the bones (especially to the long bones). On autopsy, the primary tumor was found in the right adrenal gland.

11.48

Basilar Skull Fracture

Ecchymosis of the orbit due to basilar skull fracture in a 5-year-old boy. Bilateral ecchymoses were noted on the superior and inferior aspects of the orbits. Radiographic studies of the skull demonstrated a basilar skull fracture. Orbital fractures, which can also lead to periocular ecchymoses, were ruled out.

Differential Diagnosis—Metastatic neuroblastoma may involve the orbit and produce unilateral or bilateral ecchymoses with proptosis. Other orbital tumors may have similar findings.

11.49

Suspected Child Abuse

Multiple hematomas were noted on the face and body of this 3-year-old girl. There was no evidence of bone fractures or subdural hematoma. Platelet count and coagulation studies were normal. The skin lesions could not be attributed to any disease process. Further history led to the diagnosis of suspected child abuse and neglect. The child was released after investigation of the domestic situation by social service agencies with the diagnosis of suspected child abuse.

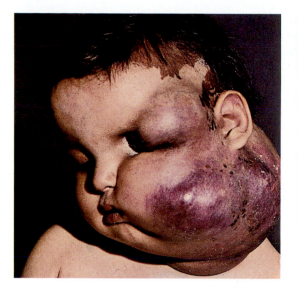
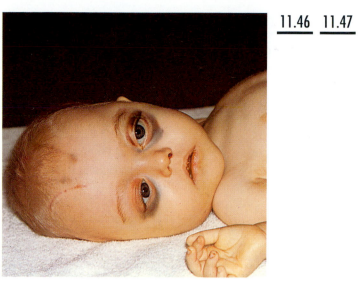

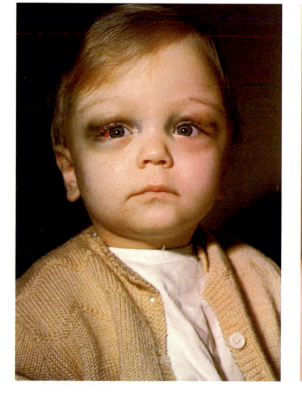
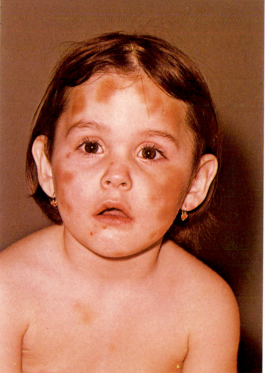

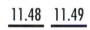

11.50

Pseudoglioma

Pseudoglioma (pseudoretinoblastoma) involving the left eye of a 2-year-old girl. Ophthalmologic examination revealed a circumscribed, light yellow opacity that obliterated the red reflex. This condition is caused by traumatic hemorrhage of the retina and vitreous body.

Differential Diagnosis—Similar opacification and loss of the red reflex may be seen in retinoblastoma, other intra-ocular tumors, retrolental fibroplasia, persistence of the primary vitreous body, organized purulent exudate of the vitreous body, and vascularization of the vitreous body after severe fetal uveitis. Leukocoria (white pupil) may be caused by cataracts, detached retina, and severe chorioretinal degeneration.

11.51

Cavernous Hemangioma

Deep cavernous hemangioma of the right lower eyelid in a 6-month-old girl. Findings included extensive, poorly defined, soft swelling of the entire lower eyelid with blue-purple discoloration of the skin.

Differential Diagnosis—Differential diagnosis includes lymphangioma, lipoma of the eyelid, and dermoid cyst of the eyelid.

11.52

Dermoid Cyst

Congenital dermoid cyst of the right upper eyelid of a 14-year-old girl. Findings included a bean sized, poorly defined, soft swelling of the lateral corner of the eye below the eyebrow. Histologic examination revealed a cyst lined by kera-tinized squamous epithelial cells containing hair follicles and sebaceous glands, confirming the diagnosis of dermoid cyst.

Differential Diagnosis—Differential diagnosis includes dermoid cysts, lipoma, lymphangioma, and hemangioma.

11.53

Retinoblastoma

Retinoblastoma in a 10-month-old girl. Findings included heterochromia of the iris and strabismus of the left eye. The lens was uneffected. The vitreous of the left eye was filled with a vascular tumor which was recognized because of its yellow-white reflection in the pupils (leukocoria). Intraocular pressure was normal, and there was no progressive enlargement of the eye (buphthalmos). Retinoblastoma may involve one or both eyes during the first year of life. In this case, a small retinoblastoma was found in the right eye. It had not penetrated the vitreous. Chromosome analysis demonstrated a deletion of the long arm of chromosome 13 (a frequent finding in bilateral retinoblastoma). The left eye was enucleated. The tumor had not yet penetrated the choroid or the optic nerve. Radiotherapy of the right eye led to complete regression of the tumor.

Differential Diagnosis—The differential diagnosis includes congenital cataracts, retrolental fibroplasia, persistent hyperplasia of the primary vitreous, retinal dysplasia, and endophthalmitis caused by nematodes.

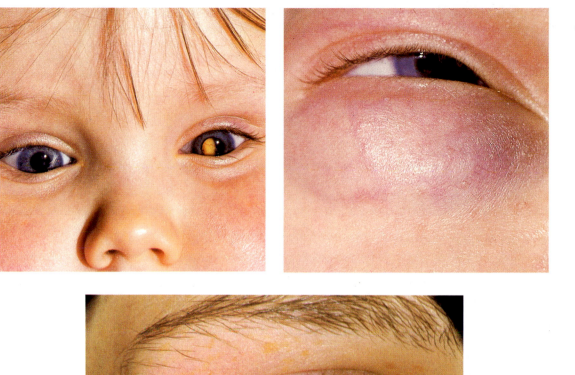

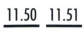

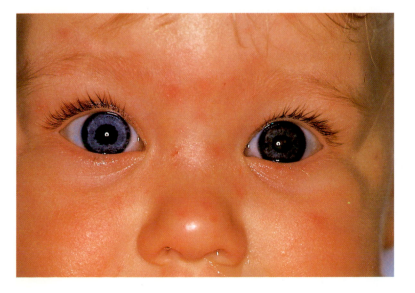

11.53

12.1
Anophthalmia

Anophthalmia and blepharophimosis (abnormal narrowing of the palpebral fissures) in a 6-week-old child. The child developed microcephaly, mental retardation, and seizures. Examination of the eyes beyond the narrow palpebral fissures revealed no rudimentary eyeballs. The child was later provided with ocular prostheses. No specific cause was found.

In cases of anophthalmia, the orbits are usually small and the eyelids are closed and concave. Anophthalmia may occur as an isolated malformation or in associated with trisomy 13 (Patau syndrome, page 84). Magnetic resonance imaging can be used to differentiate anophthalmia from marked microphthalmos.

12.2
Fetal Rubella Syndrome

Bilateral cataracts and glaucoma (as well as keratoconjunctivitis due to *Pseudomonas*) in a 5-week-old boy with fetal rubella syndrome. The infant's mother had contracted rubella during the second trimester of pregnancy. The child had many of the features of fetal rubella syndrome. Shortly after birth, the child was noted to have clinical findings of a patent ductus arteriosus (loud, continuous murmur) and congestive heart failure. Typical radiographic changes were noted in the long bones (radiographs of the proximal tibial revealed linear radiolucencies alternating with areas of increased density). Rubella-specific immunoglobulin M was noted in the child's and mother's serum. At 6 weeks of age, the child underwent surgical ligation of the ductus arteriosus. Surgery to remove the cataract was performed at 13 months of age without complication.

In fetal rubella syndrome, cataracts may develop in up to 50% of patients. Various forms of cataracts are possible within the spectrum of fetal rubella syndrome. Other anomalies of the eye related to fetal rubella syndrome include microphthalmia, corneal opacity, strabismus, and nystagmus. Glaucoma is also associated with fetal rubella syndrome. Other prenatal infections which may cause cataracts include cytomegalovirus and toxoplasmosis. For differential diagnosis of congenital cataracts, see page 214 and for differential diagnosis of glaucoma, see pages 332 and 328.

12.3
Amaurosis

Bilateral congenital amaurosis in an 8-month-old girl. No other symptoms were noted. The findings included pupils which were glassy when exposed to light and amaurotic nytagmus. The child was noted to rub her eyes frequently (oculodigital phenomenon). The cause of amaurosis was unclear. There is no family history of partial or total loss of vision.

Frequent causes of congenital blindness include microphthalmia, corneal opacification, dense lenticular opacification, atrophic chorioretinal scarring, macular colobomata, and severe hypoplasia of the optic nerve. In cases of the recessively inherited Leber's congenital retinal amaurosis, retinal degeneration may not develop until later in life (despite persistent blindness). Early diagnosis of this condition is possible with electroretinography. Often there are EEG changes, microcephaly, and other anomalies of the central nervous system.

12.4
Microphthalmia

Unilateral microphthalmia in a 3-week-old boy. The eyeball and orbit of the right eye were noted to be diminished in size since birth. This was an isolated deformity the cause of which is unknown. Microphthalmia is frequently a bilateral defect and is often associated with other occular anomalies including hyperopia, pseudophakia, microphakia, cataract, and colobomata of the iris and choroid membrane. Malformation of the anterior chamber may lead to glaucoma. Microphthalmia may be seen in cases of intrauterine infection (rubella, toxoplasmosis, cytomegalovirus), fetal alcohol syndrome, and thalidomide embryopathy. Certain chromosomal abnormalities are associated with microphthalmia (trisomy 13, page 84). Microphthalmia is observed in the following syndromes:

1. Aicardi's syndrome (agenesis of the corpus collosum)
2. Cryptophthalmos syndrome (absence of eyelids, orbits covered by skin)
3. Ectodermal syndromes (including Hallermann-Streiff syndrome, oculodentodigital syndrome)
4. Fanconi syndrome (pancytopenia)
5. Meckel-Gruber syndrome (microcephaly, genitourinary abnormalities, polydactyly)
6. Sjögren-Larsson syndrome (ichthyosis, spastic paralysis, mental retardation).

In cases of Norrie's disease (an X-linked trait), there is congenital bilateral retinal malformation and blindness which may later lead to shrinking and wasting of the eyeball (phthisis bulbi).

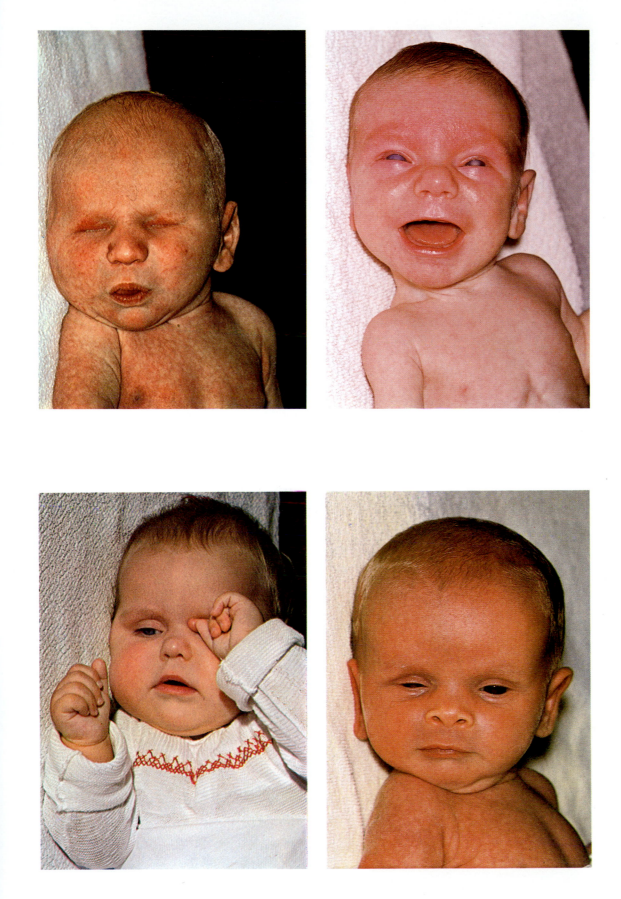

12.5 Coloboma

Congenital coloboma of the iris in a 10-month-old girl. An absent sector of the right iris gives the pupil a pear-shaped appearance. Coloboma are due to fetal malclosure of the optic cup.

A coloboma of the iris may be associated with coloboma of the fundus and optic nerve. Coloboma may be associated with chromosomal abnormalities including trisomy 13 and 18.

12.6 Gunn Syndrome

Gunn syndrome in a 6-month-old girl. The ptotic left upper eyelid was lifted rhythmically in synchrony with chewing and swallowing. The condition was due to a congenital malformation of enervation. The ptotic upper eyelid was lifted when the jaw was moved on the opposite side. Rapid lifting of the lower eyelid could be induced by talking quietly, yawning, and extension of the tongue.

Gunn syndrome is usually unilateral and may be associated with amblyopia, anisometropia, and paralysis of extraocular muscles. The syndrome is typically sporadic but may also be inherited as an autosomal dominant trait.

12.7 Microphthalmia

Microphthalmia and partial adhesion of the eyelids (ankyloblepharon) in a 1-month-old girl. Microphthalmia and bilateral shortened palpebral fissures had been noted since birth with partial adhesion of the eyelid margins between the upper and lower eyelids. The condition is caused by lack of eyelid movement during fetal development. Narrowing of the palpebral fissures may also occur in congenital blepharophimosis which can be inherited as a dominant or recessive trait.

12.8 Duane Syndrome (Type II)

Congenital Duane syndrome (type II) in a 6-year-old girl. Adduction of the right eye was restricted with intact abduction with narrowing of the palpebral fissures and retraction of the eyeball during adduction. To compensate for this defect, the girl generally turned her head toward the unaffected side to achieve binocular vision. Electromyography demonstrated coinnervation of the lateral rectus muscle in adduction which led to inhibition of adduction and retraction of the eyeball.

In Duane syndrome (type I) abduction is restricted or absent. During adduction the palpebral fissure is also narrowed and the eyeball retracted. During abduction the palpebral fissure widens. At rest, a mild convergent strabismus arises. The cause is a defect in innervation of the lateral rectus muscle in abduction and paradoxical activity during adduction.

In Duane syndrome (type III) both abduction and adduction are restricted.

Duane syndrome affects the left eye more frequently than the right eye, but may be bilateral or asymmetric. Girls are more often affected than boys. About 1% of all children with strabismus have this syndrome. Other anomalies of the eye may also be present. Surgical treatment is necessary in severe cases.

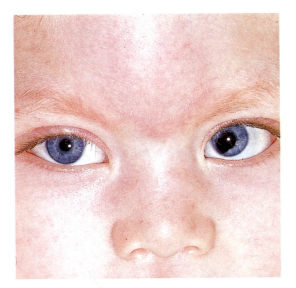

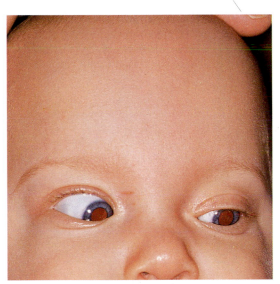
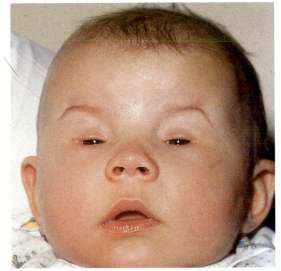

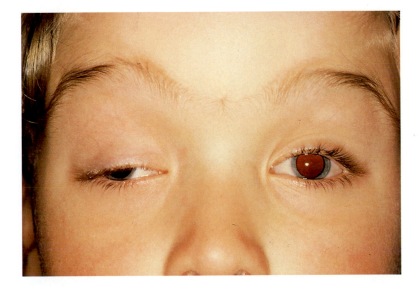

12.9

Residual Pupillary Membrane

Residual pupillary membrane in a 7-year-old boy. Several delicate strands of tissue extended from the iris to the capsule of the lens. Vision was not impaired.

Different grades or persistent pupillary membrane are possible. Small residual parts of the membrane are frequent in newborns. Larger residue, which may be detrimental to vision, are rare and may be combined with anterior cataracts. Residual pupillary membrane must be distinguished from posterior synechiae which stem from an inflammatory process in the anterior section of the eye.

12.10

Partial Aniridia

Bilateral partial aniridia in a 7-year-old girl who had poor vision and photophobia. The involved area where the iris was absent appeared black like the pupil. There were no associated anomalies such as glaucoma, cataracts, or hypoplasia of the macula and optic nerve. Wilms tumor, which may be associated with aniridia, was ruled out through sonography. Therapy included prescription of dark contact lenses.

Aniridia is usually bilateral and never truly "complete."

Isolated aniridia is an autosomal dominant trait with a frequency in the general population of 1:100,000. Sporadic aniridia is observed in conjunction with other anomalies (including microcephaly, renal or genital malformations, and hemihypertrophy). Neoplasms which may be associated with aniridia include Wilms tumor, rhabdomyosarcoma, and adrenal tumors. Deletion of the short arm of chromosome 11 is found in aniridia-Wilms tumor syndrome.

12.11

Ataxia Telangiectasia

Ataxia telangiectasia (Louis-Bar syndrome) in a 10-year-old girl who had symptoms of progressive ataxia since 2 years of age. Prominent snakelike telangiectasias of the conjunctiva as well as telangiectasias of the superior and inferior eyelids, the pinna, and the left upper arm were noted. In addition to truncal ataxia and ataxic gait, other extrapyramidal signs were noted (including nystagmus, dysarthria, and dementia). Serum IgA and IgE were decreased.

Differential Diagnosis—The differential diagnosis of conjunctival telangiectasia includes nevus flammeus of the conjunctiva, Fabry's disease (deficiency of α-galactosidase activity), telangiectasias of the conjunctiva, and conjunctivitis.

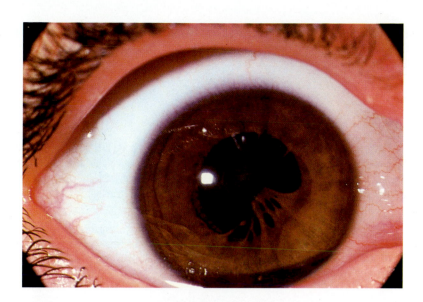

12.9

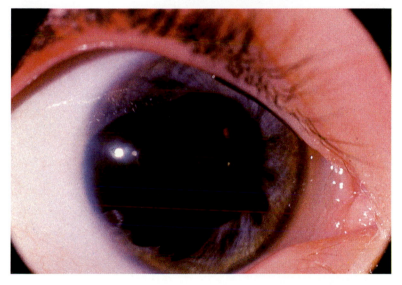

12.10

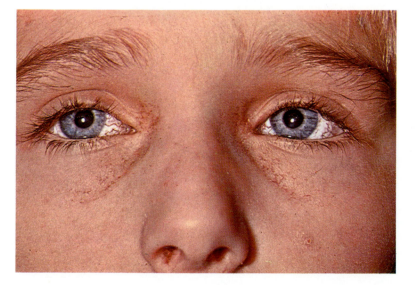

12.11

12.12

**Pigment Spots
of the Iris**

Small, bilateral pigment spots of the iris in an 8-year-old boy. Pigment spots of the iris due to an accumulation of melanocytes occur in 50% to 60% of the population. Although present at birth, pigment spots become more noticeable during puberty.

12.13

Conjunctival Nevus

Conjunctival nevus in a 12-year-old boy. A small, flat, yellow nevus was noted near the limbic area of the right eyelid. Pigmented nevi of the conjunctiva occur frequently. They are usually small, slightly raised, bright yellow to black-brown lesions, which are first noted in early childhood and may increase in size and pigmentation during puberty. They may also be found near the lacrimal duct or the edge of the eyelid. Malignant degeneration is rare.

12.14

**Dislocation
of the Lens**

Dislocation of the lens in a 20-year-old woman with Marfan syndrome. The zonular fibers, which arise in the ciliary body and insert into the lens, are visible in the lower half of the pupil.

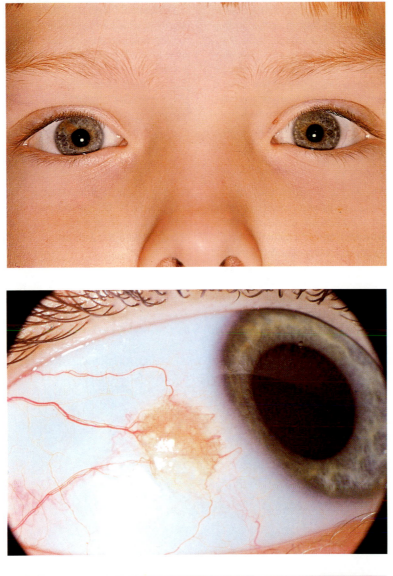

12.12

12.13

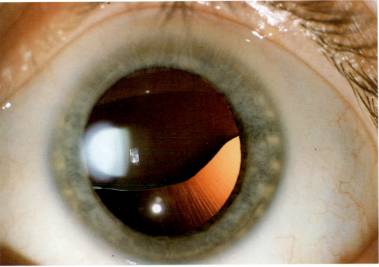

12.14

12.15
Hydrophthalmus

Hydrophthalmus in a 4-year-old boy. The enlargement of the right eye and cornea resulted from glaucoma in early childhood. Glaucoma was suspected because of the boy's excessive tearing (epiphora), sensitivity to light (photophobia), and worsening vision. No corneal opacification or Haab's band opacities (tears in Descemet's membrane) were noted, as these are seen in advanced stages of glaucoma. The cause of glaucoma was congenital obstruction of the iridocorneal angle caused by residual mesodermal tissue.

Differential Diagnosis—Differential diagnosis of an enlarged eye includes megalocornea, in which case the intraocular pressure is normal. Glaucoma may also occur secondary to other eye malformations, metabolic and inflammatory processes, tumors of the eye, trauma, as well as phakomatoses (neurofibromatosis) and Rubinstein-Taybi syndrome (page 54).

12.16
Corectopia

Corectopia (abnormal position of the pupils) in a 4-year-old boy. Findings included congenital medial displacement of both pupils. Dislocation of the lens was also noted. Dislocation of the lens (ectopia lentis) can be caused by abnormalities of the suspensory system secondary to a developmental defect or trauma. In persistent cases where there is subluxation, ectopia of the lens and pupil can lead to glaucoma. Simple ectopia of the pupil (without ectopia of the lens) is of little pathologic significance.

12.17
Albinism

Albinism limited to the eye of a 15-year-old boy. This iris was noted to be bright blue with reddened margins. The eyelashes were black. Albinism was limited to the eye. When examining the eyes, one could see the blood vessels of the choroid on the white-yellow background of the sclera. The boy was very sensitive to light and had to constantly wear sunglasses. Vision was reduced due to hypoplasia of the macula.

Lack of pigmentation in albinism affects the iris as well as the retina. Albinism is also found in patients with Chediak-Higashi syndrome, in which a defect in T-cell-mediated immunity and granulocyte function is noted.

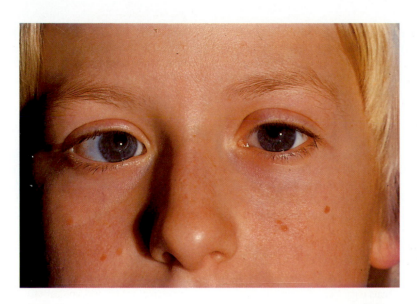

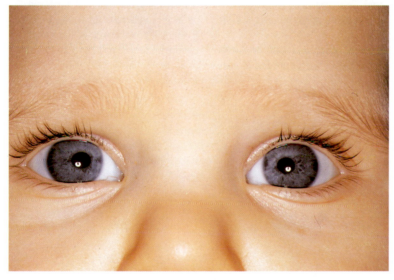

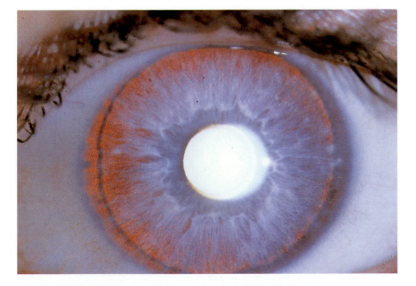

12.18

Ectropion

Congenital ectropion (eversion of the eyelid) in a 10-month-old boy. Extreme erythema of the conjunctiva of the lower eyelid was noted. Excessive tearing also occurred. Prolonged cases of ectropion allow for keratitis to develop. Congenital ectropion is due to poor development of the lateral canthal ligament. Other cases of ectropion may result from scar formation after trauma, burns, inflammation, or in conjunction with facial paralysis. Surgical correction is possible in cases of congenital ectropion.

12.19

Congenital Coloboma

Congenital coloboma of the upper eyelid in a 6-month-old boy. A triangular defect with its base in the free margin of the lid was evident on the nasal half of both upper eyelids associated with the absence of eyelashes. Congenital colobomas of the eyelid may occur as an isolated malformation or in association with other extensive facial malformation such as mandibulofacial dysostosis (Treacher-Collins syndrome, Figure 2.41) or in Goldenhar syndrome (Figure 2.55.). Acquired colobomas of the eyelid are usually due to trauma and may occur in the temporal third of the eyelid.

12.20   12.21

Megalocornea

Megalocornea in a 3-month-old girl. The diameter of the cornea was 15 mm (normal range: 10.5–12.5 mm). Intraocular pressure was not raised. This congenital, nonprogressive enlargement of the cornea leads to refractive error and visual disturbances.

  Differential Diagnosis—Megalocornea must be distinguished from progressive corneal enlargement due to congenital glaucoma. Glaucoma usually presents with photophobia, excessive tearing, and corneal opacity. Glaucoma requires immediate surgical treatment. Keratoconus (cone-shaped protuberance of the mid cornea) and keratoglobus (spherical protuberance of the cornea) usually are not seen until adolescence and can lead to visual problems.

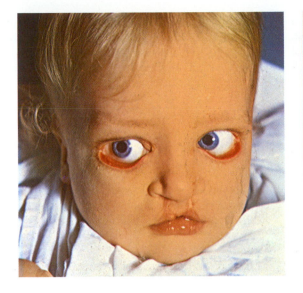

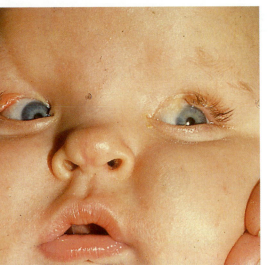

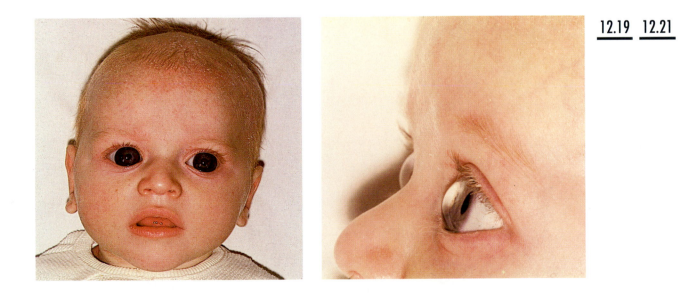

12.22
Osteopetrosis Tarda

Osteopetrosis tarda (Albers-Schonberg syndrome) in a 3-month-old boy. Initial findings included bilateral exophthalmos, which was later followed by blindness and cranial nerve paralysis (due to compression of the cranial foramina). The extent of the exophthalmos could be objectively measured with the use of an exophthalmometer. Progression of the symptoms was rapid, as is seen in the autosomal recessive form of the disease.

Differential Diagnosis—Bilateral exophthalmos may be due to neoplastic processes (tumors, histiocytosis X), vascular anomalies, and inflammatory processes. Exophthalmos may also be noted in hyperthyroidism, and cranial malformations (craniosynostosis, Down syndrome).

12.23
Hydrophthalmos

Unilateral enlargement of the eye secondary to glaucoma in a 7-day-old girl with Sturge-Weber syndrome (encephalotrigeminal angiomatosis). The left eye was reddened, larger, and firmer than the right eye. The wide pupil reacted only sluggishly to light. Fundoscopic examination demonstrated a cavernous hemangioma of the right choroid (ipsilateral to a nevus flammeus of the face). Surgical correction was undertaken to normalize the pressure of the eye. Glaucoma recurred, leading to a iridocyclitis and eventual enucleation of the eye at one year of age. The child was provided with an ocular prosthesis.

Glaucoma may cause enlargement of the eyeball during early childhood. Excessive tearing, photophobia, and blepharospasm are often the first symptoms of infantile glaucoma.

Differential Diagnosis—Traumatic injury to the eye often leads to acquired glaucoma. Other causes of glaucoma include megalocornea, aniridia, and other developmental disorders of the anterior chamber. For discussion of other causes of secondary glaucoma see page 328.

12.24
Osteogenesis Imperfecta

Osteogenesis imperfecta (type I) in a 3-month-old girl. Thinning of the sclera causes the uvea to become more apparent giving the sclera a blue appearance (also seen in Marfan syndrome and Ehlers-Danlos syndrome). Other eye anomalies include corneal opacities, hyperopia, keratoconus, and megalocornea. Blue sclera may be normal in the first weeks of life, since the cornea is relatively thin and transparent at this age. Confirmation of the diagnosis of osteogenesis imperfecta is based on clinical findings (recurrent fractures, skeletal deformities, marked hypermobility of the joints), and typical radiographic bone findings.

12.22

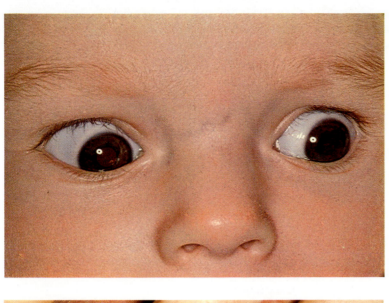

12.23

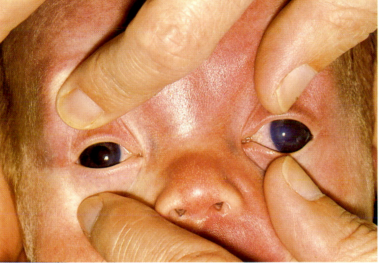

12.24

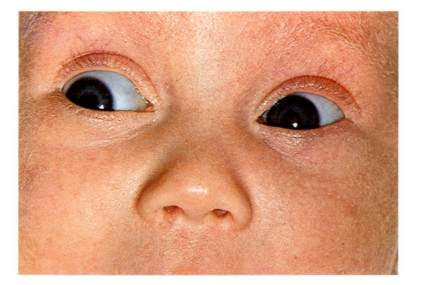

12.25
Subconjunctival
Hemorrhage

Subconjunctival hemorrhage in a 4-year-old boy with acute lymphocytic leukemia. Extensive bilateral hemorrhages were noted under the conjunctiva. In addition, vitreous hemorrhage and skin ecchymoses were noted. Laboratory investigation revealed a platelet count of less than 3,000/μL.

12.26
Proliferative
Retinopathy

Proliferative retinopathy in a 4-year-old girl. Proliferative fibrous changes in the retina and vitreous were noted after blunt trauma to the eye. Because of poor absorption of the hemorrhage, gray, white and yellow strands of scar tissue formed, which led to retinal detachment.

12.27
Cavernous
Hemangioma

Deep cavernous hemangioma of the left upper eyelid in a 1-year-old boy. The extensive raised, poorly defined blue-red hemangioma was noted under the skin. The lesion was present since birth, but had recently grown larger. Movement of the eyelid and vision were limited.

Differential Diagnosis—Differential diagnosis includes lymphangioma, lipoma, dermoid, keratoma, and plexiform neurofibroma.

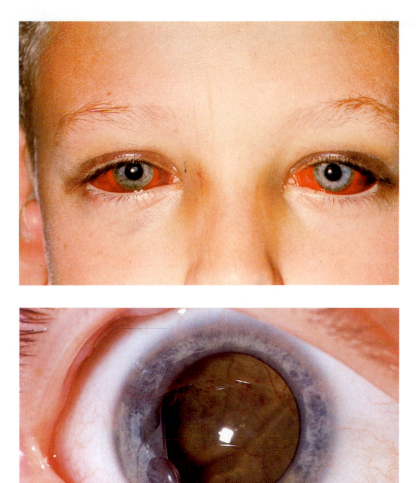

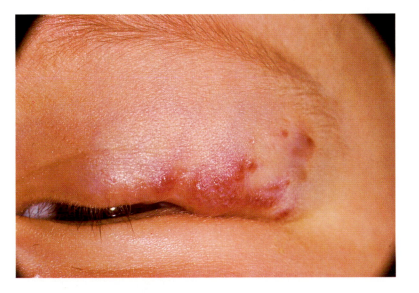

12.28

Hordeolum

External hordeolum in a 15-year-old boy. A circumscribed, painful red swelling of the lower eyelid appeared suddenly. Purulent drainage from the center of the lesion grew *Staphylococcus aureus*. This was an inflammation of the glands of Zeis.

In internal hordeolum, the meibomian glands are inflamed. In internal hordeolum, the abscess is larger, lies deeper, and ruptures through the skin or the conjunctival surface.

12.29

Chalazion

Chalazion in a 12-year-old girl. Findings included a persistent, firm, pellet-sized, painless nodule in the lower eyelid. The skin of the eyelid was easily movable. There were no signs of acute inflammation. Chalazion is a chronic, granulomatous inflammation of the meibomian glands. Visual impairment (due to astigmatism resulting from pressure on the eye) or cosmetic concerns are indications for surgical excision.

12.30

Blepharitis

Blepharitis in a 12-year-old girl. Both the upper and lower lid margins were erythematous and thickened with small crusted ulcerations. *Streptococcus pyogenes* was identified as the causative agent.

In angular blepharitis, *Moraxella* are often the cause. Secondary bacterial infections, frequently caused by staphylococci, are associated with eczema or seborrhea of the eyelids. Inflammation of the eyelids can also be caused by lice or mites. Viral infections (including herpes simplex, herpes zoster, molluscum contagiosum, or papova virus) can also cause blepharitis.

12.31

Lower Lid Abscess

Lower lid abscess in a 9-year-old boy. Findings included severe erythema and swelling of the external third of the lower right eyelid with signs of fluctuation. Abscess of the eyelid may occur after trauma, secondary to osteomyelitis of the orbital ridge, or secondary to a suppurative infection of the paranasal sinuses. Hematogenous spread from sepsis is rare. Infection of the eyelid may lead to orbital cellulitis and cavernous sinus thrombosis.

12.32

Dacryoadenitis

Acute dacryoadenitis in a 12-year-old boy. Findings included painful erythema and swelling of the outer third of the upper eyelid. The palpebral fissure was S-shaped. If the upper eyelid was lifted, one could see the enlarged lacrimal gland. Also noted were edema of the conjunctiva in the region of the lacrimal gland and preauricular lymphadenopathy. The etiology of the dacryoadenitis was unclear. Inflammation of the lacrimal gland can be caused by mumps or other viral infections. Inflammation can be secondary to infection of the conjunctiva.

12.33

Bacterial Panophthalmitis

Bacterial panophthalmitis (endophthalmitis) in a 3-year-old boy. The left eye was painful, inflamed, and swollen. Severe inflammation of the eyelids and periorbital tissue was noted. The infection was caused by a penetrating wound to the eye. The child was successfully treated with systemic antibiotics.

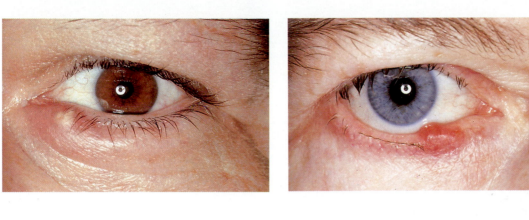

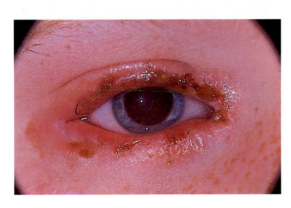
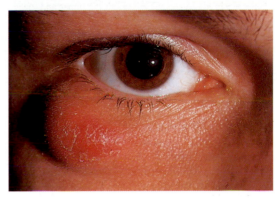

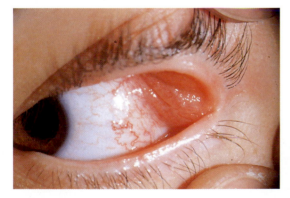
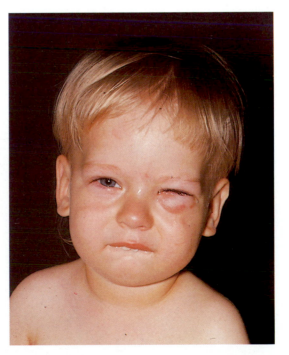

12.34
Ophthalmia Neonatorum

Ophthalmia neonatorum (due to *Neisseria gonorrhoeae*) in a newborn child. Findings included severe swelling of the eyelid and purulent drainage from the left eye. The cornea was inflamed. The illness began on the second day of life. Transmission occurred during birth, from a mother who was unaware of an intercurrent gonorrheal infection. The child developed ophthalmia neonatorum despite prophylactic eye care with silver nitrate solution. Numerous gram-negative diplococci were found in Gram stain and in culture. The child was treated with systemic and topical antibiotics and compresses.

Conjunctivitis due to gonorrhea must be differentiated from other causes of purulent conjunctivitis in the newborn, including other bacterial pathogens (staphylococci, *Pseudomonas*, *Haemophilus*). Conjunctivitis can be caused by the prophylactic eye treatment (chemical conjunctivitis). Inclusion conjunctivitis of the newborn is caused by *Chlamydia trachomatis*. Inclusion conjunctivitis does not begin until the fifth or seventh day after birth and can lead to weeks or months of purulent secretion. *Chlamydia* can be identified microscopically and by culture.

12.35
Orbital Cellulitis

Orbital cellulitis in a 12-year-old girl. The findings included redness and swelling of the left eyelid, proptosis, and limited movement of the eye. The child was febrile, and the eye was extremely painful. Orbital cellulitis was caused by an underlying ethmoid sinusitis (detected on skull radiograph). The child responded rapidly to systemic antibiotics. Causes of periorbital or orbital cellulitis include purulent blepharitis, dacryocystitis, osteomyelitis of the upper jaw, maxillary sinusitis, and hematogenous spread due to the bacterial sepsis.

Differential Diagnosis—Differential diagnosis includes cavernous sinus thrombosis, inflammation of the tear duct, and cellulitis of the eyelid.

12.36
Orbital Cellulitis

Orbital cellulitis (due to osteomyelitis of the maxilla) in a 3-month-old boy. Inflammation of the periorbital and intraorbital tissues was evident by the erythema and swelling of the eyelids, restricted movement of the eye, and systemic illness. Antibiotic therapy and surgical drainage were required.

Possible complications of orbital cellulitis include involvement of the optic nerve, cavernous sinus thrombosis, meningitis, subdural empyema, and cerebral abscess.

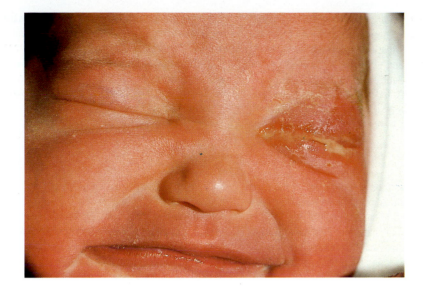

12.34

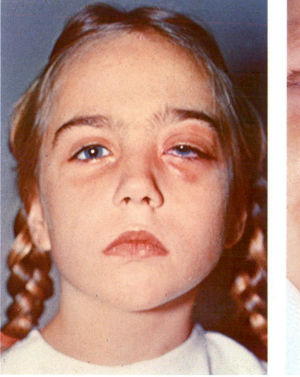

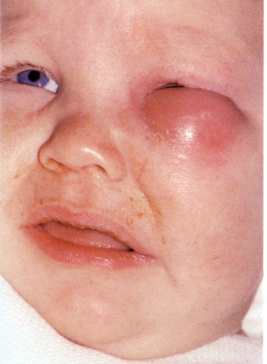

12.35   12.36

12.37
Cellulitis

Cellulitis of the lower eyelid (periorbital cellulitis) in a 4-year-old girl. The findings included painful erythema and fluctuant swelling of the right lower eyelid with narrowing of the palpebral fissure and extension of the inflammation to the cheek. Eye movement was not restricted and exophthalmos was not present (clinically differentiating this process from an orbital cellulitis). Orbital cellulitis, subperiosteal abscess, and sinusitis were ruled out by imaging procedures. *Streptococcus pyogenes* was identified as the causative agent. The cellulitis resolved rapidly with systemic antibiotic therapy. Surgical incision was not necessary.

Differential Diagnosis—An eyelid abscess may present as a circumscribed collection of pus in the skin of the eyelid and is clinically difficult to differentiate from eyelid cellulitis if severe edema is present.

12.38
Dacryostenosis

Congenital dacryostenosis (due to obstruction of the nasal lacrimal duct) in a 5-month-old boy. Mucopurulent discharge was noted to collect in the left conjunctival sac, without evidence of conjunctival inflammation. Patients with nasolacrimal duct obstruction may have secondary infection and inflammation of the nasolacrimal sac (dacryostenosis), inflammation of the surrounding tissue (pericystitis), or periorbital cellulitis.

Differential Diagnosis—Differential diagnosis of congenital dacryostenosis includes infantile glaucoma, infectious conjunctivitis, keratitis,uveitis, and other eyelid anomalies with secondary inflammation.

12.39
Conjunctivitis

Conjunctivitis caused by *Chlamydia trachomatis* (inclusion conjunctivitis) in a 10-day-old boy. Follicular conjunctivitis of the left eye began 7 days after birth. The findings included erythema and swelling of the conjunctiva and purulent exudate without involvement of the cornea. *Chlamydia* was identified as the causative organism.

Differential Diagnosis—Inclusion conjunctivitis must be differentiated from gonococcal conjunctivitis (shorter incubation time, corneal involvement, increased purulence), chemical conjunctivitis (associated with topical application of silver nitrate), and congenital dacryostenosis (obstruction of the lacrimal duct leading to collection of mucous purulent discharge in the conjunctival sac without conjunctival injection).

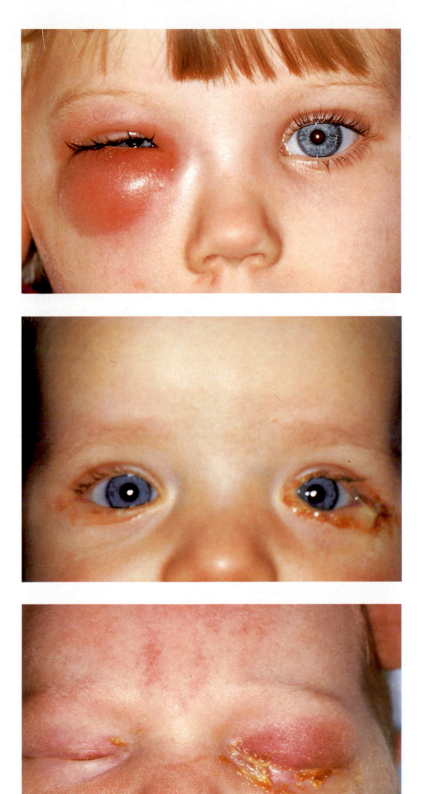

12.40

Tay-Sachs Disease

Tay-Sachs disease (GM$_2$ gangliosidosis type I) in a 7-month-old boy. In the early stages of the illness, a cherry-red spot was noted in the area of the macula; a red-brown area of the fovea surrounded by a light gray-white halo. These findings were caused by ganglioside accumulation in the retinal ganglion cells. As the illness progressed, the boy developed optic atrophy and gray-white discoloration of the entire retina.

A cherry-red spot of the macula can also occur in association with other ganglioside storage diseases such as Niemann-Pick disease, Sandhoff disease (GM$_2$ gangliosidosis type II), and type I mucolipidosis. Cherry-red spot of the macula is often observed in retinal edema associated with chorioretinitis and disturbance in retinal circulation.

12.41

Cystinosis

Cystinosis in a 2-year-old boy. Deposits of light, sparkling cystine crystals were noted in the cornea on slit lamp examination. The deposition of cystine crystals in the superficial corneal layers led to persistent photophobia. Fine pigment changes of the retina were also noted. The cystine content of the child's leukocytes was elevated.

12.42

Neurofibromatosis

Neurofibromatosis (von Recklinghausen's disease) in a 13-year-old girl. A large pigmented nevus and many smaller pigmented nevi were noted in the iris. The girl had seven large pigmented macules on the skin (cafe-au-lait spots). In addition, the child had hearing impairment and vertigo due to an acoustic neuroma.

Pigmented nevi of the iris at times can only be seen on a slit lamp examination. This finding may be important in supporting the diagnosis of neurofibromatosis. Family history of neurofibromatosis is frequently positive since the condition is inherited as an autosomal dominant trait.

12.43

Retinoblastoma

Retinoblastoma in a 2-year-old boy. The tumor mass emanated from the retina of the left eye and could be appreciated by examining the child's pupils. The white reflex (leukocoria) occurred as the tumor grew larger and moved forward. The right eye was not affected. The affected eye was enucleated.

12.44

Optic Glioma

Optic glioma in a 3-year-old boy. The findings included proptosis and loss of vision in the left eye. The intraorbital tumor originated in the optic nerve and was seen on ophthalmologic examination. Radiographs demonstrated expansion of the optic nerve foramen. Computed tomography ruled out involvement of the optic chiasm.

Tumors that cause unilateral or bilateral exophthalmos in children include rhabdomyosarcoma, neuroblastoma, neurinoma of the optic nerve, hemangioma, lipoma, and retrobulbar lymphangioma. There are also endocrine, infectious, and traumatic causes of exophthalmos.

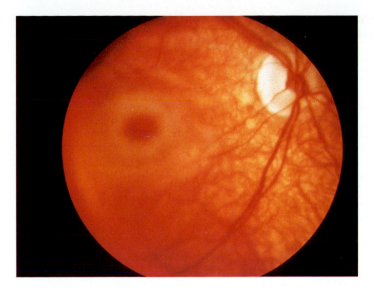

12.40

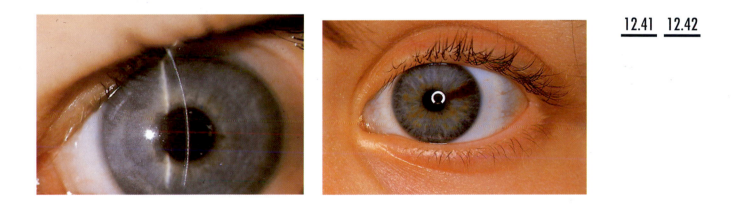

12.41   12.42

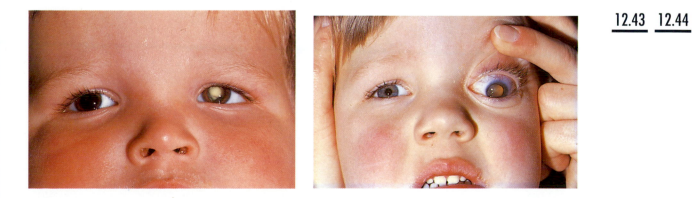

12.43   12.44

12.45 12.46

Neurofibromatosis (Type II)

Neurofibromatosis (type II) in a 30-year-old man. Findings included a central, subcapsular cataract in the right eye (Figure 12.45) and a semitransparent epiretinal membrane over the entire macula in the left eye (Figure 12.46).

12.47

Neurofibromatosis (Type II)

Neurofibromatosis (type II) in a 16-year-old girl. A hematoma of the retina and pigmented retinal epithelium were noted in the right eye. Lisch nodules (hamartomas) of the iris are only seen in neurofibromatosis type I.

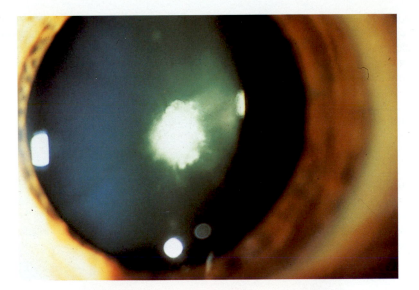

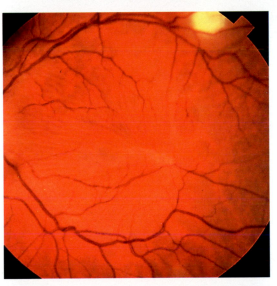

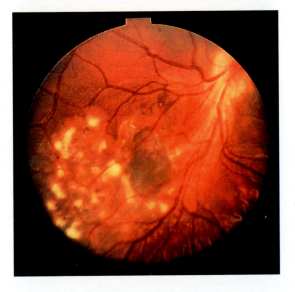

13.1

Obesity

Obesity in a 14-year-old girl. Large accumulations of adipose tissue were noted over the torso and extremities. Based on her height, the patient was 40 kg overweight. In a 6-week period (under hospital supervision), the patient lost 15 kg on a weight reduction diet. Menarche occurred at age 12; secondary sexual development was complete. Both parents were similarly obese. Pictured next to the obese girl, is a girl the same age with normal height and weight.

Differential Diagnosis—Obesity may be seen in conjunction with Frohlich syndrome, Cushing syndrome, Prader-Willi syndrome, and Bardet-Biedl syndrome (associated with obesity, polydactyly, retinopathy, hypogenitalism). Obesity seen in hypothyroidism is due to both myxedema and decreased basal metabolic rate.

13.2

Prader-Willi Syndrome

Prader-Willi syndrome in a 14-year-old boy. Findings included generalized obesity, hypogonadism, and cryptorchidism. The child was 12 cm shorter than average for his age. The syndrome is associated with learning disability. In the newborn period, the child had typical muscular hypotonia which led to asphyxia. At the age of 16 years, the child developed diabetes mellitus (a frequent complication of Prader-Willi syndrome). Deletion of the paternal chromosome 15q11-q13 and a normal maternal chromosome 15 were noted on karyotype.

13.3

Obesity

Marked obesity in a 12-year-old boy. Red "stretch" marks of the abdominal skin were noted (striae atrophicae).

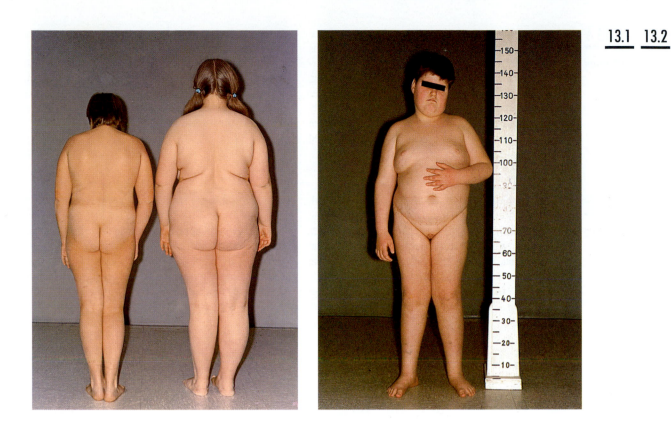

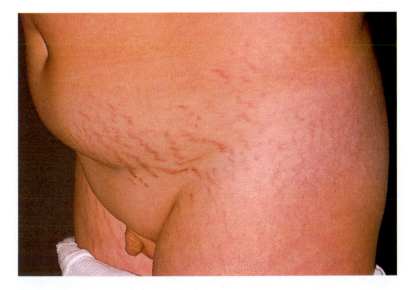

13.4
Lipodystrophy

Generalized lipodystrophy in a 13-month-old boy. Since birth, the child was noted to have decreased subcutaneous adipose tissue. The underlying musculature was easily apparent because of the lack of subcutaneous tissue. In addition, macrocephaly, "senile" facial expression, and sparse hair were noted. Growth and mental development were extremely delayed. Feeding was difficult and could be accomplished only with the use of a gastric feeding tube. The child died at 15 months of age of bronchopneumonia. Autopsy demonstrated generalized atrophy of adipose tissue.

Differential Diagnosis—Differential diagnosis for lipodystrophy includes Seip-Lawrence Syndrome (total lipoatrophy with excessive height and hypertrichosis), Miescher syndrome (acanthosis nigricans and diabetes mellitus), acquired total lipodystrophy and partial lipodystrophy.

13.5
Failure to Thrive

Failure to thrive of uncertain etiology in a 6-year-old girl. Findings included a marked paucity of subcutaneous adipose tissue and muscle development. The child was 15 cm shorter than average and had hyperpigmented skin, cutis laxa, and extreme physical and mental retardation. The symptoms were first noted at 1 month of age and progressed steadily since then. Despite exhaustive diagnostic investigations, the cause of this growth failure remained unknown. The child died at the age of 8 years.

Differential Diagnosis—Failure to thrive can occur as a result of organic disease (chronic infection, malignancy), psychiatric disorders, adrenal insufficiency (Addison's disease), and hypophyseal insufficiency (panhypopituitarism). Anorexia nervosa may also occur in older children.

13.6
Juvenile Generalized Fibromatosis

Juvenile generalized fibromatosis (Ormond syndrome) in a 10-year-old boy. The child was severely cachectic (7 kg below normal weight for age). Multiple intraperitoneal and retroperitoneal fibromas caused intestinal obstruction and displaced both ureters. In addition, there was fibromatous involvement of the mediastinum, the pleura, and the pericardium. As a result of this generalized fibromatosis, edema, ascites, urinary retention, and cardiac failure was noted. Transient improvement was noted with symptomatic treatment; however, death ensued within 5 months due to cardiac failure.

In Ormond syndrome, retroperitoneal fibrosis causes progressive compression and stenosis of the ureters which leads to hydronephrosis and, in severe cases, to uremia. Involvement of the abdominal cavity, the chest, and the mediastinum is also possible.

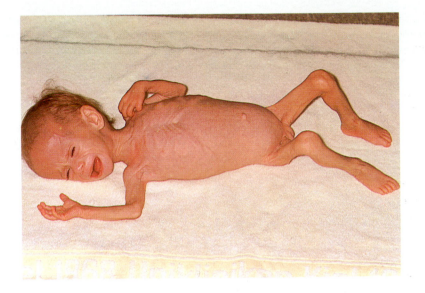

13.4

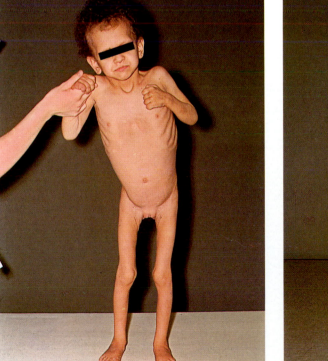

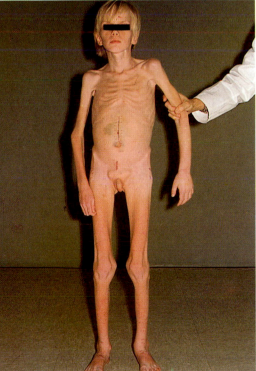

13.5   13.6

13.7

Rickets

Vitamin D deficiency rickets in a 2-year-old boy. Findings included swelling of the wrist, short stature and delayed motor development. Other findings included epiphyseal enlargement (leading to protuberance of the malleoli), rachitic rosary, and bending of the shaft of the tibia. After 3 weeks of daily vitamin D_3 treatment, there was normalization of hypocalcemia and hypophosphatemia, as well as increased calcium deposition in the bones.

13.8

Rickets

Vitamin D deficiency rickets in a 10-month-old boy. Kyphosis of the lower thoracic spine was noted. When standing, there was evidence of lordosis of the lumbar spine. Joints were hyperextensible due to relaxation of the ligaments. Treatment consisted of vitamin D supplementation and physical therapy.

13.9

Rickets

Vitamin D deficiency rickets in a 14-month-old girl. Findings included bilateral coxa vara and genu vara.

13.10

Rickets

Vitamin D deficiency rickets in a 13-year-old Turkish girl. Findings included severe bowing of the legs and short stature (height 26 cm below average for age). The figure demonstrates her condition after spontaneous fracture of the right tibia as well as fracture of the seventh and ninth ribs. Severe vitamin D deficiency was caused by a combination of environmental factors, including poor nutrition and constant confinement (due to fear of being discovered as an illegal alien). Treatment consisted of vitamin D therapy and corrective surgery.

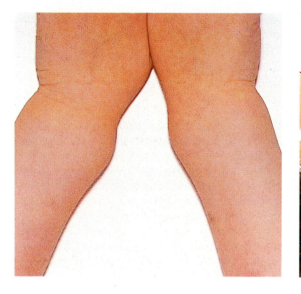 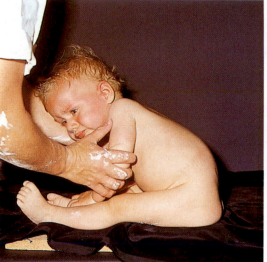

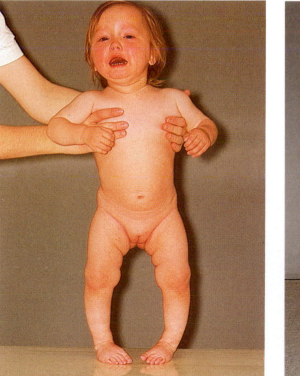 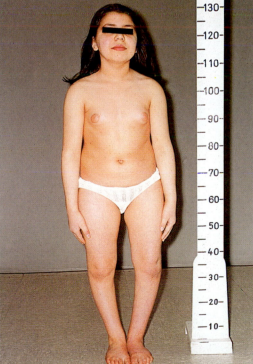

13.11

Rickets

Vitamin D deficiency rickets in a 14-month-old boy whose regular prophylactic dose of vitamin D had been discontinued. Findings included rachitic rosary (beading of ribs at the costochondral junction) and delayed gross motor development. The diagnosis was confirmed by radiographic studies and laboratory investigations (demonstrating a reduction in 25-hydroxycholecalciferol).

13.12   13.13

Pseudohypopara-thyroidism

Pseudohypoparathyroidism (hereditary osteodystrophy, Albright syndrome) in an 11-year-old girl. Findings included brachydactyly and shortening of the metacarpals (particularly the fifth metacarpal bones with corresponding malleolus bilaterally) and metatarsal bones (particularly the left fourth metatarsal). Pseudohypoparathyroidism was first noted because of failure to thrive and developmental delay. Laboratory investigation revealed hypocalcemia and hypophosphatemia. Further examinations demonstrated an elevated parathormone level as well as end organ resistance to parathormone (PTH did not raise the level of calcium or increase phosphate excretion in the urine). Trousseau sign and Chvostek sign were positive, but no tetanic seizures were observed. These laboratory abnormalities improved after high dose vitamin D therapy and calcium supplements were given.

Differential Diagnosis—Brachydactyly may be seen in 50% of the patient's with Turner syndrome. Pseudohypoparathyroidism may be inherited as an X-linked dominant trait. Shortening of the fifth finger is seen in Russell-Silver syndrome (primordial dwarfism with asymmetry of the body) and in brachydactalic syndromes. Brachydactyly may also appear as an isolated finding or as part of other syndromes (Weill-Marchesani syndrome, Biemond syndrome, Brailsford-Morquio syndrome).

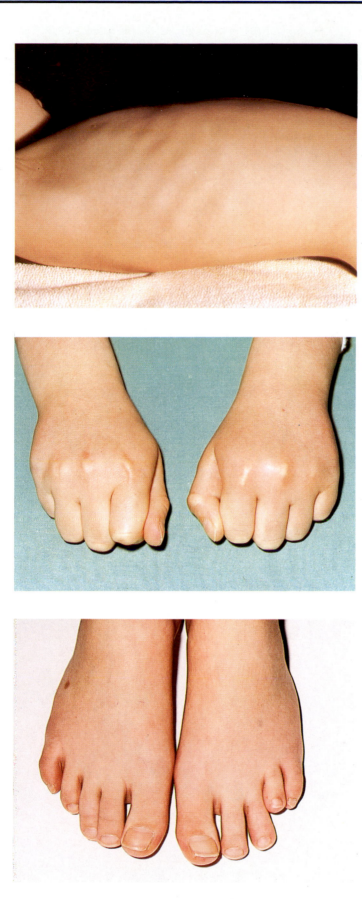

13.14 13.15

Scurvy

Scurvy in an 11-month-old girl. Findings included scorbutic rosary and "frog position" posture (flexed knees and hips with external rotation; Hampelmann's phenomenon) due to malnutrition (vitamin C deficiency). Movement of the arms and legs was extremely painful due to subperiosteal hematomas detected on skeletal radiographs. Hemorrhagic manifestations, including cutaneous and mucous membrane hemorrhage, hematuria, and melena, were absent. Rumpel-Leede test was positive. Vitamin C content in plasma and leukocytes was significantly reduced, confirming the diagnosis of scurvy. The child was effectively treated with vitamin C supplements.

Differential Diagnosis—A broad range of possible diagnoses must be considered since scurvy encompasses both skeletal abnormalities and hemorrhagic manifestations. Differential diagnosis includes arthritis, osteomyelitis, rickets, congenital syphilis, and diseases which cause cutaneous purpuric lesions including Henoch-Schonlein purpura and thrombocytopenic purpura.

13.16

Scurvy

Scurvy (vitamin C deficiency) in 12-month-old boy. The child was fed a special preparation of milk lacking vitamin C and was never given fruits or vegetables. The gums were dark red and swollen due to bleeding of the mucous membranes. The child maintained the typical "frog position" posture (Hampelmann's phenomenon). Skeletal findings included periosteal hematomas (which led to pseudoparalysis) and scorbutic rosary. Diagnosis of vitamin C deficiency was confirmed by radiographic studies and determination of the vitamin C content in blood and urine after a test dose of vitamin C.

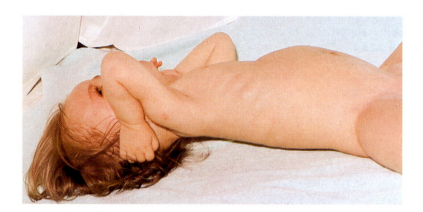

13.14

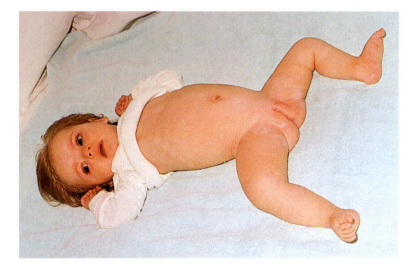

13.15

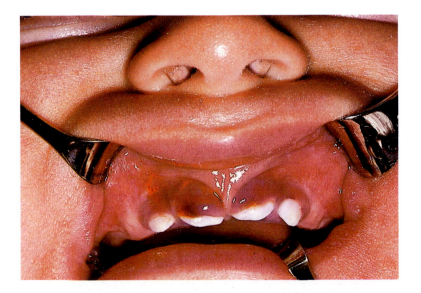

13.16

13.17
Hurler Syndrome

Hurler syndrome (mucopolysaccharidosis type 1-H) in a 10-year-old boy. Findings included coarse facial features, enlargement of the skull, swollen lips, enlarged thick tongue, coarse hair, and heavy eyebrows. The boy was also noted to have a disproportionately small body, hepatosplenomegaly, corneal opacities, and mental retardation. Further laboratory investigations demonstrated a decreased activity of α-L-idur-onidase in the child's leukocytes. In the urine, excretion of dermatan sulfate and heparan sulfate was greatly increased.

Differential Diagnosis—Differential diagnosis of Hurler syndrome includes other types of mucopolysaccharidoses and congenital hypothyroidism (for differential diagnosis of macroglossia page 82).

13.18
Protoporphyria

Protoporphyria in an 8-year-old boy. The child routinely developed an intensely pruritic and erythematous rash on parts of the body exposed to sunlight. Several small, atrophic scars resulting from chronic dermatitis following repeated sunburn were noted on the cheeks. Protoprophrinogen 9 was present in high concentrations in the plasma and erythrocytes.

Differential Diagnosis—A differential diagnosis of photosensitivity is discussed on page 186. If urticarial symptoms are present, solar urticaria must also be considered.

13.19
Hunter Syndrome

Hunter syndrome (mucopolysaccharidosis type II) in a 7-year-old boy. Findings included thick lips, heavy eyebrows, coarse facial features, hepatosplenomegaly and joint stiffness. No corneal opacities were noted. The relatively late onset of failure to thrive, hearing impairment, mental retardation, and typical bony changes were characteristic of mucopolysaccharidosis type II, which progresses more slowly than Hurler syndrome (mucopolysaccharidosis type I). Examination of fibroblasts confirmed the diagnosis (absence of L-iduronosulfate sulfatase). Although biochemically similar, Hunter syndrome can be divided into two types. This child had type A Hunter syndrome. In comparison to type A Hunter syndrome, the symptoms of type B Hunter syndrome are milder and not associated with mental retardation.

13.20
Sanfilippo Syndrome

Sanfilippo syndrome (mucopolysaccharidosis III) in a 12-year-old boy. Findings included somewhat coarse facial features, thickened skin, and heavy eyebrows. No corneal clouding was noted. The liver and spleen were slightly enlarged. Joint stiffness, decreased mobility, and typical skeletal changes (dysostosis multiplex) were present. The diagnosis was confirmed by the increased excretion of heparan sulfate in the urine and demonstration of the specific enzyme defect. In subsequent years, continued neurologic deterioration was noted, including severe dementia and the inability to walk.

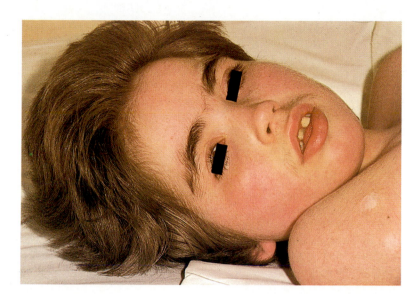

13.17

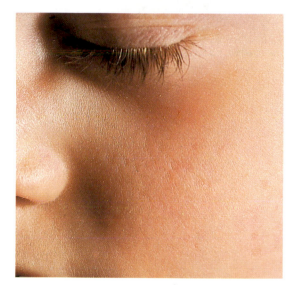

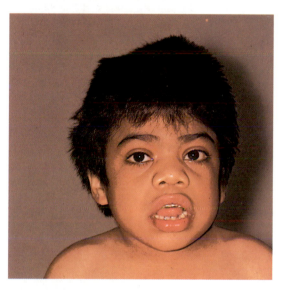

13.18   13.19

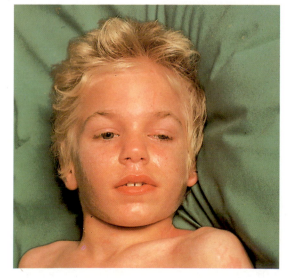

13.20

13.21   13.22
Hunter Syndrome

Hunter syndrome (mucopolysaccharidosis II) in a 5-year-old boy. Findings included the typical facial features of Hunter's syndrome: coarse facial features, depressed nasal bridge, hypertelorism, swollen lips and enlarged tongue (Figure 13.21). Other findings included macrocephaly, short neck, microsomia, paw-shaped hands (Figure 13.22), hearing impairment, and hepatosplenomegaly. No corneal opacities were noted. Laboratory investigation demonstrated an increased excretion of dermatan sulfate and heparan sulfate in the urine. In fibroblast culture, L-iduronosulfate sulfatase was decreased.

Hunter syndrome may be differentiated from other types of mucopolysaccharidoses by specific enzyme assays. Hunter's syndrome may be differentiated from Hurler syndrome by the absence of corneal opacities.

13.23   13.24
Mucolipidoses (ML-1)

Mucolipidoses (ML-1) in a 12-year-old boy. The child was first brought for medical attention at one year of life because of delayed psychomotor development and was seen again at age 1½ years because of skeletal deformities. Findings included a relatively short trunk and neck, protrusion of the anterior chest wall, and long extremities and hands. Joint mobility was not restricted. The child was noted to have coarse facial features, depressed nasal bridge, and deafness. On ophthalmologic examination, a cherry-red spot was noted in the area of the macula. Corneal opacities were later appreciated. The liver was slightly enlarged and no splenomegaly was noted. Skeletal radiographs detected changes similar to those seen in Hurler syndrome. Laboratory investigations demonstrated vacuolated lymphocytes on the peripheral blood smear, and excretion of sialic acid-containing oligosaccharide in the urine. Cells obtained in fibroblast culture demonstrated deficient glucoprotein-sialidase activity.

Differential Diagnosis—The differential diagnosis of a cherry-red spot on the macula includes Tay-Sachs disease, GM-1 gangliosidosis, infantile Niemann-Pick disease, and metachromatic leukodystrophy. Similar skeletal changes can be seen in other mucopolysaccharidoses.

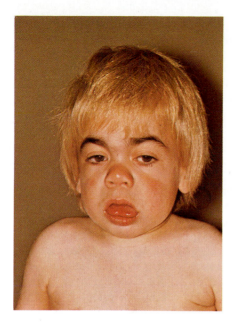

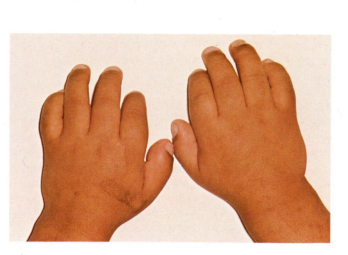

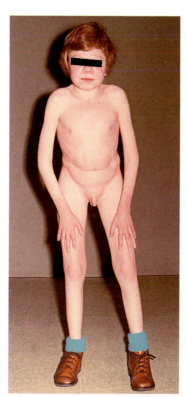

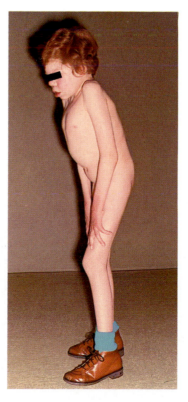

13.25

Hyperlipoproteinemia type IIa

Hyperlipoproteinemia type IIa (familial idiopathic hypercholesterolemia) in a 14-year-old girl. Of note was an arcus lipoides (cholesterol deposits in a gray ring at the margin of the cornea). Laboratory evaluation demonstrated increased plasma cholesterol, increased low density lipoprotein (LDL), and normal plasma triglyceride. The child's father had died at the age of thirty because of a myocardial infarction. This child's high plasma cholesterol (700–1,000 mg/dl) indicated homozygosity, which carries an unfavorable prognosis (leaking to early atherosclerosis and myocardial infarction). A diet containing low cholesterol and polyunsaturated fats was prescribed. The child was also treated with oral cholestyramine and nicotinic acid.

13.26

Type I Hyperlipidemia

Type I hyperlipidemia in a 15-year-old boy. The findings included tuberous xanthomas (red-yellow nodules of varying size) that were found under the extensor surface of the elbow. These easily movable nodes had been noted since three years of age. Similar xanthomas were found on the knees and the heels. The child came for medical attention because of severe abdominal pain accompanied by fever, leukocytosis, and hepatosplenomegaly. Laboratory investigation demonstrated that the serum was cloudy, serum triglyceride level was high, and the cholesterol content was slightly elevated. Lipoprotein electrophoresis demonstrated a wide chylomicron band. An intravenous injection of heparin did not lead to clearing of the serum, demonstrating a lack of lipoprotein lipase.

In other cases of type I hyperlipidemia, xanthomas may be found over the face and mucous membranes (particularly in the mouth). Xanthomas may be papular or nodular. They are often found on the extensor surfaces of the extremities near the joints.

Differential Diagnosis—Differential diagnosis of xanthoma includes hyperlipidemia type II (hypercholesterolemia), biliary cirrhosis, diabetes mellitus, Seip-Lawrence syndrome, and renal disease (including chronic renal failure and nephrotic syndrome). Xanthomas without hypercholesterolemia are seen in Letterer-Siwe disease (histiocytosis X) and Niemann-Pick disease. Disseminated xanthoma and juvenile xanthogranuloma are not associated with hypercholesterolemia. Xanthomas may be seen in Wolman disease (primary familial xanthomatosis) associated with failure to thrive, hepatosplenomegaly, and adrenal calcification.

13.27

Xanthelasma

Xanthelasma in a 35-year-old man. Findings included flat, yellow indurations of the skin caused by cholesterol deposition. Serum cholesterol and triglyceride levels were elevated. In this case, the underlying cause was biliary cirrhosis.

Xanthelasma refers to xanthomas that are localized to the eyelids. Usually they are bilateral, soft, yellow, velvety nodules or plaques. Xanthelasmas also occur in healthy people, but seldom before the age of twenty years. Hyperlipoproteinemia and diabetes mellitus should be considered in the differential diagnosis.

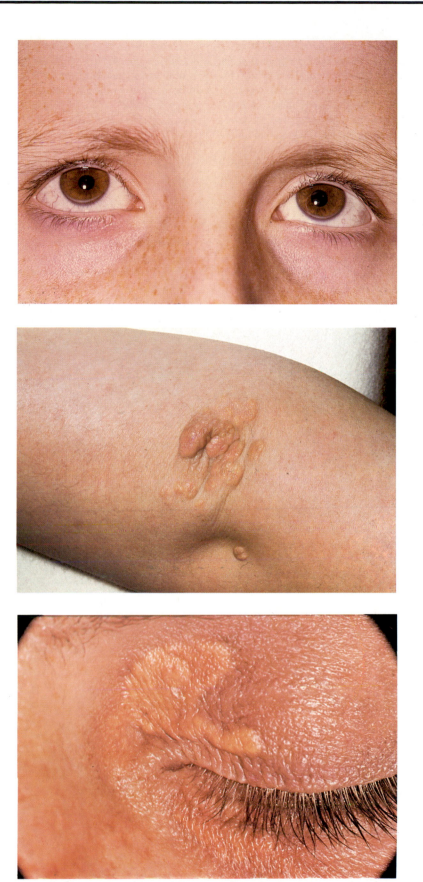

13.28

Wilson's Disease

Wilson's disease (hepatolenticular degeneration) in a 17-year-old boy. A Kayser-Fleischer corneal ring (blue-green or yellow ring at the corneal margin) could be detected with a slit lamp. The diagnosis of Wilson's disease was made at the age of 11 years when the child came to the clinic with hepatomegaly and jaundice. Laboratory investigation revealed decreased serum copper and ceruloplasmin levels. Liver biopsy demonstrated increased deposition of copper.

Kayser-Fleischer corneal ring is seen in the peripheral segments of the cornea and is usually 1–3 mm wide. It can appear red, olive-green, or yellow in color. These findings can regress after therapy for Wilson's disease. Red-brown corneal discoloration has been noted in copper workers or in cases where a person is chronically exposed to copper (penetrating injury with a copper-containing foreign body). Keratin deposits may occur in the cornea of healthy people. Other heavy metals can be deposited in the cornea, including gold (during systemic treatment), iron (due to intraocular blood or foreign body), and silver (due to local application).

13.29

Wilson's Disease

Wilson's disease (hepatolenticular degeneration) in a 7-year-old boy. Because of copper storage in the tissue, a Kayser-Fleischer corneal ring was visible. In addition, gray-brown pigmentation of the skin and mucous membranes was evident, particularly on the gums and mucous membranes of the lips.

Differential Diagnosis—The differential diagnosis includes heavy metal intoxication (Burton's lines), patchy gingival hyperpigmentation seen in some black individuals, hyperpigmentation of the mucous membranes in Addison's disease (page 376), pigmented lesions of Peutz-Jeghers syndrome, and "amalgam" tattoo from dental procedures.

13.30

Menke Kinky Hair Syndrome

Menke kinky hair syndrome in a 6-month-old boy. The scalp hair was short, brittle, depigmented and twisted. Reduced levels of serum ceruloplasmin and copper were noted.

13.31a 13.31b

Menke Kinky Hair Syndrome

Menke kinky hair syndrome in a 9-month-old boy. Sparse scalp hair was brittle, partially depigmented, and disheveled. On microscopic examination, the hair appeared twisted and brittle (pili torti, page 258). At first, the child's hair had appeared normal, but as the child grew, changes in the hair were noted. Gross motor and mental development was delayed. Radiographs demonstrated skeletal findings similar to those seen in scurvy. Laboratory investigation demonstrated a low serum ceruloplasmin and copper level.

Menke kinky hair syndrome is an X-linked recessively inherited disorder of copper metabolism, which can lead to severe cerebellar degeneration.

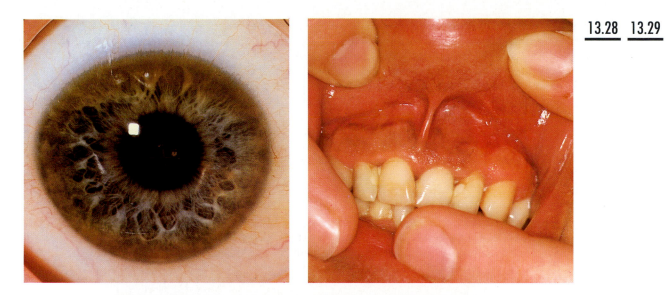

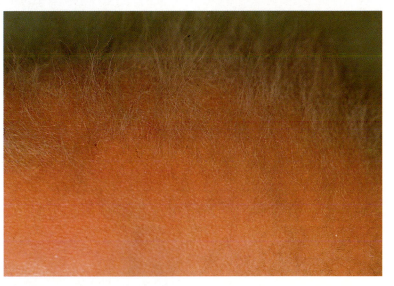

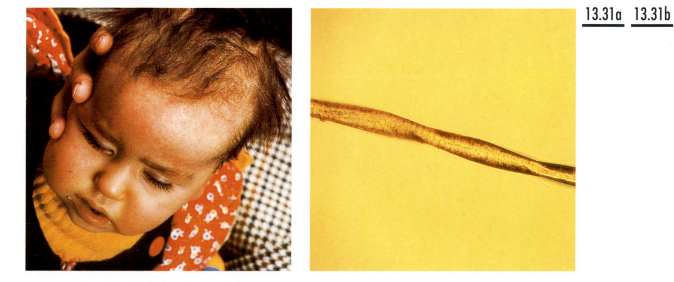

13.32 13.33
Acrodermatitis Enteropathica

Acrodermatitis enteropathica in a 10-month-old girl. Extensive, sharply outlined erythematous areas of skin, which were partially covered with crusts and scales, were noted in the perioral region, the nares, the anogenital area, the knees, the lower legs, and the distal extremities (toes and fingers). The oral and intestinal mucosa was also involved. Of note was the symmetrical distribution of the skin lesions as well as the preference for the distal extremities. At first, the skin changes were vesicular or bullous in nature. Hair loss and nail dystrophy, which occur in acrodermatitis enteropathica, were not noted initially. Later, the child had severe episodes of diarrhea. Further testing revealed a low serum zinc level. Regular oral doses of zinc relieved all symptoms and prevented a relapse.

Differential Diagnosis—Similar skin lesions (vesicles, scales, or crusts) must be distinguished from epidermolysis bullosa, psoriasis, or impetigo. Secondary infections with *Candida* occur frequently in cases of acrodermatitis enteropathica.

13.34
Seborrheic Dermatitis

Seborrheic dermatitis in a 7-month-old girl. Of note were partially confluent erythematous scaly lesions of varying size. The lesions were nonpruritic and involved the anogenital area, the legs, and the face. The lesions had been noted during the first week of life. Despite intensive treatment, several relapses occurred.

Differential Diagnosis—See page 178.

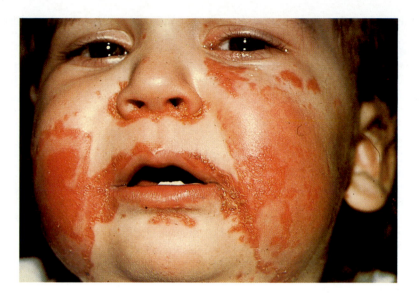

13.32

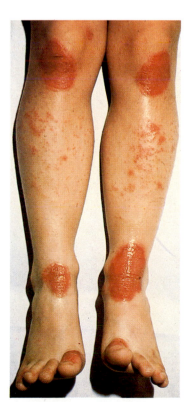

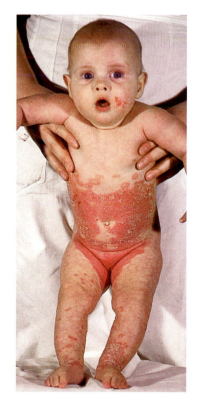

13.33   13.34

13.35   13.36

Histiocytosis X

Histiocytosis X (Hand-Schuller-Christian syndrome) in a 3-year-old boy. Cutaneous findings included numerous macular, papular, and nodular red-brown lesions on the face, neck, axilla, and groin. The lesions were scaly or partially covered by crusts. The child has been referred to the clinic because of polydipsia and polyuria (indicating diabetes insipidus).

Radiographs of the skull revealed numerous osteolytic lesions. Skin biopsy revealed typical histiocytes (foamy histiocytes).

Differential Diagnosis—The differential diagnosis of the skin lesions in histiocytosis X must be distinguished from primary seborrheic dermatitis.

13.37   13.38

Histiocytosis X

Histiocytosis X (Letterer-Siwe syndrome) in a 9-month-old boy. Findings included many closely grouped maculopapular lesions of the trunk and extensive nonpruritic lesions on the lower half of the face. Petechiae and ecchymoses, which may be seen in Letterer-Siwe syndrome, were not found in this case. Two weeks earlier, the child presented with sudden onset of high fever and shortness of breath. Hepatosplenomegaly and generalized lymphadenopathy were noted. Chest radiograph demonstrated pulmonary infiltrates frequently seen in Letterer-Siwe syndrome. Bone marrow aspirate demonstrated proliferating histiocytes.

Differential Diagnosis—Scaly papular skin lesions seen in histiocytosis X are often mistaken for seborrheic dermatitis. Erythema and swelling of the gingiva and ulceration of the mucous membrane may be present causing gingivostomatitis (pages 106 and 148) to be considered in the differential diagnosis.

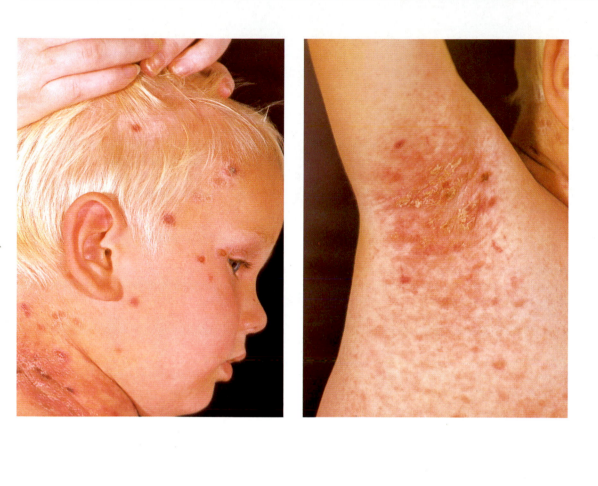

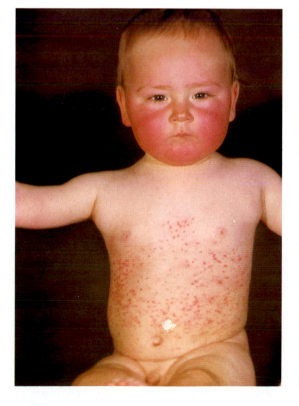

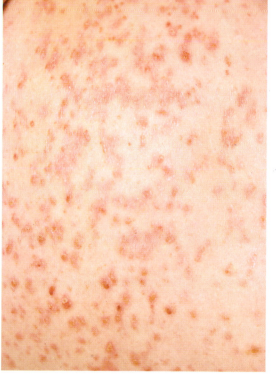

13.39

Histiocytosis X

Histiocytosis X (eosinophilic granuloma) in a 15-year-old girl. Several grouped papules of varying size were noted on the anterior chest wall. These lesions were initially yellow, but later became reddened due to hemorrhage. Because of persistent pain in her thigh, radiographs of the femur were obtained, which demonstrated the typical osteolytic lesions seen in eosinophilic granuloma. Spontaneous remission can occur and therapy is often not necessary.

13.40

Histiocytosis X

Histiocytosis X (Hand-Schuller-Christian syndrome) in a 6-year-old girl. Numerous yellow, slightly scaling papules were noted on both eyelids and on the scalp, trunk, and thighs. Exophthalmos, which occurs in 10% of cases, was not noted. Radiographs of the skull demonstrated multiple osteolytic lesions. Diabetes insipidus, which is seen in 50% of patients with Hand-Schuller-Christian syndrome, developed three months later. The child was treated with DDAVP (for diabetes insipidus) and chemotherapy.

13.41

Histiocytosis X

Histiocytosis X (Hand-Schuller-Christian syndrome) in an 8-year-old boy. Elongated, red-yellow, xanthomatous plaques were found on the conjunctiva.

Mucous membrane lesions may be found in the oral cavity of patients with histiocytosis X (including gingival hypertrophy, necrotizing gingivitis, and stomatitis). A wide range of cutaneous findings may occur including seborrhea-like lesions on the scalp and external auditory canal, maculopapular rashes with vesicle formation, intertrigo, xanthomas, petechiae, and ecchymoses.

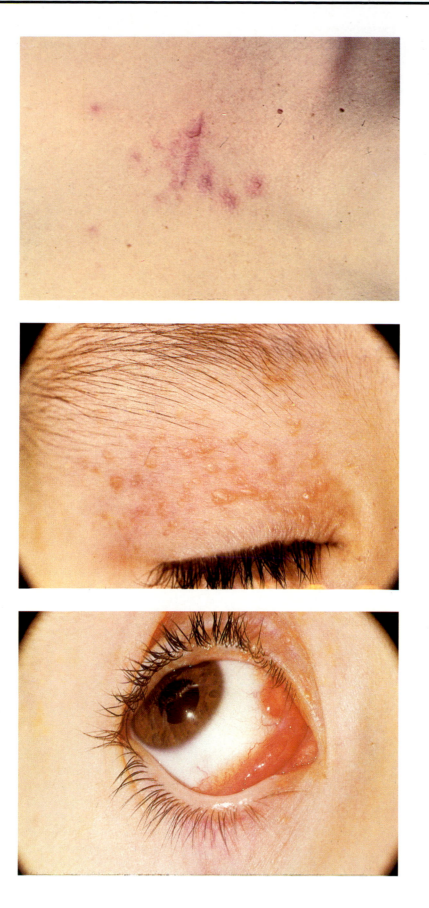

14.1 14.2
Hypothyroidism

Congenital primary hypothyroidism in a 4-year-old girl. Newborn screening for hypothyroidism was not routinely done at the time of this child's birth. During the first year of life, the parents noted lethargy, difficulty feeding, constipation, and delayed motor development. At 4 years of age, the child had significant growth retardation (height 10 cm below average), dry, bristly hair, depressed nasal bridge, and myxedema of the face and dorsum of the hands. The child's mental development appeared normal for age. Laboratory evaluation demonstrated low levels of T_3 and T_4 with elevated TSH. The child responded well to exogenous thyroid hormone.

Differential Diagnosis—Primary congenital hypothyroidism must be distinguished from acquired hypothyroidism seen in older children. In secondary hypothyroidism (as seen in cases of craniopharyngioma), the plasma TSH level is low.

14.3
Congenital Goiter

Congenital goiter in a 6-week-old girl whose mother had taken potassium iodide during pregnancy (as a treatment for bronchial asthma). The exposure to large amounts of iodide in utero caused enlargement of the child's thyroid gland and disturbed thyroid hormone synthesis leading to hypothyroidism. The enlarged gland did not cause airway obstruction at birth. The symptoms gradually regressed with thyroxine treatment.

Congenital goiter can also occur when there is an defect in thyroid hormone synthesis (because fetal TSH stimulates increased intrauterine thyroid growth), or in cases of maternal Grave's disease (due to LATS antibody crossing the placenta).

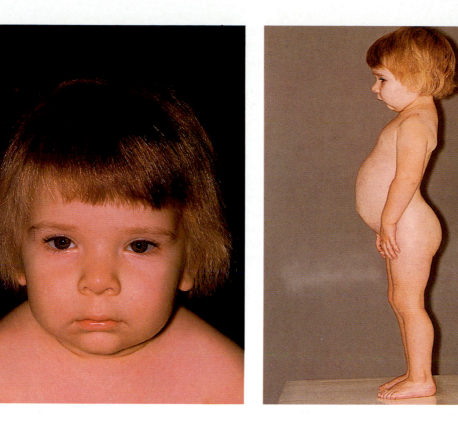

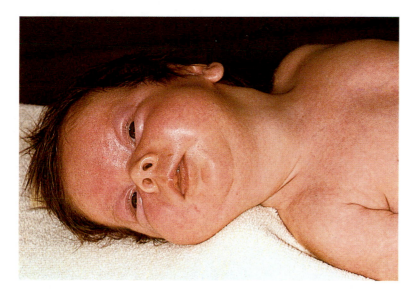

14.4
Primary Hypothyroidism

Primary hypothyroidism in a 1-year-old girl. Findings included coarse facial features, macroglossia, thick lips, and nonpitting edema (myxedema) of the face, the supraclavicular region, the dorsum of the hands, and the external genitalia. Significant growth retardation (length 2 cm below the third percentile) and delayed gross motor development are noted. T_3 (triiodothyronine) and T_4 (thyroxin) were low. TSH (thyroid-stimulating hormone) was elevated. Technetium scan demonstrated an ectopically placed thyroid gland in the submandibular region. Biopsy of the submandibular thyroid gland (to rule out possible malignancy) demonstrated normal thyroid tissue. Continued treatment with thyroxine led to improvement of the symptoms.

14.5
Hyperthyroidism

Hyperthyroidism in a 10-year-old girl. Findings included diffuse goiter, exophthalmos, increased height (21 cm taller than average), sinus tachycardia, and moist skin. The child had difficulty with upward gaze and could not wrinkle her forehead (failure of the frontalis muscle to contract normally). She was originally brought to the clinic because of easy fatigability and a systolic cardiac murmur in order to rule out possible congenital heart disease. Laboratory evaluation demonstrated elevated T_3 and T_4. After treatment with propylthiouracil, the symptoms resolved.

Other eye symptoms seen in hyperthyroidism include retraction of the upper eyelid and infrequent blinking (Stellwag sign), impairment of convergence (Möbius sign), lagging of the upper eyelid with downward gaze (Graefe sign), and tremor of the eyelids when closed (Rosenbach sign). The cause of exophthalmos in hyperthyroidism is uncertain. Exophthalmos can be more pronounced on one side or entirely unilateral. For the differential diagnosis of exophthalmos, see page 332.

14.6
Simple Goiter

Simple goiter in a 15-year-old girl. A diffuse symmetric enlargement of the thyroid gland which had begun during puberty had progressed during the last few months. Thyroxine and TSH levels were normal. Technetium scan was normal. Autoantibodies against thyroid tissue were not detected. Thyroid hormone therapy was begun in order to prevent the goiter from increasing in size.

Simple goiter, or colloid goiter, has a familial occurrence, leading to the theory that it is caused by a genetic limitation of enzyme production. However, the increased occurrence of simple goiter in iodine-deficient areas, and the low incidence of simple goiter in the areas that use iodide salt, suggests that iodine deficiency may contribute to the cause of simple goiter (similar to endemic goiter). The frequent occurrence of simple goiter during puberty indicates that there is an influence of sex hormones as well as iodine metabolism.

14.7
Simple Goiter

Simple goiter in a 14-year-old girl. A goiter had been noted since 1 year of age. The thyroid was diffusely enlarged with a 2.5×1.5 cm firm nodule in the right lobe of the thyroid gland. There were no clinical signs of thyroid dysfunction and laboratory evaluations of thyroid function (T_3, T_4, TSH) were normal. Technetium scan was normal. Neither carcinoma nor thyroiditis was microscopically detected on biopsy of the enlarged lobe of the thyroid gland. The goiter regressed after thyroxine administration. Simple goiter can be asymmetric or nodular. In cases of extreme nodular changes, technetium scan and biopsy are necessary in order to rule out thyroid gland carcinoma.

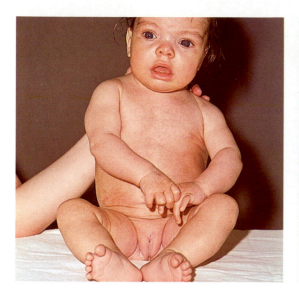

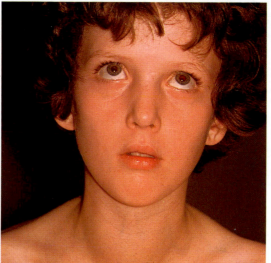

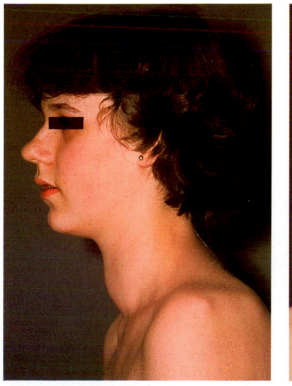

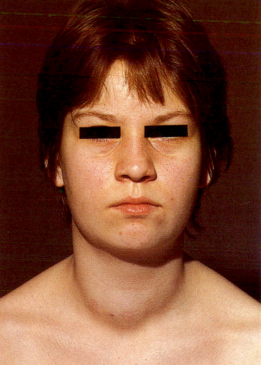

14.8

Cushingoid Syndrome

Cushingoid syndrome due to long-term corticosteroid therapy for nephrotic syndrome in a 6-year-old boy. Findings include "full moon" facies and generalized obesity. The clinical manifestations are the same as those seen in Cushing syndrome (caused by tumor or hyperplasia of the adrenal glands).

14.9

Cushingoid Syndrome

Cushingoid syndrome in the same child as in Figure 14.8. Skin atrophy and red stretch marks (striae distensae) of the thighs are demonstrated.

14.10 14.11

Cushingoid Syndrome

Cushingoid syndrome caused by long-term corticosteroid treatment for juvenile rheumatoid arthritis in a 4-year-old boy. The findings included the typical "full moon" face, hirsutism, and "buffalo hump." Hypertension was also noted.

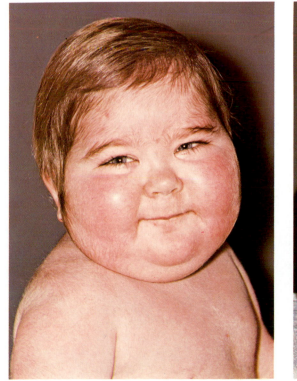

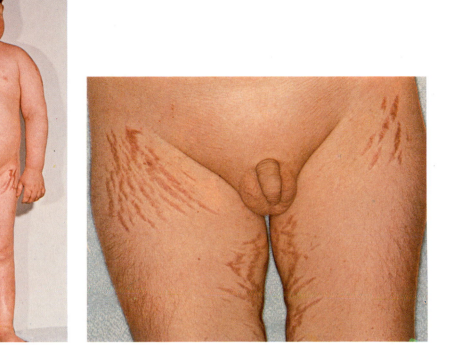

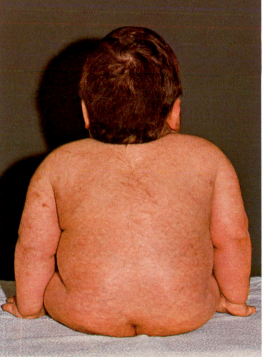

14.12 14.13 14.14
Addison's Disease

Addison's disease (adrenal insufficiency) in a 10-year-old boy. Findings included increased pigmentation of the skin and mucous membranes. Pigmentary changes were particularly marked on the face, the palms, the joints, in the anogenital region, and on the nipples and naval. Brown pigment spots were noted on the oral mucous membranes and thumbs. The increase in pigmentation is due to increased melanocyte stimulating hormone released from the pituitary gland.

The child had experienced fatigue and weakness for some time prior to hospitalization. He came to medical attention due to an acute episode of diarrhea, vomiting, and symptoms of shock. Laboratory investigation demonstrated concurrent hyponatremia, hyperkalemia, and hypoglycemia (typical of Addisonian crisis). Plasma cortisol level was low.

14.12

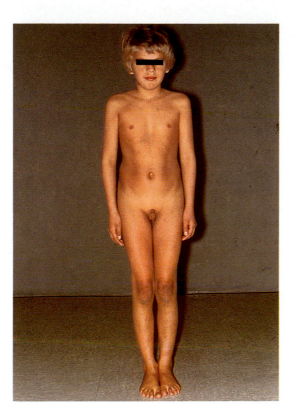

14.13   14.14

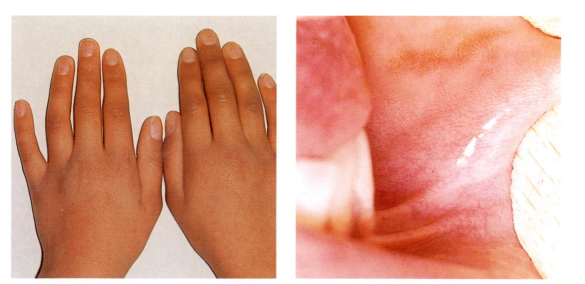

14.15

Congenital Adrenal Hyperplasia

Congenital adrenal hyperplasia (congenital adrenogenital syndrome) in a 14-year-old boy. The child was short (height 17 cm below average). Secondary sexual characteristics were fully developed. Radiographic examination of the long bones demonstrated premature closure of the epiphyses (due to androgen overproduction in the adrenal glands). Laboratory evaluation demonstrated elevated serum levels of 17-hydro-xyprogesterone (due to congenital 21-hydroxylase deficiency).

Early diagnosis can be made in boys with congenital adrenal hyperplasia (non salt-losing type), if the signs of premature pubertal development are noted during the course of regular medical evaluation.

14.16

Congenital Adrenal Hyperplasia

Congenital adrenal hyperplasia in a 7-month-old girl. Despite early diagnosis and treatment, the child died at nine months of age due to an acute adrenal crisis. Physical examination revealed that the clitoris was extremely enlarged, the labia majora appeared wrinkled (like the scrotum), and the vagina shared a common opening with the urethra (urogenital sinus). Autopsy demonstrated hyperplasia of the adrenal cortex as well as severe enterocolitis.

Differential Diagnosis—The differential diagnosis of conditions causing clitoral hypertrophy include defects of steroid biogenesis, carcinoma or adenoma of the adrenal cortex, administration of exogenous male hormones during pregnancy, androgen producing ovarian or adrenal cortical tumors in pregnant women, and syndromes including Beckwith-Wiedemann syndrome.

14.17

Adrenogenital Syndrome

Acquired adrenogenital syndrome due to an adenoma of the adrenal glands in an 8-year-old girl. Physical findings were predominantly those associated with virilization of a female child. Signs of virilization had been present since one year of age, including hypertrophy of the clitoris, abnormal hair growth around the genitalia and underarms, deepened voice, and acne vulgaris. Premature breast development was not noted. Urinary excretion of 17-ketosteroids was increased. A fist-sized tumor was palpable in the left upper abdomen. The adenoma was surgically removed after which time no other treatment was necessary. The voice became higher and the acne disappeared. Clitoral hypertrophy was surgically corrected at a later date.

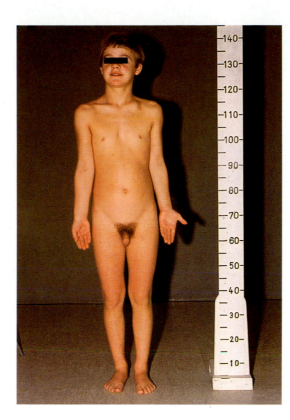

14.15

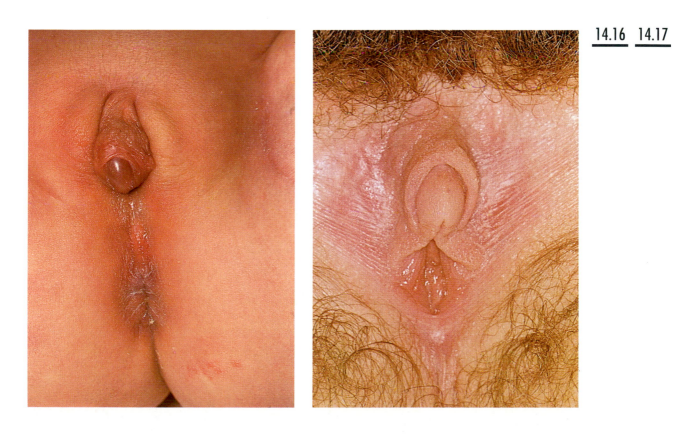

14.16   14.17

14.18

Bardet-Biedl Syndrome

Bardet-Biedl syndrome in a 14-year-old boy. The findings included hypogonadism (hypoplasia of the penis) with otherwise normal secondary sexual characteristics. Other findings included short stature, obesity, retinitis pigmentosa, polydactyly, and mental retardation.

Differential Diagnosis—The differential diagnosis of hypogonadism includes Froehlich syndrome (prune belly syndrome), Prader-Willi syndrome, Fanconi syndrome, and pituitary dwarfism.

14.19

Hermaphroditism

True hermaphroditism in a 6-month-old child. The genitalia were ambiguous. The karyotype was 46XX. Further examination demonstrated that there was an ovary on one side and a testicle on the other. In true hermaphroditism, both ovarian and testicular tissue are present.

14.20

Pseudohermaphroditism

Male pseudohermaphroditism in a 4-month-old boy. Findings included incomplete virilization of the external genitalia (underdeveloped penis and scrotum). The testes were present and the karyotype demonstrated the child to be of the male sex. Further laboratory investigations demonstrated elevated levels of androstendione and low levels of testosterone leading to the presumptive diagnosis of 17-betahydroxysteroid dehydrogenase deficiency.

Differential Diagnosis—The differential diagnosis includes other defects in the synthesis of testosterone.

14.21

Pseudohermaphroditism

Female pseudohermaphroditism (virilization of the external genitalia) in a 2-month-old girl. The findings included clitoral hypertrophy and fusion of the labia majora and the urogenital sinus (common opening of the urethra and the vagina). In this case, the virilization was due to estrogen and progesterone treatment during the mother's pregnancy.

Differential Diagnosis—Differential diagnosis of female pseudohermaphroditism includes other virilizing conditions such as congenital adrenal hyperplasia (due to 21-hydroxylase deficiency).

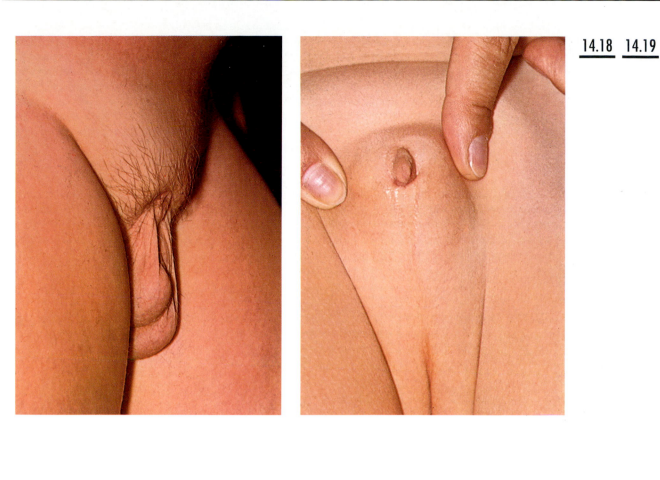

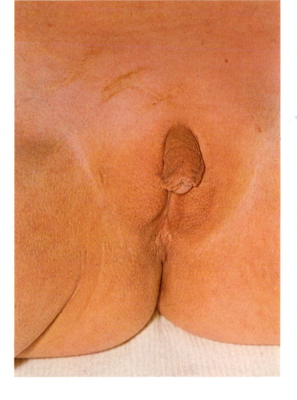

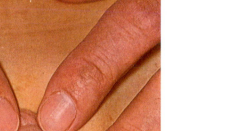

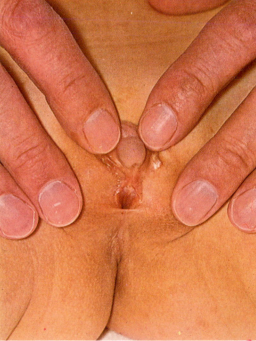

14.22

Premature Thelarche

Premature thelarche (development of the breasts) in a 1-year-old girl. The child had grown to a normal height for her age. External and internal genitalia were normal; there was no pubic or axillary hair noted. Vaginal smear demonstrated columnar epithelium, which was normal for this age. Plasma FSH and LH were not elevated; urinary excretion of ketosteroids and hydroxysteroids were slightly increased. There was no other evidence of hypothalamic disease, central nervous system tumor, or other tumors that could secrete gonadotropin-like substances (chorion epithelioma of the ovary). Spontaneous regression of the symptoms occurred within the year (benign form of premature thelarche). In this case, premature thelarche was probably due to a slight disruption in the normal function of the hypothalamic-pituitary-ovarian axis.

14.23

Precocious Puberty

Precocious puberty in a 2-year-old boy. Findings included enlargement of the penis and testicles as well as premature growth of pubic hair. Other symptoms included increased height (16 cm taller than average), muscular build, and deep voice. Plasma FSH and LH levels were elevated. Osseous maturation was advanced, as demonstrated by an increased bone age. After neoplastic processes and certain central nervous system diseases were ruled out as a cause of precocious puberty, treatment with LH-RH analogues was considered.

14.24

Klinefelter Syndrome

Klinefelter syndrome in a 15-year-old boy. Asymmetric breast enlargement (left greater than right) and delayed development of secondary characteristics led to the diagnosis. Other physical findings included small right testicle and absent left testicle. Karyotype was 46XXY.

14.25

Pubertal Gynecomastia

Pubertal gynecomastia in a 13-year-old boy. Findings included slight asymmetric enlargement of the breasts, right greater than the left, without associated endocrine abnormalities. Spontaneous regression was noted after 2 years.

Pubertal gynecomastia may occur in upward of 60% of adolescent males. It is usually noted between the ages of 14 and 15. Breast enlargement may last a few months and seldom greater than 1 to 2 years. Pubertal gynecomastia may be related to a decreased ratio of testosterone to estradiol.

Differential Diagnosis—Gynecomastia may occur in association with Klinefelter syndrome, Leydig cell tumors, feminizing adrenal gland tumors, and cirrhosis of the liver. Medications such as ACTH and human chorionic gonadotropin (HCG) may cause gynecomastia. Gynecomastia may also be an isolated hereditary abnormality.

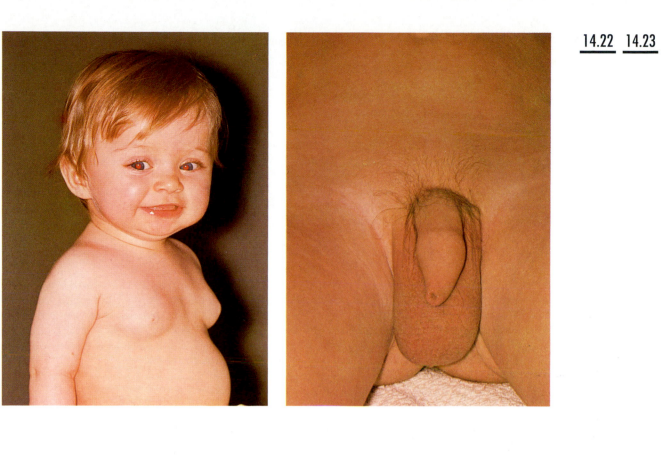

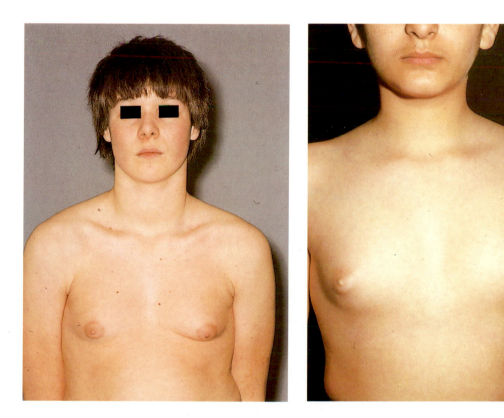

14.26

Precocious Puberty

Precocious puberty in a 12-year-old boy. The findings included increased height (18 cm above average), premature development of secondary sexual characteristics (since age 3), and deepened voice. Of particular note was the increased head circumference and widened third ventricle due to a supracellar tumor (craniopharyngioma). The cranial pharyngioma required surgical excision. In addition, a ventricular shunt had to be placed due to hydrocephalus. After 4 years, there were no signs of renewed growth of the craniopharyngioma, and no further endocrine abnormalities were noted.

14.27

Acromegaly

Acromegaly in a 19-year-old girl. Findings included coarse facial features with enlargement of the lower jaw, the ears, the nose, and the mouth. In addition, the hands and feet appeared enlarged. The cause of these symptoms was an eosinophilic adenoma of the anterior pituitary, which led to overproduction of growth hormone (GH). The child had the typical abnormal response to glucose load testing; hyperglycemia induced by glucose loading did not cause the normal suppression of growth hormone.

14.28

Beckwith-Wiedemann Syndrome

Beckwith-Wiedemann syndrome in a 1-week-old boy. Findings included macroglossia, visceromegaly, and macrosomia. The child was brought to the hospital because of hypoglycemic seizures. Initial therapy included intravenous glucose infusions. At a later date, the child required an operation for a large umbilical hernia.

Differential Diagnosis—The differential diagnosis of macroglossia includes congenital hypothyroidism, acromegaly, Down syndrome, Hurler syndrome, glycogen storage disease type II (Pompe's disease), primary amyloidosis, thyroglossal duct cyst, hemangioma, lymphoma, rhabdomyoma of the tongue, and neurofibromatosis (in cases where the fibroma is localized to the tongue).

14.29

Hypothyroidism

Congenital primary hypothyroidism in a 4-month-old boy. Findings included an enlarged tongue, broad nose, and depressed nasal bridge. The child's growth was delayed. The anterior fontanel was wide (3 × 4 cm). Other signs of hypothyroidism were absent. Thyroxine (T_4) was significantly reduced and TSH was elevated. Screening for hypothyroidism (which is the standard of care today), did not exist when this child was born.

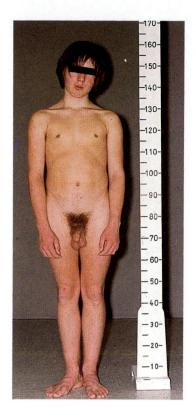

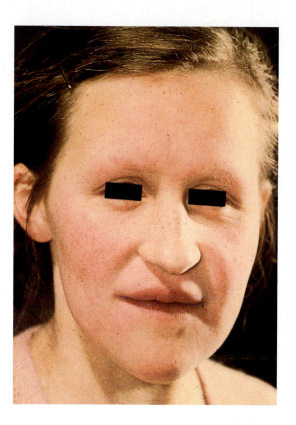

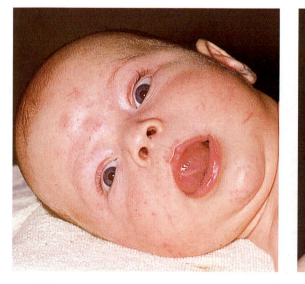

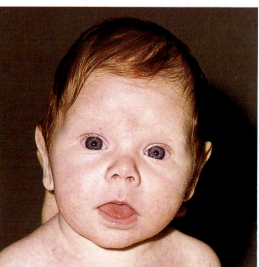

14.30

Pituitary Dwarfism

Pituitary dwarfism (due to deficiency of growth hormone) in a 5-year-old girl. She is shown standing next to a normal child of the same age. The girl is 17 cm below average height and is otherwise normally proportioned (ratio of head and torso length to the length of the legs). At birth and during the first year of life, the child's growth was noted to be normal. After the second year of life, growth was noted to slow down. Skeletal radiographs demonstrated delayed osseous maturation. The growth hormone level was low and did not respond to insulin induced hypoglycemia or arginine infusion.

    Differential Diagnosis—The differential diagnosis for growth failure includes:

1. Intrauterine growth retardation (congenital growth failure with normal growth hormone production) and other constitutional bone diseases (achondroplasia, osteogenesis imperfecta)
2. Constitutional delayed development (body length, bone maturity, and puberty are 2 to 4 years delayed)
3. Familial short stature (present when skeletal maturity proceeds in step with age and other family members have short stature)
4. Hormonal diseases such as primary hypothyroidism, precocious puberty, Cushing disease, and congenital adrenal hyperplasia
5. Chromosomal aberrations such as Turner syndrome and Down syndrome
6. Malnutrition and metabolic disease such as kwashiorkor, rickets, and Hurler syndrome

14.31

Fetal Alcohol Syndrome

Fetal alcohol syndrome in a 2½-year-old girl. The child's mother was an alcoholic who drank liquor daily during pregnancy. Findings included growth failure which had been noted since birth (at birth 8 cm shorter than average, currently 13 cm below average height), microcephaly, and typical facies (short palpebral fissures, maxillary hypoplasia, thin upper lip—see page 80). Mental development was delayed. The child exhibited behavioral problems including hyperactivity. For discussion of congenital heart disease in fetal alcohol syndrome, see page 96.

14.32

Diastrophic Dwarfism

Diastrophic dwarfism (Maroteaux-Lamy syndrome) in a 4½-year-old boy. Findings included disproportionate dwarfism (abnormal shortness of the proximal segments of the limbs), club feet, and widening between the first and second toes ("sandal gap"). The big toes were abducted and the thumbs were hyperextensible and hyperabductable (hitchhiker thumbs). Mental development was normal. Radiographic examination of the long bones demonstrated spreading of the metaphyses as well as delayed closure and deformation of the epiphyses (especially of the proximal femoral epiphysis).

    Diastrophic dwarfism is related to a special form of generalized osteochondral dysplasia, an autosomal recessive condition which is evident at birth. It leads to severe kyphoscoliosis, which may cause significant physical handicap and require extensive orthopedic care.

    Disproportionate microsomia also occurs in Down syndrome, congenital hypothyroidism, achondroplasia, and other micromelic lethal dwarfism syndromes. It occurs in cases of Hurler syndrome, pyknodysostosis syndrome, Melnick-Needles syndrome (osteodysplasia), and Robinow-Silver syndrome.

14.33

Pituitary Dwarfism

Pituitary dwarfism (growth hormone deficiency) in a 14½-year-old girl. Proportionate microsomia (28 cm below average height) was noted despite growth hormone treatment since the child's second year of life. The child's height had only increased 12 cm in 3 years. No growth hormone rise was noted after insulin induced hypoglycemia or arginine infusion. Other causes were ruled out. The child's obesity is caused by growth hormone deficiency due to inadequate lipolysis.

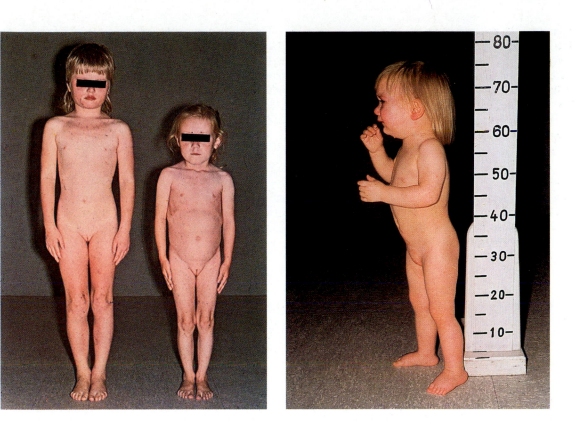

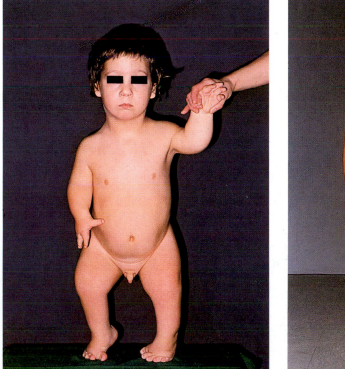

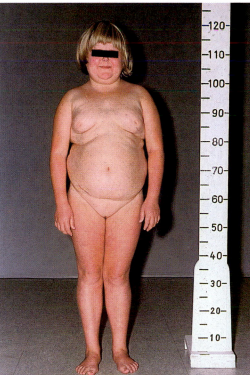

15.1 Measles

Typical measles exanthem on the face of a 3-year-old boy. The illness began with fever, rhinitis, and conjunctivitis 7 days prior to the onset of the rash. The rash consisted of maculopapular lesions that were patchy, poorly defined, and partially confluent. At first, the lesions were light red but later became dark red and light brown. The rash began on the head and then spread down the torso and the extremities. The rash faded in the same sequence as it had appeared.

The rash seen in rubella spreads in a similar fashion. Maculopapular rashes appear in other viral illnesses (including Coxsackievirus, echovirus, and adenovirus), in infectious mononucleosis, and in exanthem subitum. Maculopapular rashes are also seen with penicillin allergy and other drug rashes. Similar rashes may also be seen in meningococcemia, scarlet fever, congenital syphilis, and listeriosis.

15.2 Measles

Koplik's spots seen on the inner aspect of the cheek in a 3-year-old girl. These spots were noted on the third day of illness. The lesions consisted of white spots surrounded by a red halo. At first, the lesions were localized opposite the lower molars; later, the lesions were noted to spread over the remaining oral mucosa. As is typical in measles, Koplik's spots were no longer visible after the second day of the exanthem stage.

15.3 Measles

Severe hemorrhagic measles in a 12-year-old girl. The child was unconscious due to encephalitis. Hemorrhagic changes occurred in the measles lesions (black measles) and in the mucous membranes (on the palate and on the nasal mucosa).

15.4 Infectious Mononucleosis

Pleomorphic skin rash (partially maculopapular, partially urticarial with isolated petechial hemorrhages) in a 2-year-old girl with infectious mononucleosis. The clinical presentation of infectious mononucleosis included prolonged persistent fever, generalized lymphadenopathy, hepato-splenomegaly, and abdominal pain. Peripheral blood smear demonstrated the typical changes seen in mononucleosis (leukocytosis and atypical lymphocytes). A bone marrow aspirate was performed and leukemia was ruled out. The child recovered over several weeks.

15.5 Penicillin Allergy

Penicillin allergy in a 12-year-old boy with congenital heart disease. The child had been treated with penicillin as prophylaxis for bacterial endocarditis. On the second day of penicillin treatment, the child demonstrated a generalized maculopapular rash over the entire body. The rash was pruritic. Skin test with benzylpenicilloylpolylysine was positive. Penicillin-specific IgE was detected in serum (RAST test).

The most frequent reaction in a patient who is allergic to penicillin in an urticarial rash (page 168). In some cases, one can see Henoch-Schoenlein purpura, Lyell syndrome, or other drug-related skin rashes.

15.6 Ampicillin Rash

Ampicillin rash (after 9 days of treatment with antibiotics) in a 9-year-old girl with urinary tract infection. Maculopapular, nonpruritic lesions were noted over the entire body. No fever was noted. The rash disappeared after ampicillin treatment was discontinued. The child had not previously received ampicillin.

Ampicillin rashes may occur in 5–10% of children ex-posed to ampicillin. Unlike other allergic conditions, renewed exposure to ampicillin does not lead to a rash. In over 90% of patients with infectious mononucleosis, a nonurticarial rash may appear after administration of ampicillin. If urticaria are seen in association with ampicillin, it is almost always a true allergic reaction. Frequently, these patients may also have an allergic response to other penicillin drugs.

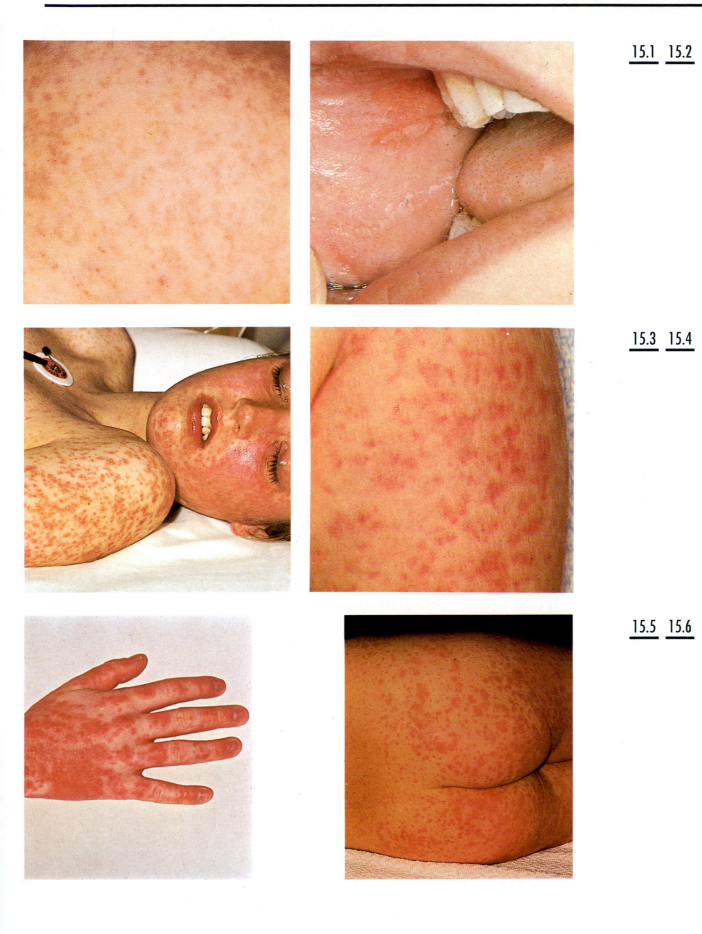

15.7–15.10

Scarlet Fever

Scarlet fever in a 3-year-old child. The child became acutely ill with fever, vomiting, and pharyngitis. On the second day of illness, a diffuse, erythematous rash appeared on the chest (Figure 15.7) and quickly spread over the trunk and extremities. The rash consisted of closely grouped papules the size of pinheads and had the appearance of sandpaper. Rash and petechial hemorrhages were noted on the palate and palatopharyngeal arches (Figure 15.8).

After scraping off the white coating on the tongue, one could clearly see red, edematous papillae (strawberry tongue, Figure 15.9). Lamellar and circular desquamation was found on the palms (Figure 15.10) and over the entire body during the third week of illness. The clinical diagnosis was confirmed by detection of group A β-hemolytic streptococci on throat culture, as well as demonstrating a significant rise in serum anti-streptolysin O (ASO) titer. The condition resolved after 10 days of treatment with penicillin.

Differential Diagnosis—Scarlet fever must be differentiated from many other conditions including viral diseases (measles, rubella, enterovirus, Coxsackievirus, echovirus, infectious mononucleosis), Henoch-Schoenlein purpura, and drug eruptions.

15.11

Rubella

Typical rash of rubella noted behind the ears of a 1-year-old child. The measles-like maculopapular rash began in the retroauricular area and quickly spread down the rest of the body. The prodromal phase was associated with mild symptoms compatible with an upper respiratory tract infection. This child had no prodromal symptoms. The rash appeared on the first day of illness together with mild fever and painful cervical lymphadenopathy.

The rash seen in rubella fades within two to three days; more quickly than the exanthem of measles. The exanthem of measles may leave a brown discoloration as it fades.

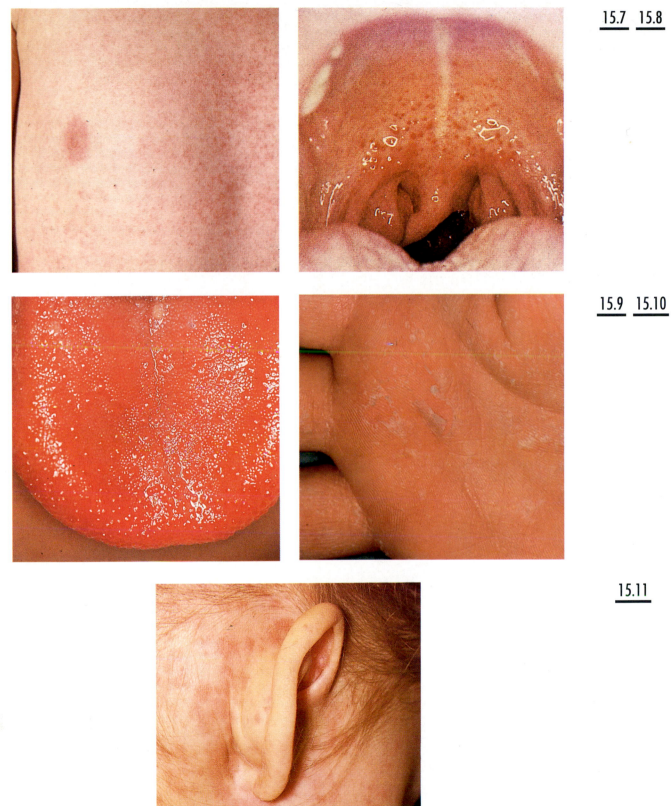

15.12a 15.12b

Erythema Infectiosum

Erythema infectiosum (Fifth disease) in a 3-year-old girl. The first sign of illness was a butterfly-shaped erythematous rash with slightly raised borders noted over both cheeks. The rash regressed after 2 to 3 days. Afterward, a maculopapular, lacy, reticulated rash, which frequently changed in appearance, was noted over the torso and the extremities. The rash was nonpruritic and no fever was noted.

A butterfly-shaped facial rash can also occur in erythema multiforme (page 170), Gianotti-Crosti syndrome (page 248), and systemic lupus erythematosus (page 272).

15.13

Exanthem Subitum

Exanthem subitum (roseola infantum) in a 10-month-old girl. After 3 days of fever associated with no other symptoms, a light-red, maculopapular exanthem appeared over the torso and spread to the face and extremities. The child's fever dropped with the appearance of the rash. On peripheral blood smear, neutropenia and relative lymphocytosis were noted. The rash was noted for one day and then disappeared.

Differential Diagnosis—Differential diagnosis of exanthem subitum includes other viral diseases such as rubella and rubeola, and allergic drug reactions.

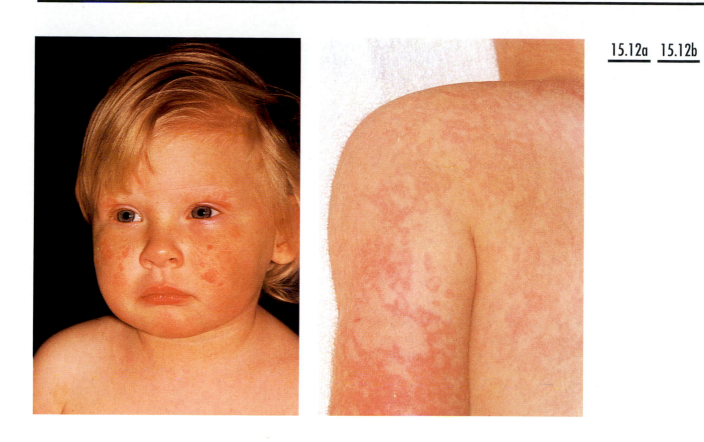

15.12a   15.12b

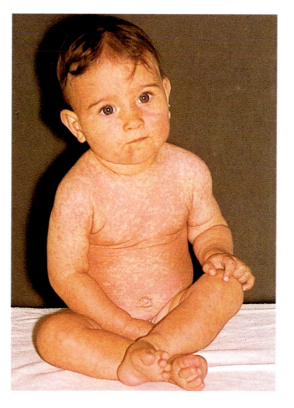

15.13

15.14

Varicella

Impetiginized varicella (chickenpox with secondary bacterial infection) in a 4-year-old boy. The findings included numerous pruritic papules and vesicles which were partially excoriated and crusted over the entire body and scalp. Many of these lesions had purulent drainage due to secondary bacterial infection. In the mouth, several ulcerated vesicles were present. The lesions first began on the trunk, then spread to the face and the parts of the extremities close to the trunk; the palms and the soles were less affected. New crops of lesions continued to appear for the first 4 days; all stages of the disease were therefore present concurrently.

Differential Diagnosis—Differential diagnosis of varicella (chickenpox) includes herpes zoster, herpes simplex, Coxsackie hand-foot-and-mouth disease (page 246), impetigo contagiosa, pemphigoid, papular urticaria (strophulus), scabies, insect bites, intercontinentia pigmenti, other vesicular dermatitides (i.e., dermatitis herpetiformis), and drug rashes.

15.15

Impetigo Contagiosa

Impetigo contagiosa on the face of a 3½-year-old boy. Findings included small, nonpruritic vesicles and pustules covered with yellow crusts. *Staphylococcus aureus* was detected on culture. For differential diagnosis see page 240.

15.16   15.17

Varicella

Varicella in a 4-year-old boy. Findings included numerous vesicles on the mucous membranes of the mouth, as well as lesions over the torso. The rash was extremely pruritic. During this time, the child was febrile and ill-appearing. For differential diagnosis of vesicular stomatitis see page 246.

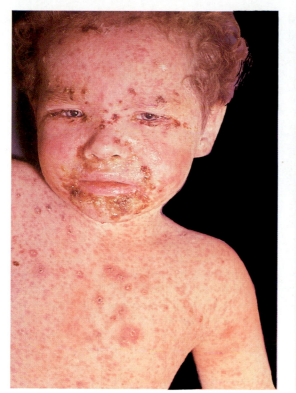

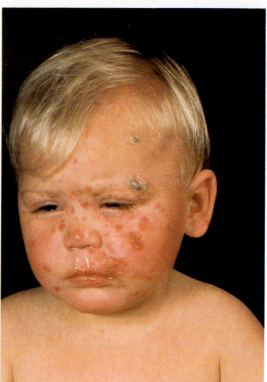

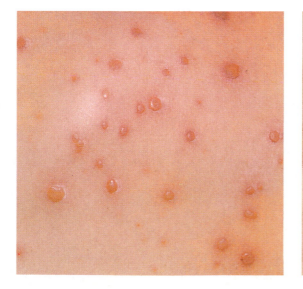

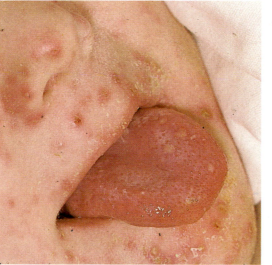

15.18

Acute Cervical Lymphadenitis

Acute cervical lymphadenitis in a 1½-year-old child. Findings included a 6-cm, painful, fluctuant, erythematous swelling of the lymph nodes on the right side of the neck. Surgical incision drained a yellow pus which grew *Staphylococcus aureus*.

15.19

Bronchogenic Cyst

Solitary lateral bronchogenic cyst of the neck in a 2-year-old boy. The findings included painless swelling of the right side of the neck which had been noted for a year. This soft, cystic tumor was the size of a small egg and could be easily moved. No erythema was noted. The tumor was excised surgically and was noted to contain fluid. Histologic examination demonstrated a bronchogenic cyst lined with epithelial cells.

15.20–15.22

Infectious Mononucleosis

Infectious mononucleosis in a 2-year-old boy. Findings included swollen, but only slightly painful cervical and submandibular lymphadenopathy (Figure 15.21) and erythematous enlarged tonsils with a gray-white exudate (Figure 15.20). Hemogram demonstrated a white blood count of 30,000 cells/mm³. These cells were mostly lymphocytes, among which there were many atypical lymphocytes with oval or bean-shaped, eccentrically placed nuclei and basophilic staining cytoplasm (Figure 15.22). Serum IgM antibodies against Epstein-Barr virus were detected.

Persistent fever, generalized or localized lymphadenopathy, and tonsillitis (with or without exudate) are typical symptoms of infectious mononucleosis. The diagnosis can be confirmed through serologic testing. Other causes of cervical lymphadenopathy (such as leukemia) or membranous tonsillitis (such as diphtheria) must be ruled out.

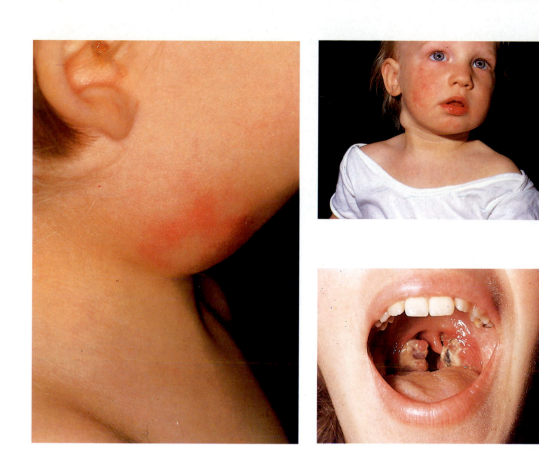

15.18   15.19

15.20

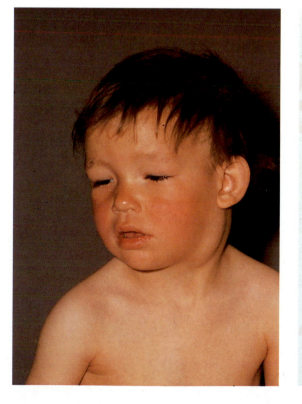

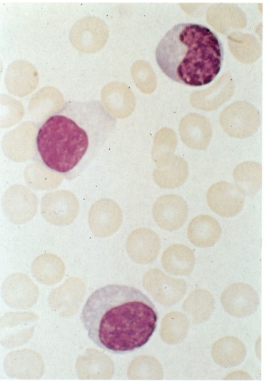

15.21   15.22

15.23

Meningococcal Sepsis

Meningococcal sepsis in a 2½-year-old girl. Petechial and purpuric skin lesions over the arms and legs developed at the time the child became ill with fever and vomiting. Peripheral blood smear demonstrated leukocytosis (white cell count 38,000 cells/mm³). Blood culture was positive for meningococcus. Platelet count was normal and there was no evidence of disseminated intravascular coagulation. The skin lesions were due to vasculitis and hypoprothrombinemia (due to hepatic dysfunction). These skin lesions are not pathognomonic of meningococcal infection. Similar findings are possible in sepsis due to other causes, rickettsial disease (Rocky Mountain spotted fever), and viral illnesses including Coxsackievirus and echovirus infections.

15.24

Typhoid Fever

Typhoid fever in a 5-year-old girl. Maculopapular erythematous skin lesions approximately 3–4 mm in diameter were noted on the abdomen and lower third of the thorax. The rash appeared during the second week of illness and disappeared after 2 days. During this time, the child had high fever, lethargy, splenomegaly, and diarrhea (pea soup-like stools). Blood culture demonstrated *Salmonella typhosa*. The child was successfully treated with a combination of sulfamethoxazole and trimethoprim.

Differential Diagnosis—Similar skin lesions may be seen in roseola and bacterial infections including meningococcal sepsis, Rocky Mountain spotted fever, and brucellosis.

15.25

Cutaneous Leishmaniasis

Cutaneous leishmaniasis (Old World cutaneous leishmaniasis) in a 13-year-old Greek girl. Several red nodules, 3–5 mm in diameter, were noted over both lower legs (at the location of sandfly bites). These nodules were partially ulcerated and scab covered. The nodules later attained the size of 1–2 cm in diameter and healed without forming a scar. These lesions were caused by an infection with *Leishmania tropica*, a protozoan seen in Mediterranean countries, Asia, Africa, and parts of South America. Human beings become infected with this protozoan through sandfly bites. The parasite may be detected microscopically in tissue taken from the edge of the ulcer.

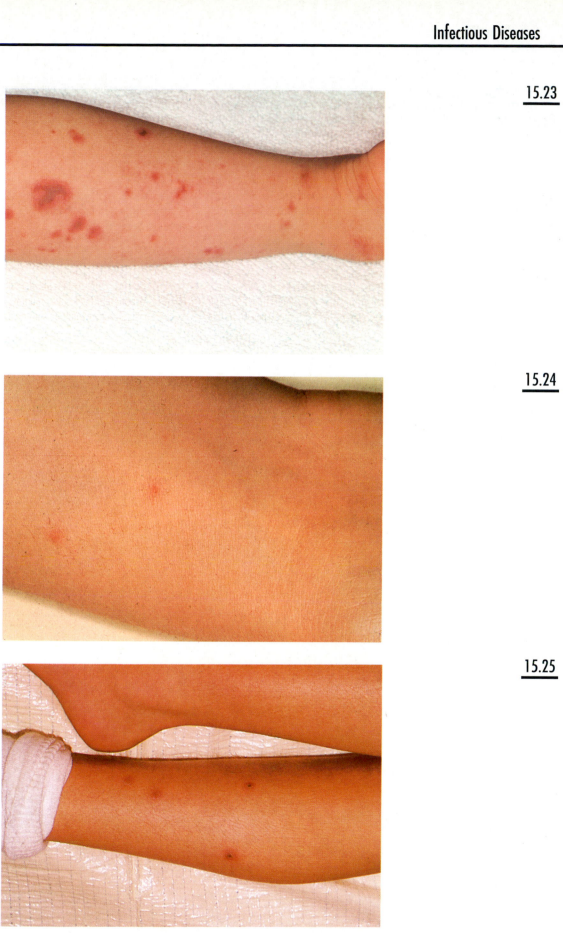

15.23

15.24

15.25

15.26
Osler's Nodes

Osler's nodes due to postoperative endocarditis in a 2-year-old boy. Several pea-sized, red, firm nodules were noted on the palms of the hands (particularly on the thumb). These appeared together with high fever and other symptoms of bacterial endocarditis shortly after surgical correction of an intracardiac defect. *Staphylococcus aureus* was identified in blood cultures.

15.27   15.28
Meningococcal Sepsis

Meningococcal sepsis in a 2½-year-old girl. Numerous ecchymoses were found on the dorsum of the hands (Figure 15.27), arms, legs, and trunk. Several erythematous patches, 1–2 mm in size, were found in the chest and abdomen (caused by bacterial microemboli, Figure 15.28). Meningococci were identified in blood culture.

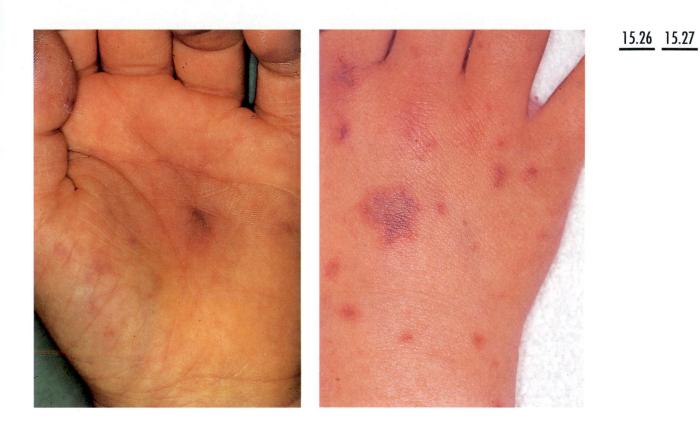

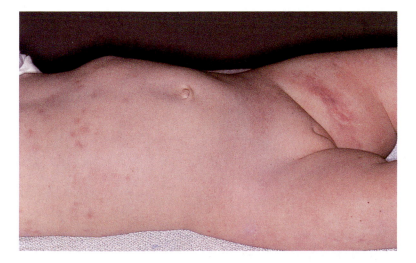

15.29

Erysipelas

Erysipelas in a 15-year-old girl. Extensive, painful, edematous, erythematous swellings were noted over the left half of the face, originating from two skin wounds infected with group A β-hemolytic streptococci. The child had high fever and regional lymphadenpathy. The infection responded to seven days of penicillin treatment. Complications of this infection include nephritis, abscess formation, and septicemia.

Differential Diagnosis—The differential diagnosis includes cellulitis and abscess from other bacterial organisms.

15.30

Dog Bite

Pasteurella multocida infection caused by a dog bite in a 9-year-old boy. Findings included extensive erythema and swelling of both cheeks with scab formation at the wound site. The pathogenic agents which caused the wound infection are almost invariably found in the oral cavities of cats and dogs. Penicillin treatment may aid in wound healing.

15.31

Erysipelas

Erysipelas in a 12-year-old boy. An intense, poorly demarcated, erythematous swelling was noted over the dorsum of the right foot. The swelling and erythema spread to the lower leg. The condition was accompanied by tenderness, regional lymphadenopathy, and high fever. The site of entry for the group A β-hemolytic streptococci was not determined. Because of the danger of abscess formation and the potential for sepsis, treatment for penicillin was immediately started.

15.32

Breast Enlargement

Bilateral breast enlargement in a 5-day-old boy. Palpable and visible enlargement of breast tissue (as well as mild secretion from the mammary glands) in the newborn is caused by exposure to transplacentally acquired maternal hormones. The condition regressed without any treatment after 1 week.

15.33

Mastitis

Mastitis in a 2-week-old female child. Findings included marked swelling and erythema of the right breast, which did not respond to antibiotic treatment alone. After one week, the area was incised and drained, at which time abundant purulent material was drained. Culture of the purulent material revealed an infection with *Staphylococcus aureus*. The abscess resolved after incision and drainage and antibiotic therapy.

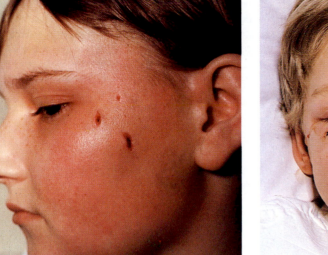

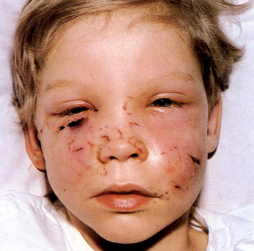

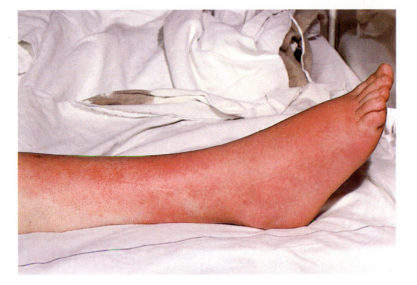

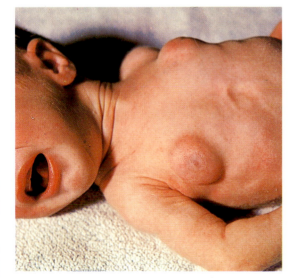

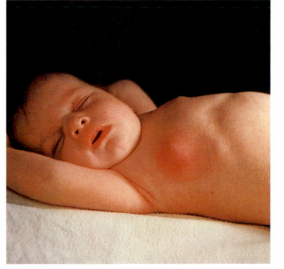

15.34

Necrotizing Ulcerative Gingivitis

Necrotizing ulcerative gingivitis (Vincent's angina fusobacteria infection) in a 6-year-old boy. Findings included an ulcer of the left tonsil and painful swelling of the ipsilateral mandibular lymph nodes. Other findings included halitosis. The child was afebrile. Microscopically, a swab from the ulcer demonstrated abundant fusiform bacilli. The child was treated with penicillin.

Differential Diagnosis—In cases of tonsillar diphtheria, a thin, gray, adherent exudate can be found on the tonsils (which extends to part of the soft palate). In infectious mononucleosis, inflamed swollen tonsils are partially covered by a gray-white diphtheria exudate. The exudate is restricted to the tonsils and can easily be wiped off. With infectious mononucleosis, the peripheral blood smear demonstrates leukocytosis and atypical lymphocytes.

15.35

Secondary Syphilis

Secondary syphilis in a 16-year-old girl. Eight weeks after the primary infection, the patient developed a generalized macular rash (primarily on the trunk) and generalized lymphadenopathy. Both tonsils were swollen and covered with many gray-white papules and plaques (mucous patches). Similar gray-white lesions were found along the buccal mucosa. The diagnosis of secondary syphilis was confirmed by detection of serum specific antibodies; a positive *Treponema pallidum* hemagglutination assay (TPHA-TP) and a positive fluorescent treponemal antibody-absorption test (FTA-ABS).

15.36

Oral Thrush

Oral thrush (*Candida stomatitis*) in a 10-year-old boy with acute lymphocytic leukemia. Gray-white, partially confluent, firmly attached deposits were noted on the buccal mucosa and the tongue. After scraping off the thrush deposits, punctate hemorrhages were noted on an inflamed base. On microscopic examination, one could detect yeastlike cells and filaments confirming the diagnosis of *Candida* infection.

15.37

Adenoidal Hypertrophy

"Adenoid facies" in a 2-year-old boy due to obstruction of nasal breathing secondary to adenoidal hypertrophy. Findings included dry lips, dry oral mucous membranes, and nasal voice. The child was noted to have loud snoring during sleep, persistent rhinitis, and recurrent otitis media with persistent middle ear infusions causing hearing difficulty. Treatment included adenoidectomy and myringotomy.

Differential Diagnosis—Obstruction of nasal breathing can be caused by foreign bodies in the nose, nasal septal deviation, intranasal polyps, and high palate.

15.38

Subconjunctival Hemorrhage

Acute bilateral subconjunctival hemorrhage in a 9-year-old boy caused by pertussis-like cough and bronchopneumonia. The superficial nature and intense red color were typical. Platelet count and coagulation studies were normal. The hemorrhage completely regressed within 2 weeks.

Subconjunctival hemorrhages often result from rupture of conjunctival vessels and, in less extensive cases than the one pictured, are sharply outlined and surrounded by normal conjunctiva. Unilateral or bilateral subconjunctival hemorrhages may be seen in cases of orbital contusions, orbital fracture, rupture of the posterior sclera, leukemia, hypertension, viral conjunctivitis (adenovirus), and from lifting heavy loads.

15.39

Tuberculous Meningitis

Tuberculous meningitis in a 16-year-old girl with oculomotor paralysis of the left eye. When the normal right eye fixed on an object, the paralyzed left eye deviated outward due to predominance of the abducens nerves. To avoid diplopia, the head was usually turned to the opposite side.

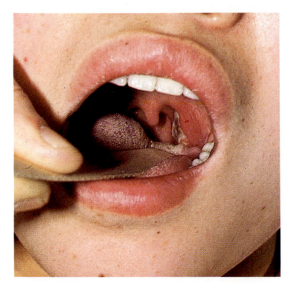

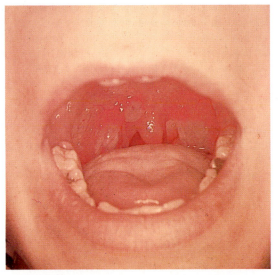

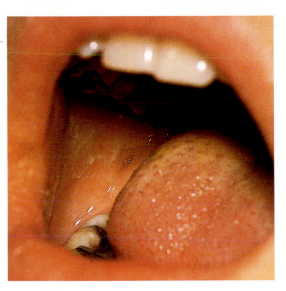

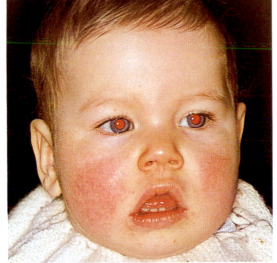

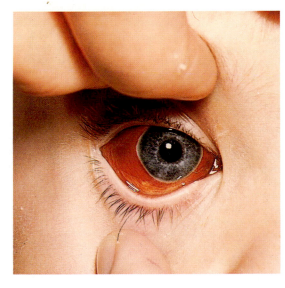

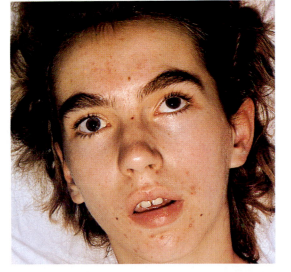

15.40

Phlyctenular Keratoconjunctivitis

Phlyctenular keratoconjunctivitis in an 8-year-old girl with tuberculosis. The inflamed conjunctiva and cornea were jelly-like in appearance with small, yellow, slightly elevated nodules noted at the edge of the cornea (phlyctenules). The girl had continuous flow of tears and spasms of the eyelids.

Ulceration of the cornea and secondary bacterial infection may occur. Phlyctenular keratoconjunctivitis is a nonspecific hypersensitivity reaction in the eye, which may be treated topically with corticosteroids.

15.41   15.42

Papulonecrotic Tuberculid

Papulonecrotic tuberculid in a 10-year-old girl with a persistent case of tuberculosis. Numerous groups of purple papules of varying size were noted on the extremities and trunk. These lesions had central necrosis and crust formation. Skin biopsy demonstrated an area of central necrosis surrounded by an inflammatory infiltrate with epithelioid and giant cells.

Acid fast bacteria were not detected. The tuberculin skin test was strongly positive. The lesions healed after 2 to 3 weeks leaving behind pigmented scars.

Differential Diagnosis—Differential diagnosis includes insect bites, ptyriasis lichenoides, and Mucha-Habermann disease (page 220).

15.43

Lupus Vulgaris

Lupus vulgaris in a 14-year-old boy. The lesions began as small erythematous papules that evolved into nodules and irregular plaques. The lesion pictured is penny-sized, slightly scaling, brown-red nodule with central ulceration. The lesion was located on the face. The lesion had an apple-jelly color when pressure from a spatula was applied. Prominent swelling of the regional lymph nodes was noted (preauricular lymphadenopathy). Although somewhat resistant to treatment, the condition slowly responded to tuberculostatic therapy, leaving an atrophic scar.

The lesions of lupus vulgaris are usually solitary and frequently located on the face and neck. These lesions can be caused by cutaneous innoculation of tuberculous bacillus, or through drainage of an affected node. A disfiguring scar may develop. Today, this form of tuberculous disease is extremely rare.

Differential Diagnosis—Depending on the stage of the infection, the following conditions must be differentiated: lymphocytoma, juvenile melanoma, discoid lupus erythematosus, mycotic skin infection, and sarcoidosis.

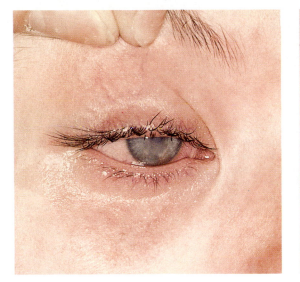

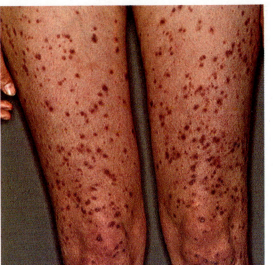

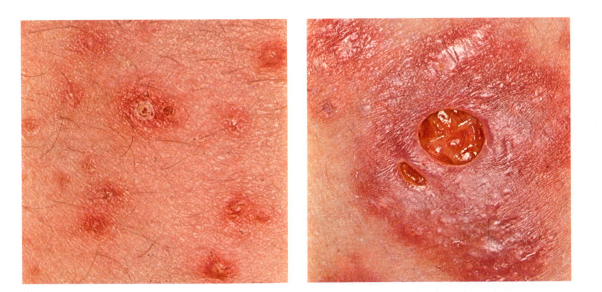

15.44 15.45
Positive Tuberculosis Skin Test

Positive tuberculosis skin test (Moro). Of note was the appearance of several red nodules 48–72 hours after rubbing a tuberculin salve into the skin over the chest.

15.46
Positive Tuberculin Reaction

Positive tuberculin reaction (Mantoux test). Of note was the appearance of local inflammation (8 cm in diameter), erythema, and central necrosis after intracutaneous injection of 0.1 ml of purified protein derivative (5 tuberculin units). This reaction is typical of delayed type hypersensitivity (greatest reaction seen after 3 to 4 days with resolution over 2 to 3 weeks).

If the suspicion of tuberculosis infection is strong, a weak concentration of tuberculin solution should be used (1 tuberculin unit), due to the danger of severe reaction. For routine testing, 5 tuberculin units are used. In cases where the use of BCG vaccine is being considered, skin testing should first be demonstrated to be negative.

15.47
"Positive" Tine Test

Tuberculosis skin testing may be accomplished with the use of the tine test, a disposable testing unit with four small blades that have been dipped in old tuberculin concentrate. The appearance of papules, diffuse reddening, and infiltration at the site of inoculation within 48 to 72 hours is considered "positive." Inadequate inoculation may produce false negative results.

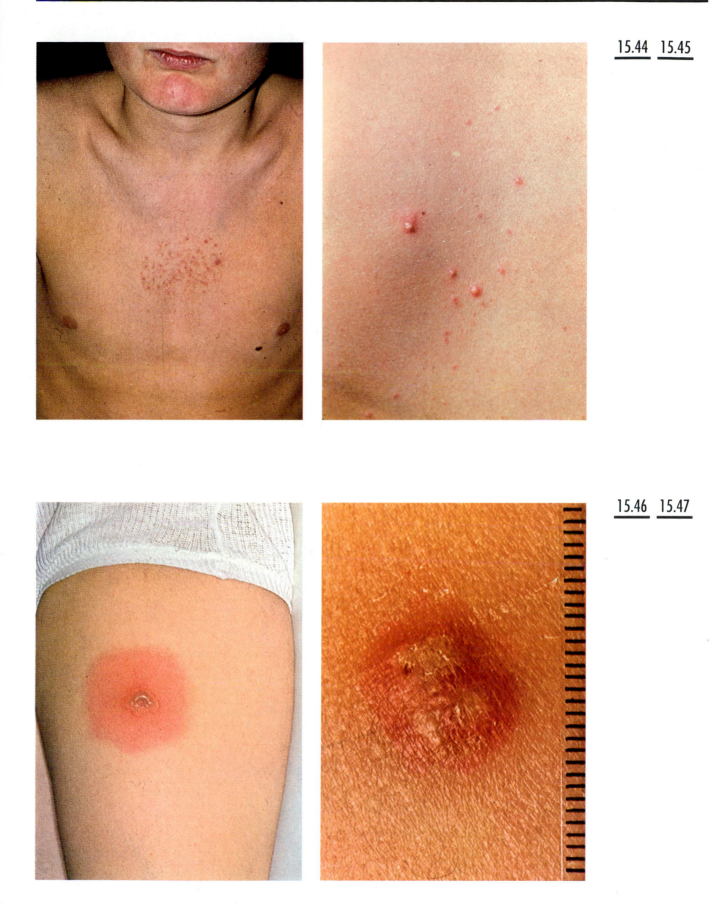

15.48

Smallpox Vaccination

A 13-month-old boy 9 days after active vaccination with smallpox. Several pearl-gray, fluid-filled vesicles with central indentation were noted on an erythematous base. The condition resulted from spread of virus from the site of inoculation on the upper arm. Healing occurred without scar formation.

15.49

Vaccinia Gangrenosa

Vaccina gangrenosa after smallpox vaccination in an 8-month-old infant. The findings included extensive palm-sized lesions on the upper right arm with pustular formation, necrosis, and early gangrene. Several pustules were also noted on the back, the axilla and the face (due to hematogenous spread). The lesions healed, leaving numerous scars.

15.50   15.51

Roseola Vaccinosa

Roseola vaccinosa (reaction to smallpox vaccination) 7 days after vaccination of a 15-month-old boy. Findings included maculopapular erythematous skin lesions over the entire body, including the back and face. Certain individual lesions had central clearing. The lesions resolved spontaneously without treatment within 5 days. There was a normal reaction at the site of vaccination in the upper right arm.

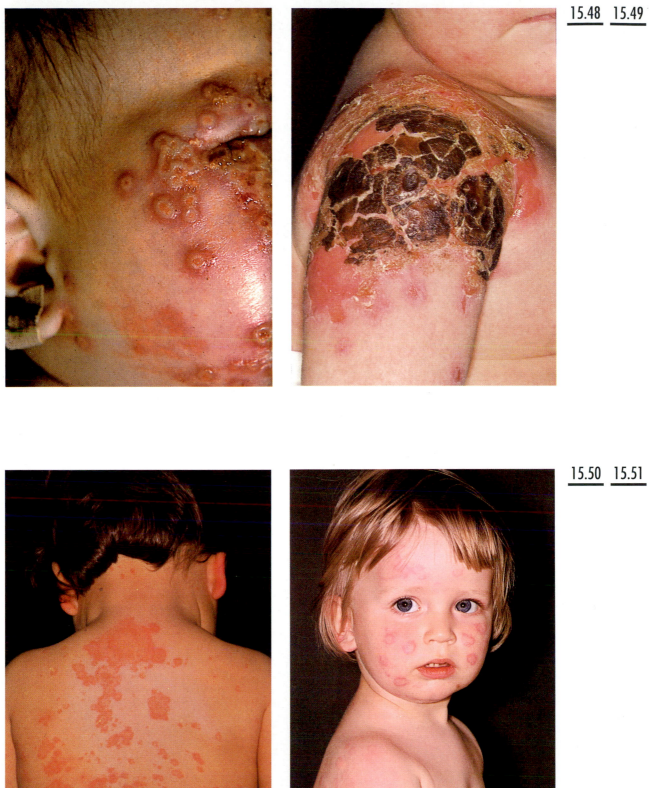

Index